Imaging for Clinicians

Series Editors:

$\bar{}$ Ribes • P.R. Ros

María I. Martínez-León
Antonio Martínez-Valverde
Luisa Ceres-Ruiz

(Editors)

Imaging for Pediatricians

100 Key Cases

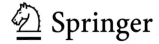 Springer

María I. Martínez-León
Department of Radiology
Pediatric Radiology Unit
Hospital Materno-Infantil del
Hospital Regional Universitario
Carlos Haya
Málaga
Spain

Antonio Martínez-Valverde
Full Professor of Pediatrics
Head of Department of Pediatrics
Hospital Materno-Infantil
Hospital Regional Universitario
Carlos Haya
Málaga
Spain

Luisa Ceres-Ruiz
Department of Radiology
Pediatric Radiology Unit
Hospital Materno-Infantil del
Hospital Regional Universitario
Carlos Haya
Málaga
Spain

ISBN 978-3-642-28628-5   ISBN 978-3-642-28629-2 (e-Book)
DOI 10.1007/978-3-642-28629-2

Springer Heidelberg New York Dordrecht London

Library of Congress Control Number: 2012939491

Cover design: eStudioCalamar, Figueres/Berlin

Printed on acid-free paper

9 8 7 6 5 4 3 2 1

Springer is part of Springer Science+Business Media (www.springer.com)

To my son, SSS, my life.

To Ramón, ILANY, TPAL.

María I. Martínez-León

To Dora, our children and our grandchildren.

Antonio Martínez-Valverde

To my children Carmen and Pedro the best of my life, and to Octavi.

Luisa Ceres-Ruiz

Contents

8 Emergency Imaging

Contributors

ALBERTO ACOSTA MENDOZA
Department of Radiology
Hospital Universitario
Materno-Infantil de Canarias
Las Palmas de Gran Canaria
Spain

NATALIA AGUILAR PÉREZ
Radiologist
Family Physician Hospital Costa del Sol
Marbella
Málaga
Spain

GUSTAVO ALBI RODRÍGUEZ
Pediatric Radiologist
Hospital Infantil del Niño Jesús
Madrid
Spain

JAVIER ALONSO HERNÁNDEZ
Department of Pediatric Orthopaedics
Hospital Infantil Universitario
Niño Jesús
Madrid
Spain

ALEJANDRO ARANDA MORA
Neonatology Unit
Hospital Materno-Infantil del
Hospital Regional
Universitario Carlos Haya
Málaga
Spain

BEATRIZ ASENJO GARCÍA
Radiologist
Head of the Department of Radiology
Hospital Regional Universitario
Carlos Haya
Málaga
Spain

RAFAEL AVILA SUÁREZ
Department of Radiology
Hospital Universitario
Materno-Infantil de Canarias
Las Palmas de Gran Canaria
Spain

DANIEL AZORÍN CUADRILLERO
Department of Pathology
Hospital Infantil Universitario
Niño Jesús
Madrid
Spain

CARMEN BALLESTEROS-GUERRERO
Radiologist
Family Physician
Hospital Regional Universitario
Carlos Haya
Málaga
Spain

IGNACIO BARBER MARTÍNEZ
DE LA TORRE
Department of Pediatric Radiology
Hospital Universitario
Materno-Infantil Vall d'Hebron
Barcelona
Spain

DANIELA BINAGHI
Radiologist
Department of Imaging
Neurosciences Institute
Favaloro University
Buenos Aires
Argentina

CRISTINA BRAVO BRAVO
Department of Radiology
Pediatric Radiology Unit
Hospital Materno-Infantil del
Hospital Regional Universitario
Carlos Haya
Málaga
Spain

LINA CADAVID ÁLVAREZ
Department of Pediatric Radiology
Hospital Universitario
Vall d' Hebron - AMI
Barcelona
Spain

SUSANA CALLE RESTREPO
Department of Radiology
Hospital Universitario San Ignacio
Bogotá
Colombia

PILAR CARO AGUILERA
Department of Pediatrics
Pneumology Unit
Hospital Materno-Infantil del
Hospital Regional Universitario
Carlos Haya
Málaga
Spain

GERMAINE CARTIER VELÁZQUEZ
Radiologist
Hospital Regional Universitario
Carlos Haya
Málaga
Spain

AMPARO CASTELLOTE ALONSO
Department of Pediatric Radiology
Hospital Universitario
Vall d'Hebron - AMI
Barcelona
Spain

LUISA CERES RUIZ
Department of Radiology
Pediatric Radiology Unit
Hospital Materno-Infantil del
Hospital Regional Universitario
Carlos Haya
Málaga
Spain

MARÍA CULIÁÑEZ-CASAS
Radiology Department
Pediatric and Gynecological Unit
Hospital Universitario
Virgen de las Nieves
Granada
Spain

MARIANO DEL VALLE DIÉGUEZ
Pediatric Radiology
Hospital General Universitario
Gregorio Marañón
Madrid
Spain

DOLORES DELGADO
Pediatric Surgery
Hospital Maternoinfantil
Universitario 12 de Octubre
Madrid
Spain

IGNACIO DELGADO ÁLVAREZ
Department of Pediatric Radiology
Hospital Universitario
Vall d'Hebron - AMI
Barcelona
Spain

ANABEL DOBLADO LÓPEZ
Radiologist
Hospital Regional Universitario
Carlos Haya
Málaga
Spain

RODRIGO DOMÍNGUEZ
Department of Pediatric Radiology
Randall Children's Hospital at
Legacy Emanuel
Portland, Oregon
USA

MARÍA DOLORES DOMÍNGUEZ-PINOS
Radiologist
Family Physician
Hospital Regional Universitario
Carlos Haya
Málaga
Spain

ERNESTO DOMÉNECH ABELLÁN
Department of Radiology
Pediatric Radiology Unit
Hospital Universitario
Virgen de la Arrixaca
Murcia
Spain

CARMINA DURAN FELIUBADALÓ
Department of Pediatric Radiology
UDIAT-CD
Corporació Sanitàriao i
Universitària Parc Taulí
Sabadell
Spain

CONXITA ESCOFET SOTERAS
Department of Pediatric Neurology
Hospital de Sabadell
Corporació Sanitària i
Universitària Parc Taulí
Sabadell
Spain

MARÍA GRACIA ESPINOSA
FERNÁNDEZ
Neonatologist
Department of Neonatology
Hospital Materno-Infantil del
Complejo Hospitalario Universitario
Carlos Haya
Málaga
Spain

CAROLINA FERNÁNDEZ-CREHUET
Department of Radiology
Hospital Universitario
Virgen de la Victoria
Málaga
Spain

CARMEN GALLEGO HERRERO
Department of Pediatric and
Interventional Radiology
Hospital Maternoinfantil
Universitario 12 de Octubre
Madrid
Spain

PASCUAL GARCÍA-HERRERA
TAILLEFER
Department of Radiology
Pediatric Radiology Unit
Hospital Materno-Infantil del
Hospital Regional Universitario
Carlos Haya
Málaga
Spain

MABEL GARCÍA-HIDALGO
Pediatric Radiologist
Hospital Virgen de la Salud
Toledo
Spain

MARTA GARCÍA RAMÍREZ
Pediatric Department
Hospital Materno-Infantil del
Hospital Regional Universitario
Carlos Haya
Málaga
Spain

PILAR GARCÍA-PEÑA
Department of Pediatric Radiology
Universitary Hospital
Vall d'Hebron - AMI
Barcelona
Spain

Celestino Gómez Rebollo
Department of Radiology
Hospital Universitario
Virgen de la Victoria
Málaga
Spain

Inmaculada González
Almendros
Department of Radiology
Family Physician
Hospital Regional Universitario
Carlos Haya
Málaga
Spain

Isabel Gordillo Gutiérrez
Department of Radiology
Pediatric Radiology Unit
Hospital Materno-Infantil del
Hospital General Universitario
Gregorio Marañón
Madrid
Spain

Sofía Granja
Department of Pediatric Cardiology
Hospital São João
Madrid
Spain

Pediatric Cardiology
Hospital General Universitario
Gregorio Marañón
Porto
Portugal

Mark J. Hogan
Pediatric Radiology
Department of Radiology
Nationwide Children's Hospital
Columbus, OH
USA

Antonio J. Jiménez
Department of Cell Biology,
Genetics, and Physiology
University of Malaga
Málaga
Spain

Antonio Jurado Ortiz
Head of Department of Pediatrics
Hospital Materno-Infantil del
Complejo Hospitalario
Universitario Carlos Haya
Málaga
Spain

Alvaro Lassaletta Atienza
Department of Pediatric Oncology
Hospital Infantil Universitario
Niño Jesús
Madrid
Spain

Roberto Llorens Salvador
Pediatric Radiology Unit - Medical
Imaging Area
Hospital Universitario y
Politécnico La Fe
Valencia
Spain

María López Díaz
Pediatric Surgeon
Hospital Maternoinfantil
Universitario 12 de Octubre
Madrid
Spain

Miguel A. López Pino
Department of Radiology
Hospital Infantil Universitario
Niño Jesús
Madrid
Spain

Begoña Losada
Pediatric Rheumatologist
Hospital Virgen de la Salud
Toledo
Spain

Javier Lucaya
Department of Pediatric Radiology
Hospital Universitario
Vall d'Hebron
Barcelona
Spain

CARLOS MARÍN
Pediatric Radiology
Hospital General Universitario
Gregorio Marañón
Madrid
Spain

PAUL MARTEN
Department of Pediatric Radiology
Randall Children's Hospital at
Legacy Emanuel
Portland, Oregon
USA

CÉSAR MARTÍN MARTÍNEZ
Department of Pediatric Radiology
UDIAT-CD, Corporació Sanitària i
Universitària Parc Taulí
Sabadell
Spain

SERGIO MARTÍNEZ ÁLVAREZ
Department of Pediatric
Orthopedics
Hospital Infantil Universitario
Niño Jesús
Madrid
Spain

ALBA MARTÍNEZ BROQUETAS
Department of Radiology
Hospital Infanta Elena
Huelva
Spain

MARÍA I. MARTÍNEZ LEÓN
Department of Radiology
Pediatric Radiology Unit
Hospital Materno-Infantil del
Hospital Regional Universitario
Carlos Haya
Málaga
Spain

MARÍA ISABEL MARTÍNEZ MARÍN
Pediatrician
Centro de Salud Alameda-Perchel
Department of Pediatric Emergency
Hospital Materno-Infantil del
Hospital Regional Universitario
Carlos Haya
Málaga
Spain

ANTONIO MARTÍNEZ VALVERDE
Full Professor of Pediatrics
Head of Department of Pediatrics
Hospital Materno-Infantil del
Hospital Regional Universitario
Carlos Haya
Málaga
Spain

ENRIQUE MAROTO
Pediatric Cardiology
Hospital General Universitario
Gregorio Marañón
Madrid
Spain

ENRIQUE MEDINA BENÍTEZ
Pediatric Gastroenterology
Hospital Maternoinfantil
Universitario 12 de Octubre
Madrid
Spain

CONSTANCIO MEDRANO
Pediatric Cardiology
Hospital General Universitario
Gregorio Marañón
Madrid
Spain

AMPARO MORENO FLORES
Pediatric Radiology
Unit - Medical Imaging Area
Hospital Universitario y
Politécnico La Fe
Valencia
Spain

ALBERTO MUÑOZ GONZÁLEZ
Neuroradiologist
Full Professor of Radiology
Department of Radiology
School of Medicine
Universidad Complutense
de Madrid
Madrid
Spain

JAMES W. MURAKAMI
Pediatric Radiologist
Nationwide Children's Hospital
Columbus, Ohio
USA

DOLORES MURO VELILLA
Medical Imaging Area
Pediatric Radiology
Hospital Universitari i Politécnic
La Fe, Valencia
Spain

FÁTIMA NAGIB RAYA
Department of Radiology
Hospital Regional Universitario
Carlos Haya
Málaga
Spain

ISIDORO NARBONA ARIAS
Department of Obstetrics and
Ginecoloy
Hospital Materno-Infantil del
Hospital Regional Universitario
Carlos Haya
Málaga
Spain

VÍCTOR NAVAS LÓPEZ
Department of Pediatrics
Gastroenterology Unit
Hospital Materno-Infantil del
Complejo Hospitalario
Universitario Carlos Haya
Málaga
Spain

PEDRO NAVIA
Interventional Neuroradiology
Radiodiagnostic Service
Hospital 12 de Octubre
Madrid
Spain

LAURA ORTIZ TERÁN
Post-Doctoral Research Fellow
Department of Radiology
Massachusetts General Hospital
Athinoula A. Martinos Center
for Biomedical Imaging
Boston, Massachusetts
USA

ANGELES PALOMO BRAVO
Hematology Service
Hospital Materno-Infantil del
Hospital Regional Universitario
Carlos Haya
Málaga
Spain

ELENA PASTOR-PONS
Radiology Department
Pediatric and Gynecological Unit
Hospital Universitario
Virgen de las Nieves
Granada
Spain

VÍCTOR PÉREZ CANDELA
Department of Radiology
Hospital Universitario
Materno-Infantil de Canarias
Las Palmas de Gran Canaria
Spain

ALMUDENA PÉREZ LARA
Department of Radiology
Hospital Regional Universitario
Carlos Haya
Málaga
Spain

FRANCISCO JAVIER PÉREZ-FRÍAS
Department of Pediatrics
Pneumology Unit
Hospital Materno-Infantil del
Hospital Regional Universitario
Carlos Haya
University of Málaga
Málaga
Spain

ESTELA PÉREZ RUIZ
Department of Pediatrics
Pneumology Unit
Hospital Materno-Infantil del
Hospital Regional Universitario
Carlos Haya
University of Málaga
Málaga
Spain

SARA PICÓ ALIAGA
Medical Imaging Area
Pediatric Radiology Section
Hospital Universitari i Politectnic
La Fe, Valencia
Spain

JOAQUIM PIQUERAS
Department of Pediatric Radiology
Hospital Universitario
Vall d'Hebron - AMI
Barcelona
Spain

ANA PLÁ
Interventional Neuroradiology
Radiodiagnostic Service
Hospital 12 de Octubre
Madrid
Spain

CRISTIAN QUEZADA JORQUERA
Department of Pediatric Radiology
Universitary Hospital
Vall d'Hebron - AMI
Barcelona
Spain

ANA RAMÍREZ BARRAGÁN
Department of Orthopedic and
Trauma Surgery
Hospital Infantil Universitario
Niño Jesús
Madrid
Spain

SUSANA RAMÍREZ JIMÉNEZ
Pediatrician
Centro de Salud
Miraflores de los Angeles
Málaga
Spain

LUIS RIERA SOLER
Department of Pediatric Radiology
UDIAT-CD, Corporació Sanitària i
Universitària Parc Taulí
Sabadell
Spain

YOLANDA RUIZ MARTÍN
Department of Pediatric Radiology
Hospital Universitario
Gregorio Marañón
Madrid
Spain

FERMÍN SÁEZ GARMENDIA
Pediatric Radiology
Hospital Universitario de Cruces
Cruces
Barakaldo
Bizkaia

RICARDO SAN ROMÁN MANSO
Vascular and Interventional
Radiology
Hospital Universitario 12 de Octubre
Madrid
Spain

ÁNGEL SÁNCHEZ-MONTAÑEZ
Department of Pediatric Radiology
Hospital Universitario
Vall d'Hebron - AMI
Barcelona
Spain

CINTA SANGÜESA NEBOT
Medical Imaging Area
Pediatric Radiology
Hospital Universitari i Politécnic
La Fe, Valencia
Spain

CRISTINA SEGOVIA VERJEL
Pediatrician Radiologist
Department of Radiology
Hospital Universitario
Virgen del Rocío, Sevilla
Spain

CRISTINA SERRANO GARCÍA
Department of Radiology
Pediatric Radiology Unit
Hospital Universitario
Virgen de la Arrixaca
Murcia
Spain

SARA INMACULADA SIRVENT CERDÁ
Department of Radiology
Hospital Infantil Universitario
Niño Jesús
Madrid
Spain

MARIANO SOCOLOVSKY
Neurosurgeon
Peripheral Nerve Unit
Department of Neurosurgery
University of Buenos Aires
School of Medicine
Buenos Aires
Argentina

FRANCISCO SOLDADO CARRERA
Pediatric Upper Extremity
and Microsurgery Unit
Hospital Universitario
Materno-Infantil Vall d'Hebron
Barcelona
Spain

INÉS SOLÍS MUÑIZ
Department of Radiology
Hospital Infantil Universitario
Niño Jesús
Madrid
Spain

PEDRO TORRES RUBIO
Department of Radiology
Hospital Infantil Universitario
Niño Jesús
Madrid
Spain

AGNIES M. VAN EEGHEN
Department of Radiology
Herscot Center for TSC
Massachusetts General Hospital
Boston, Massachusetts
USA

ÉLIDA VÁZQUEZ MÉNDEZ
Department of Pediatric Radiology
Hospital Universitario
Vall d'Hebron - AMI
Barcelona
Spain

MARÍA VIDAL DENIS
Department of Radiology
Hospital Materno-Infantil del
Hospital Regional Universitario
Carlos Haya
Málaga
Spain

Ana María Viegas Sainz
Department of Obstetrics
& Gynecology
Hospital NISA – Aljarafe
Castilleja de la Cuesta
Sevilla
Spain

José Luis Zunzunegui
Pediatric Cardiology
Hospital General Universitario
Gregorio Marañón
Madrid
Spain

María I. Martínez-León

Contents

M.I. Martínez-León et al., *Imaging for Pediatricians*, Imaging for Clinicians,
DOI 10.1007/978-3-642-28629-2_1, © Springer-Verlag Berlin Heidelberg 2012

Case 1: Congenital Hydrocephalus

María Dolores Domínguez-Pinos and Antonio J. Jiménez

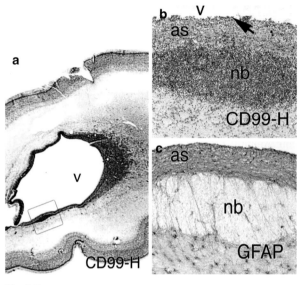
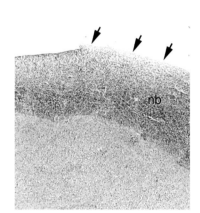

Fig. 1.1

Fig. 1.2

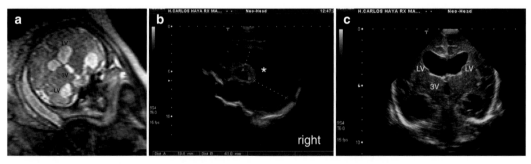

Fig. 1.3

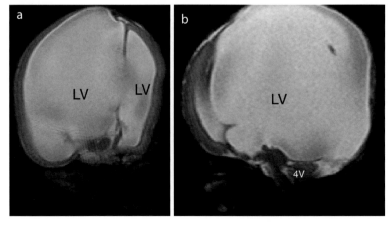

Fig. 1.4

Hydrocephalus is an active distension of the ventricular system of the brain resulting from inadequate passage of cerebrospinal fluid (CSF) from its point of production within the cerebral ventricles to its point of absorption into the systemic circulation. This leads to a net increase of CSF in the cranial cavity and to an increase in the size of the ventricle. It can be originated during the development, with genetic or acquired origins. When there is blockage within the ventricular system, hydrocephalus is called obstructive or non-communicating. In children with hydrocephalus, enlarged ventricles are associated with compression of cortical areas and correlated with cognitive impairment. However, in fetuses with moderate communicating hydrocephalus, the germinal neuroepithelium has been shown to be altered and has also been associated with an abnormal migration of neuroblasts.

Congenital hydrocephalus is detected early in gestational controls by ultrasound. Atrium size greater than 9 mm or ventricular enlargement >1.5 mm on serial examinations and high biparietal diameter are signs of hydrocephalus. Associated findings can also be evaluated with ultrasound and MRI.

Young infant presents irritability, lethargy, vomiting, a full fontanel, and increased head circumference. After 12 months of age, the head circumference changes more slowly, and the diagnosis is based on clinical symptoms.

Insertion of a ventriculoperitoneal shunt represents a lifetime commitment for the child and family. However, the presence of ventriculomegaly alone does not necessarily indicate the need for treatment.

Comments

(Fig. 1.1a–c). Section of the telencephalon immunostained with an anti-CD99 and counterstained with hematoxylin (CD99-H). Ventriculomegaly is present in the lateral ventricle (v). The area framed in (a) is detailed in (b and c). Neuroblasts (nb) accumulate near the ventricle and can be present in the surface (*arrow*), which lacks ependyma. Instead of ependyma, the surface is covered with a thick layer of astrocytes (as) that are labeled with anti-CD99 antibodies and glial fibrillary acidic protein (GFAP).

(Fig. 1.2). Section of the telencephalon stained with hematoxylin-eosin showing the existence of areas lacking ependyma (*arrows*). Neuroblasts (nb) have accumulated near the surface denuded of ependyma. (Fig. 1.3a). Hydrocephalus due to aqueductal stenosis: coronal view of fetal MRI: there is enlargement of the lateral ventricles, with the third ventricle almost normal. (Fig. 1.3b, c). Sagital and coronal views of cranial ultrasound show dilated lateral ventricles with a 19.4-mm caudothalamic cleft. (Fig. 1.4a, b). Coronal and sagittal views of MRI showing significant cortical thinning with severe dilatation of the ventricles. The fourth ventricle is normal. Findings suggestive of aqueductal stenosis.

Imaging Findings

Case 2: Tuberous Sclerosis Complex

Laura Ortiz Terán and Agnies M. Van Eeghen

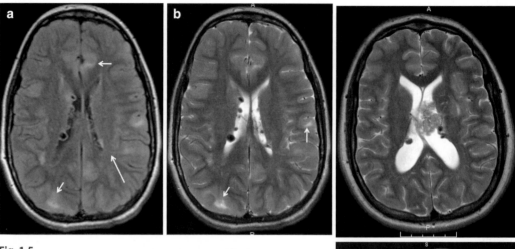

Fig. 1.5

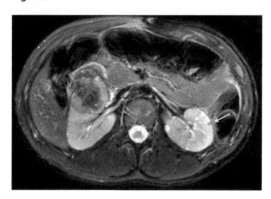

Fig. 1.6

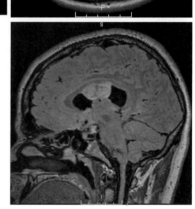

Fig. 1.7

DIAGNOSTIC CRITERIA

Table 1: Revised Diagnostic Criteria for Tuberous Sclerosis Complex

Major Features	Minor Features
Facial angiofibromas or forehead plaque	Multiple randomly distributed pits in dental enamel
Non-traumatic (peri) ungual fibroma	
Hypomelanotic macules (>3)	Hamartomatous rectal polyps
Shagreen patch (connective tissue nevus)	Bone cysts
Multiple retinal nodular hamartomas	Cerebral white matter migration lines
Cortical tuber	Gingival fibromas
Subependymal nodule	Non-renal hamartoma
Subependymal giant cell astrocytoma	Retinal achromic patch
Cardiac rhabdomyoma, single or multiple	"Confetti" skin lesions
Lymphangiomyomatosis	Multiple renal cysts
Renal angiomyolipoma	

Definite TSC: Either 2 major features or 1 major feature with 2 minor features
Probable TSC: One major feature and one minor feature
Possible TSC: Either 1 major feature or 2 or more minor features

Roach ES et al. J Child Neur. 2004

Fig. 1.8

A 13-year-old girl with a history of developmental delay, infantile spasms, refractory partial-complex epilepsy, and autistic features.

Comments

Tuberous sclerosis complex (TSC) is an autosomal dominant disorder resulting from mutations in the TSC1 or the TSC2 gene. Incidence is estimated to be 1 in 6,000.

TSC is a multisystem disorder characterized by the formation of hamartomas in multiple organ systems, most commonly the brain, skin, kidneys, and eyes (Fig. 1.8).

Neurologic manifestations were first described by D. M. Bourneville in 1880 and later by H. Vogt in 1908. Vogt described what is known as the "classic triad" of symptoms: seizures, mental retardation, and adenoma sebaceum (angiofibromas). However, studies have demonstrated that less than 30% of patients have these three symptoms.

Seizure disorders occur in 70–90% of patients and often develop within the first year of life. Developmental and behavioral disorders, including autism spectrum disorders, are also frequently diagnosed. Subependymal nodules (SEN), radial migration lines (RML), and subependymal giant cell tumors (SGCT) are the most commonly described neuroradiological features in TSC.

Renal manifestations include angiomyolipomas (AML) and cysts. AML, present in 75% of patients, are a major criterion in TSC, whereas the presence of cysts is not specific for TSC. Fetal cardiac rhabdomyomas and rhabdomyosarcomas are increasingly seen as the first presenting sign in TSC.

Of all the manifestations involving TSC, seizures, SGCT, renal failure, and lymphangioleiomyomatosis contribute the most to morbidity and mortality. However, complications can be minimized by early diagnosis, lifelong monitoring, and proactive treatments such as mTOR (mammalian target of rapamycin) inhibitors, involved in tumor reduction, especially SGCT and AML.

Imaging Findings

(Fig. 1.5a, b). FLAIR and T2-weighted images showing periventricular nodules consistent with SEN, a hyperintense RML in the left occipital horn (*long arrow*) and several hyperintense subcortical and cortical lesions known as tubers (*short arrows*). (Fig. 1.6). A well-defined, fat-containing mass located in the superior pole of the right kidney and another T2 dark focus in the lateral aspect of the interpolar region of the left kidney (*arrow*), both consistent with AML. Subcentimeter cysts are seen in both kidneys. (Fig. 1.7a, b). Axial T2 and sagittal FLAIR images show a large heterogeneous mass adjacent to the foramen of Monro with displacement of the septum to the right consistent with a SGCT. Several periventricular SEN are also noted. (Fig. 1.8). Diagnostic criteria for tuberous sclerosis complex (Roach and Sparagana (2004)).

Case 3: Pediatric Human Immunodeficiency Virus Encephalopathy

María Dolores Domínguez-Pinos and María I. Martínez-León

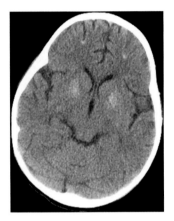

Fig. 1.9

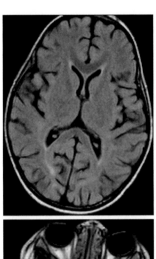

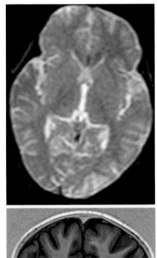

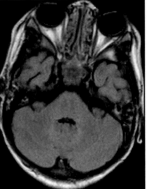

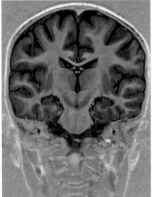

Fig. 1.10

Fig. 1.11

Lessions	Disease	
Difuse white matter disease	HIV encephalopathy (HIVE) Diffuse CMV encephalitis	
Patchy white matter disease	HIVE Progressive multifocal leucoencephalopathy (PML) Herpes viral infection Non-specific white matter T2 hyperintense	
Focal mass with enhancement	Toxoplasmosis Lymphoma (PCNSL) Cryptococcoma	Mycobacterial infection Cytomegalovirus
Focal mass without enhancement	Pseudocysts and cyptococcomas Toxoplasmosis Atypical PCNSL	
Focal lesion no mass with enhancement	Toxoplasmosis Cerebral infartion Viral encephalitis	Bacterial cerebritis PML
Focal lesion no mass without enhancement	Unifocal PML Diffuse infiltrative form of PCNSL	

Fig. 1.12

A 4-year-old African girl with neonatal human immunodeficiency virus (HIV) infection.

Comments

Maternal-fetal transmission (vertical) is the main route of transmission of infection in childhood. Twenty-three percent of infected infants will develop AIDS (acquired immune deficiency syndrome) in the first years of life.

A viral DNA polymerase chain reaction (PCR) test is performed at 48th day of life for the diagnosis in blood, detecting 40% of infected infants. It is repeated within 2 weeks for negative cases. In cases in which the central nervous system (CNS) is involved, it could be performed in the cerebrospinal fluid (CSF).

CNS disease includes the primary effects of HIV (progressive encephalopathy and static encephalopathy), opportunistic infections (toxoplasm, cytomegalovirus, cryptococcus, etc.), neoplasms (lymphoma), and vascular disease (cerebrovascular ischemic accidents or hemorrhage).

Clinical findings are nonspecific and range from mild cognitive impairment to frank neurological deficit or coma.

Magnetic resonance imaging (MRI) has high sensitivity for the detection of lesions in HIV encephalopathy. White matter disease (predominantly frontal) and cerebral atrophy (central, generalized, or encephalomalacia) are common findings.

Calcifications appear in 33% in basal ganglia in 33% of cases (bilateral and symmetrical), in subcortical frontal white matter, and in the cerebellum.

The coexistence of multiple pathologies has been described in up to 30% of autopsies.

Current treatment with HAART (high active antiretroviral therapy) has transformed the prognosis of HIV infection and reduces malignancies and opportunistic infections.

Imaging Findings

(Fig. 1.9). Cranial CT without contrast, showing calcifications in both pale nucleus and in subcortical white matter of bilateral frontal lobes.

(Fig. 1.10). MRI brain FLAIR-weighted axial sequence showing generalized supratentorial atrophy. Anatomy of the cerebellum is preserved, and the difference with temporal lobe atrophy can be observed.

(Fig. 1.11). Although basal ganglia calcification is evident on CT, in T2-weighted gradient echo sequence, it is not identified (very sensitive to magnetic susceptibility), possibly because the signal from surrounding tissue masks the calcium signal. The same happens in the T1-weighted inversion recovery sequence (see de la Iglesia et al. (2006)).

(Fig. 1.12). Summary table of CNS findings in pediatric HIV (*Modified from Sibtain and Chinn (2002)*).

Case 4: Acute Cerebellitis Secondary to Rotavirus Infection (ACSRI)

Alberto Muñoz González

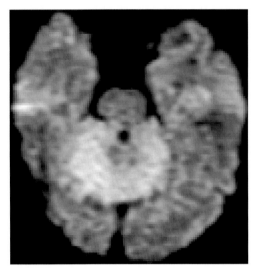

Fig. 1.13

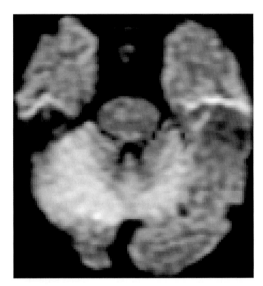

Fig. 1.14

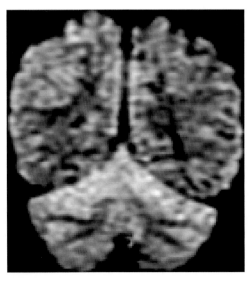

Fig. 1.15

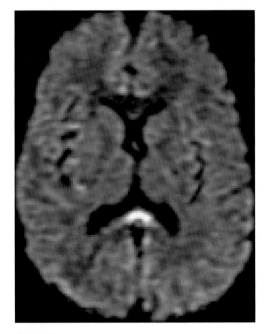

Fig. 1.16

This 5-year-old girl presented with acute onset of ataxia, tremor, nystagmus, dysmetria, and dysarthria following mutism. Two days before, she experienced a serious episode of gastroenteritis with fever. Basic blood tests showed leukocytosis and mild anemia.

Comments

Acute cerebellitis is considered an inflammatory syndrome and is clinically defined as fever, nausea, headache, and an altered mental status in conjunction with acute onset of cerebellar symptoms. Rotavirus is one of the most common pathogens causing gastroenteritis among children. Neurologic manifestations range from benign convulsions with gastroenteritis to lethal encephalitis or encephalopathy, and occur in approximately 2–5% of patients with rotavirus gastroenteritis. In addition, rotavirus is associated with acute cerebellitis, acute necrotizing encephalopathy (ANE), and mild encephalitis/ encephalopathy with a reversible splenial lesion (MERS).

The diagnosis is usually made by demonstrating a positive antigen title for rotavirus from a stool sample. CSF analysis usually reveals pleocytosis with normal glucose and protein.

Initial MR imaging between days 4 and 6 usually shows transient lesions with reduced diffusion in the cerebellar white matter/nuclei and in the splenium of the corpus callosum during the acute stage of the illness, between days 5 and 7. These disappeared on the follow-up MR imaging, with an interval of 3–9 days. In contrast, lesions in the vermis or cerebellar cortex were seen in the acute-to-chronic stages (day 5 to 1 year).

In the acute stage of other postinfectious cerebellitis, MR imaging may show severe cerebellar swelling that has compressed the brain stem or caused tonsillar herniation. However, this is rarely reported in enterovirus cerebellitis infection.

Both clinical and radiological patients with ACSRI show almost identical clinical symptoms and radiological findings. The pathophysiology of CNS involvement in patients with rotavirus gastroenteritis is not fully understood. It is often explained as direct CNS invasion by the rotavirus. Marked elevation of interleukin-6 was reported in the CSF of a patient with rotavirus cerebellitis, suggesting CNS inflammation with or without direct rotavirus invasion. However, there have been no reports explaining why rotavirus might affect the cerebellum more than the cerebrum.

Imaging Findings

Diffusion-weighted images in axial (Figs. 1.13 and 1.14) and coronal (Fig. 1.15) planes show thickening and restricted diffusion involving the vermis and upper regions of the cerebellar hemispheres, as well as the splenium of the corpus callosum (Fig. 1.16).

Case 5: Moyamoya Disease

Élida Vázquez Méndez and Ángel Sánchez-Montañez

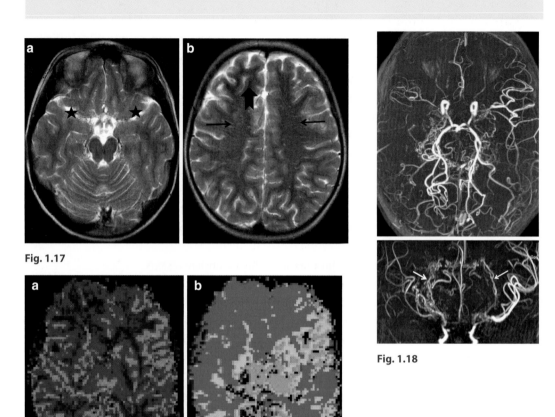

Fig. 1.17

Fig. 1.18

Fig. 1.19

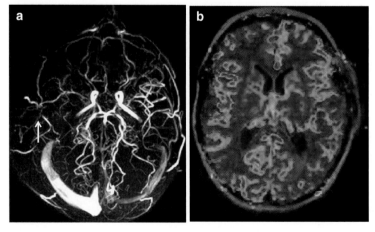

Fig. 1.20

A 4-year-old boy was examined by cranial MR imaging to investigate headaches. Family history was negative for neurofibromatosis or vascular diseases.

Moyamoya disease, a condition characterized primarily by angiographic findings, is a progressive cerebrovascular disease of uncertain etiology that involves the supraclinoid internal carotid arteries with prominent collateral arterial formation. According to the diagnostic criteria of the Japanese Cooperative Research Committee, only cases with bilateral lesions are diagnosed as "definite." It mainly affects Japanese or Koreans, although it also has been reported in other ethnic groups, with the highest incidence in the first decade of life. Clinical onset includes recurrent transient ischemic attacks or strokes, epileptic attacks, or headaches, although some patients are asymptomatic. Prevention of recurrent ischemia relies on surgical revascularization procedures: encephaloduroarteriosynangiosis (EDAS) is the external carotid artery (ECA)-to-ICA bypass.

Main imaging techniques may be used to evaluate cerebral hemodynamics in moyamoya disease. MRI has been widely used in assessing moyamoya disease because of its capacity to illustrate anatomic vascular details. Progressive arterial stenosis results in exuberant recruitment of collaterals, forming a cloudy angiographic appearance named puff of smoke ("moyamoya" in Japanese). Perfusion MRI has been found to be effective in estimating cerebral hemodynamics in moyamoya disease and evaluating changes after bypass surgery. New MRI perfusion methods, such as dynamic susceptibility contrast (DSC)-weighted bolus-tracking and arterial spin labeling (ASL), are now available for quantitative hemodynamic analyses. TTP and CBV perfusion maps can depict hemodynamic status before and after surgery and can be used to predict clinical outcomes after revascularization procedure.

(Fig. 1.17a). Axial T2-weighted images show the absence of both middle cerebral arteries (*asterisks*), (b) multiple enlarged perivascular spaces within the white matter (*long arrows*), and an ischemic lesion in the right frontal lobe (*short arrow*). (Fig. 1.18). MRA with TOF (time-of-flight) 3D sequence, axial and coronal, demonstrate severe ICA narrowing, with involvement of proximal middle cerebral arteries, and enlarged collateral lenticulostriate arteries with a "puff of smoke" pattern (*arrows*). (Fig. 1.19). Preoperative DSC reveals (a) decreased perfusion in both hemispheres, more prominent on the right side on relative cerebral blood volume (rCBV) map, and (b) prolonged time to peak enhancement (TTP) map in the right hemisphere and left frontal lobe. (Fig. 1.20). Patient underwent EDAS, first on the right side. (a) A patent bypass between the right STA-MCA is well depicted on axial MRA image (*arrow*). (b) The same revascularization procedure was then performed in the left hemisphere with excellent clinical outcome. Postoperative ASL demonstrates increased perfusion in both temporal lobes.

Case 6: Pediatric Multiple Sclerosis Revisited

Beatriz Asenjo García

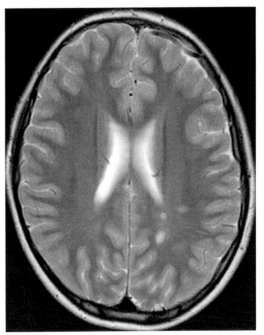

Fig. 1.21

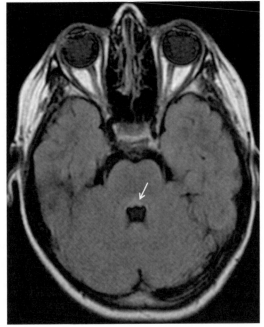

Fig. 1.22

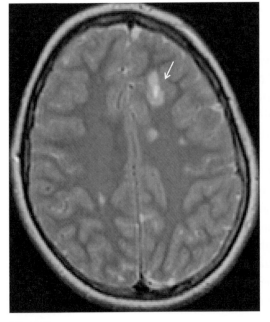

Fig. 1.23

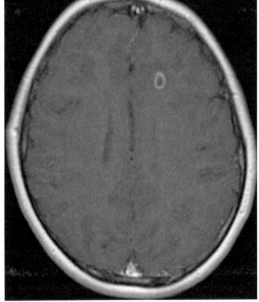

Fig. 1.24

An 11-year-old boy presents with acute onset of paralysis of both III and VII right cranial nerves.

Multiple sclerosis (MS) is a chronic inflammatory demyelinizing disease with an extremely variable clinical course. Up to 85% of patients start with a clinically isolated syndrome that includes optic neuritis and involvement of other cranial nerves and spinal cord.

The diagnosis work-up of MS includes conventional magnetic resonance (MR) imaging that demonstrates lesion dissemination in time and space. The topic of MR imaging criteria was revisited in 2010 by an expert group (MAGNIMS, Magnetic Imaging in MS). They considered periventricular and juxtacortical white matter, posterior fossa, and spinal cord as characteristic locations for lesions.

MS lesions appear as focal areas of hyperintensity on dual-echo and FLAIR imaging. On T1-weighted images, lesion characteristics are variable. They can be isointense or hypointense in respect to normal white matter. Gadolinium-enhanced T1-weighted images can differentiate active from inactive lesions, given that uptake contrast is related to the rupture of the blood–brain barrier or increased permeability associated with inflammatory processes. Lesions persistently hypointense on T1, with and without contrast, are associated with severe tissue damage such as axonal loss ("black holes").

Unfortunately, MR imaging is a highly sensitive test for detection of white matter lesions, but with a low specificity. Edema, inflammation, and other pathological lesions can present the same radiological appearance.

Modern MRI techniques such as magnetization transfer or spectroscopy can help to monitorize the disease, but they are not routinely included in the diagnosis in clinical practice.

First, MRI diagnosis: axial T2-weighted (Fig. 1.21) and FLAIR (Fig. 1.22) MR images on the clinically isolated syndrome event show hyperintense ovoid lesions located on periventricular left parietal white matter close to the IV ventricle (*arrow*). None of these lesions uptake contrast on T1-weighted images (not shown).

Three months later, axial T2 (Fig. 1.23) and T1 (Fig. 1.24) weighted images demonstrate new lesions on left frontal white matter associated to edema (*arrow*) and contrast-ring enhancement, meaning the disease is active and progressing.

Case 7: Cystic Craniopharyngioma

Germaine Cartier Velázquez and María I. Martínez-León

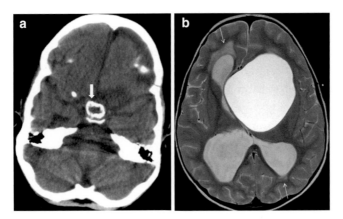

Fig. 1.25

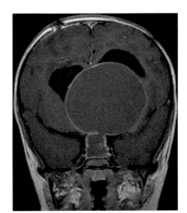

Fig. 1.26

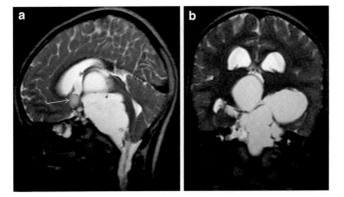

Fig. 1.27

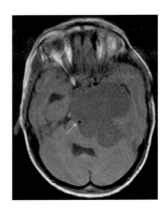

Fig. 1.28

Case 1 (Figs. 1.1 and 1.2): A 4-year-old girl with symptoms of headache, vomiting, bilateral convergent strabismus of nerve VI, and secondary hypothyroidism.

Case 2 (Figs. 1.7 and 1.8): A 9-year-old boy with neurological impairment and reduced bilateral vision.

Comments

Craniopharyngiomas are the most common tumors of the sellar region in childhood, representing up to 50% of tumors, with a similar incidence in both sexes and two peaks of age of onset: 5–10 years and 60–70 years of age.

With extra-axial location and slow growth, they typically sit in the midline and are classified as WHO grade I. They are composed of squamous epithelium derived from remnants of Rathke's pouch and can be solid, cystic, or mixed. They have two main variants: adamantinomatous, typical of pediatric age groups, and squamous-papillary. Up to 9% are considered "giant cystic craniopharyngiomas," prevalence of tumors with cystic components that reach large diameters.

Clinically, they may present with neurological, endocrinological, and visual symptoms; vision loss is the most common symptom.

Calcifications seen on CT can appear as ring-shaped, thick or thin, as eggshells, and with popcorn forms; they appear in up to 90% of cases and are the "hallmark of adamantinomatous craniopharyngiomas." Magnetic resonance imaging (MRI) T1- and T2-weighted images show that the signal of the cystic component varies according to the contents of the cyst, describing different semiological patterns: protein, fluid, blood, and fat. They exhibit heterogeneous enhancement of the solid component, generally in the sellar location, and wall enhancement of the cystic component, usually suprasellar.

Treatment possibilities include total or subtotal resection with adjuvant radiation therapy, drainage of cystic component, intracavitary instillation of RT and, ultimately, QT (intracystic bleomycin).

Imaging Findings

(Fig. 1.25). (a) CT without contrast shows ring calcification (*thick arrow*). (b) MRI Axial T2-weighted image: hyperintensity of the cyst with a signal greater than the CSF; CSF transependymal migration (*thin arrows*) caused by obstruction of the Monroes.

(Fig. 1.26). MR coronal T1-weighted images: thin enhancement of the cystic wall of the tumor, peripheral enhancement of the solid component.

(Fig. 1.27a, b). MR sagittal and coronal T2-weighted images: middle fossa tumor extension of the cystic component, posterior (retroclival) and anterior (pre-hypothalamic). Solid nodular component of small size (*long arrow*).

(Fig. 1.28). MR axial T1-weighted images: basilar artery (*arrow*) is encased 270° by the tumor and is displaced laterally and posteriorly by the cystic component. The signal of the cyst is hypointense, but higher than CSF.

Case 8: Obstetric Brachial Plexus Injuries and Magnetic Resonance Imaging

Daniela Binaghi and Mariano Socolovsky

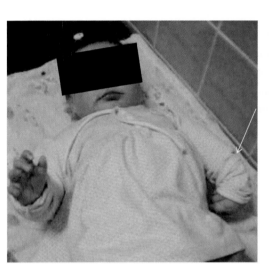

Fig. 1.29

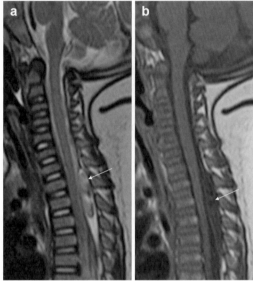

Fig. 1.30

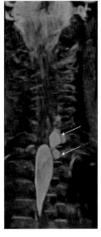

Fig. 1.31

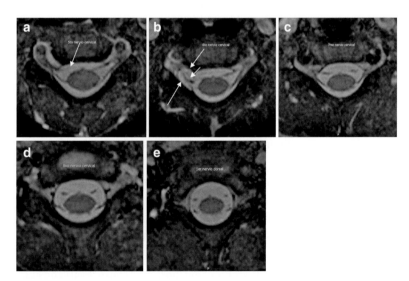

Fig. 1.32

A 4-month-old infant with flaccid paralysis of the left upper extremity present at birth (Fig. 1.29).

The brachial plexus (BP), which in the majority of individuals is formed by the ventral rami of spinal nerves C5 to T1, with or without minor branches from C4 and T2, supplies the upper extremities with motor and sensory functions.

Obstetric brachial plexus palsy, one of the most complex peripheral nerve injuries, is defined as flaccid paralysis of an upper extremity caused by traction to the BP during labor; such injury is observed in up to three per 1,000 births. The majority of these children recover with either no deficit or a minor functional deficit, but 20–30% fail to regain adequate limb function. To optimize results, a detailed evaluation is essential for treatment planning.

The degree of nerve root injury ranges from neurapraxia, which is damage to the nerve root without axonal tear that often heals spontaneously over time, to avulsion, which is a preganglionic tear. The upper BP is most commonly affected (Erb palsy), with resultant injury to the C5 and C6 roots. Isolated injury to the lower plexus (C8 and T1), as described by Déjerine-Klumpke, is rare and is suggested to originate from complete plexus palsy with resolution of the upper plexus component.

Magnetic resonance (MR) imaging is increasingly becoming the choice modality with which to assess infants and young children, in many cases replacing CT myelography. MRI allows for direct visualization of the spinal cord, roots, ligaments, and vertebral body. It also avoids radiation exposure and is much less invasive.

The image shows a 4-month-old infant with flaccid paralysis of the left upper extremity (*arrow*) (Fig. 1.29). Sagittal T2- and T1-weighted MR imaging (Fig. 1.30a, b) reveals a longitudinal posterior epidural hematoma from D1 to D5 (*arrow*) compressing the spinal cord. Its appearance may vary with time and may exhibit no characteristic intensity. However, it is not a common birth-related injury. On MR myelography (Fig. 1.31), a traumatic meningocele is a common finding (*arrows*) after nerve root avulsion; however, the absence of pseudocysts does not necessarily rule out preganglionic injury. In up to 30% of avulsions – mainly partial avulsions – no pseudocysts are detected. MR myelography should be reinforced by axial T2-balanced imaging to ensure the proper diagnosis. Another patient (Fig. 1.32), a 6-month-old infant with a typical Erb's palsy, exhibits partial avulsion of the right ventral root of C5 (Fig. 1.32a) and complete avulsion of C6 (*short arrow*) (Fig. 1.32b), with pseudomeningocele formation (*long arrows*). The right C7, C8, and T1 roots (Fig. 1.32c–e) are normal.

Case 9: Intradural Lipoma

Carmen Ballesteros-Guerrero and María I. Martínez-León

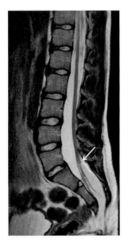
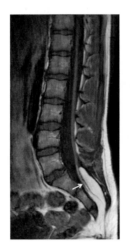
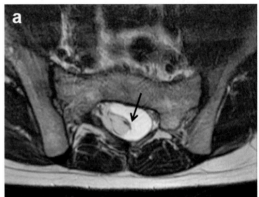
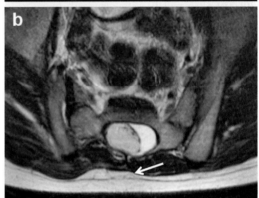

Fig. 1.33   **Fig. 1.34**

Fig. 1.35

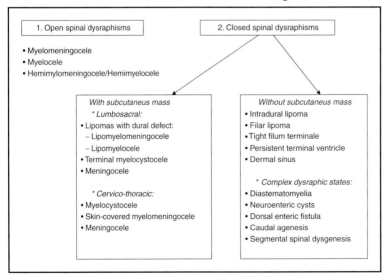

1. Open spinal dysraphisms	2. Closed spinal dysraphisms

• Myelomeningocele
• Myelocele
• Hemimylomeningocele/Hemimyelocele

With subcutaneus mass	*Without subcutaneus mass*
* Lumbosacral:	• Intradural lipoma
• Lipomas with dural defect:	• Filar lipoma
– Lipomyelomeningocele	• Tight filum terminale
– Lipomyelocele	• Persistent terminal ventricle
• Terminal myelocystocele	• Dermal sinus
• Meningocele	
	* Complex dysraphic states:
* Cervico-thoracic:	• Diastematomyelia
• Myelocystocele	• Neuroenteric cysts
• Skin-covered myelomeningocele	• Dorsal enteric fistula
• Meningocele	• Caudal agenesis
	• Segmental spinal dysgenesis

Fig. 1.36

A 12-year-old boy with incontinence of sphincters.

Spinal dysraphism includes a heterogeneous group of disorders caused by an incomplete closure of the neural tube during spinal cord development in early states of embryogenesis. Intradural lipoma is a closed spinal dysraphism without subcutaneous mass. In these patients, the presence of a subcutaneous mass on the baby's back and the identification of cutaneous markers facilitate an early diagnosis before neurological symptoms become apparent.

Comments

Prompt detection and rapid neurosurgical correction can prevent permanent neurological damage. In this context, imaging plays an important role, especially magnetic resonance imaging (MRI), as well as spinal ultrasound (SUS) at neonatal age.

The initial step is to perform a clinical examination to determine if the malformation is exposed to air or if there is skin coverage. These disorders are divided into open and closed depending on whether the underlying malformation has skin coverage or not. Closed spinal dysraphisms are further categorized based on the association with subcutaneous mass (Fig. 1.36, from Rossi's classification).

Taking into account the age of the patients and the availability of this technique, SUS is a very effective tool in primary screening. However, MRI is key to the classification and treatment planning of these abnormalities.

In our case, intradural lipoma is a closed spinal dysraphism without subcutaneous mass, the most frequent group in older children without dysraphism stigmata. Intradural lipomas are collections of adipose tissue located in the intradural space without communication with the subcutaneous fat. They are commonly situated at the lumbosacral level and usually present with tethered cord syndrome, which involves traction on a low-lying conus medullaris with progressive neurological deterioration. These lipomas are contained within an intact dural sac and can lie along the midline in the groove formed by the dorsal surface of the unapposed fold of the placode or displace the cord laterally. When they occur at the cervicothoracic level, they usually produce signs of medullar compression.

Sagittal T2-weighted (Fig. 1.33) and sagittal T1-weighted (Fig. 1.34) MRI show the lipoma (*long arrow*) as a sacral mass that extends from S1 to S5 levels within the spinal canal, isointense with subcutaneous fat, and the low-lying spinal cord tethered to the anterior surface of the sacral lipoma (*short arrow*). Axial T2-weighted (Fig. 1.35a, b) MRI shows the placode-lipoma interface lateral at S1 level (*black arrow*), and the closed dysraphism with no connection with the subcutaneous fat (*white arrow*). Scheme of open and closed spinal dysraphisms (Fig. 1.36).

Imaging Findings

Case 10: Dumbbell Neuroblastoma

Susana Ramírez Jiménez

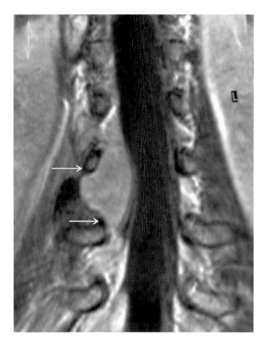

Fig. 1.37

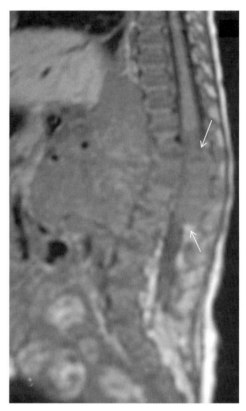

Fig. 1.39

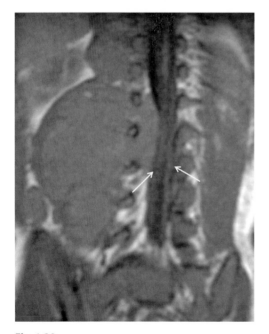

Fig. 1.38

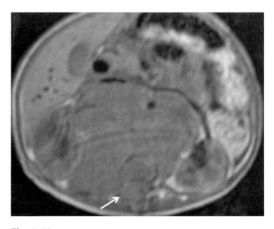

Fig. 1.40

Three patients aged 3, 1, and 10 months, respectively, with acute onset of lower extremity weakness.

Neuroblastoma (NB) occurs in very young children; the medium age at diagnosis is 17 months. Epidural compression (EC) of the tumor happens in approximately 5% of cases and is called dumbbell neuroblastoma (DNB). Localized NB are often asymptomatic, and diagnosis is made accidentally. However, EC caused by NB is usually symptomatic. Neurological impairment is present in 96% of children at diagnosis. The severity of motor deficit represents the most important risk factor for any type of sequelae, thus pointing to the importance of a high suspicion index.

Strong prognostic factors can predict whether children have a "good" or "bad" disease. Age at diagnosis (cutoff point <18 months) and stage of the disease, as formulated in the International Neuroblastoma Staging System (INSS), are considered the most important prognostic markers. Children >18 months with stage 4 (stage M) disease are at high risk of death (5-year survival <50%). In contrast, infants <18 months with localized tumors are almost always cured (survival rates >90%). Children with EC NB have localized disease more frequently and are <1 year old. In 2009, the International Neuroblastoma Risk Group (INRG) proposed a new staging system to stratify risk group patients at diagnosis before any treatment, based on preoperative imaging. INSS is based on the extension of tumor removal and lymph node status, so that excision of the primary tumor is a prerequisite for assigning patients to a stage. The INRGSS includes two stages of localized disease, which are dependent on whether image-defined risk factors are present or not at the time of diagnosis.

DNB cases represent true oncological emergencies, but there remains some controversy regarding what type of immediate intervention is best. Localized tumors are generally chemotherapy responsive, and some reports have documented equivalent neurological outcome for patients treated with chemotherapy or laminectomy. Due to the orthopedic consequences of laminectomy, most researchers recommend emergent chemotherapy as the intervention of choice for symptomatic EC by DNB.

Comments

(Fig. 1.37). Patient 1. MR localized coronal T1-weighted image shows NB that inserts into the spinal lumbar canal, remodeling and expanding the interpeduncular space (*arrows*). (Fig. 1.38). Patient 2. MR coronal T1-weighted image shows a large right adrenal DB NB with intraspinal extension. Roots are displaced (*arrows*). (Figs. 1.39 and 1.40). Patient 3. MR sagittal and axial T1-weighted images: the spinal component of the DB NB is higher, and there is compression of the medullar conus (*arrows*).

Imaging Findings

Further Reading

Case 1: Congenital Hydrocephalus

Book

Cinalli G, Maixner WJ, Sainte-Rose C (eds) (2005) Pediatric hydrocephalus, 1st edn. Springer, New York

Web Link

International Society for Hydrocephalus and Cerebrospinal Fluid Disorders: http://www.ishcsf.com/

Articles

Blaas HGK, Eik-Nes SH (2009) Sonoembryology and early prenatal diagnosis of neural anomalies. Prenat Diagn 29:312–325

David GH (2003) Fetal hydrocephalus. Clin Perinatol 30:531–539

Domínguez-Pinos MD, Páez P, Jiménez AJ, Weil B, Arráez MA, Pérez-Fígares JM, Rodríguez EM (2005) Ependymal denudation and alterations of the subventricular zone occur in human fetuses with a moderate communicating hydrocephalus. J Neuropathol Exp Neurol 64:595–604

Erickson K, Baron IS, Fantie BD (2001) Neuropsychological functioning in early hydrocephalus: review from a developmental perspective. Child Neuropsychol 7:199–229

Kestle JRW (2003) Pediatric hydrocephalus: current management. Neurol Clin 21:883–895

Oi S, Inagaki T, Shinoda M, Takahashi S, Ono S, Date I et al (2011) Guideline for management and treatment of fetal and congenital hydrocephalus: center of excellence-fetal and congenital hydrocephalus Top 10 Japan guideline 2011. Childs Nerv Syst 27:1563–1570

Rekate HL (2009) A contemporary definition and classification of hydrocephalus. Semin Pediatr Neurol 16:9–15

Rizvi R, Anjum Q (2005) Hydrocephalus in children. J Pak Med Assoc 55:502–507

Vazquez E, Mayolas N, Delgado I, Higueras T (2009) Fetal neuroimaging: US and MRI. Pediatr Radiol 39(Suppl 3):422–435

Wang KC, Lee JY, Kim SK, Phi JH, Cho BK (2011) Fetal ventriculomegaly: postnatal management. Childs Nerv Syst 27:1571–1573

Case 2: Tuberous Sclerosis Complex

Book

Kwiatkowski DJ, Whittemore VH, Thiele EA (eds) (2010) Tuberous sclerosis complex: genes, clinical features and therapeutics. Wiley-Blackwell, Weinheim

Web Link

http://www2.massgeneral.org/livingwithtsc/

Articles

Baskin HJ Jr (2008) The pathogenesis and imaging of the tuberous sclerosis complex. Pediatr Radiol 38:936–952

Casper KA, Donnelly LF, Chen B, Bissler JJ (2002) Tuberous sclerosis complex: renal imaging findings. Radiology 225:451–456

Evans JC, Curtis J (2000) The radiological appearances of tuberous sclerosis. Br J Radiol 73:91–98

Franz DN, Bissler JJ, McCormack FX (2010) Tuberous sclerosis complex: neurological, renal and pulmonary manifestations. Neuropediatrics 41:199–208, Epub 2011 Jan 5

Gallagher A, Grant EP, Madan N, Jarrett DY, Lyczkowski DA, Thiele EA (2010) MRI findings reveal three different types of tubers in patients with tuberous sclerosis complex. J Neurol 257:1373–1381

Goh S, Butler W, Thiele EA (2004) Subependymal giant cell tumors in tuberous sclerosis complex. Neurology 63:1457–1461

Kalantari BN, Salamon N (2008) Neuroimaging of tuberous sclerosis: spectrum of pathologic findings and frontiers in imaging. AJR Am J Roentgenol 190:304–309

Roach ES, Sparagana SP (2004) Diagnosis of tuberous sclerosis complex. J Child Neurol 19:643–649

Staley BA, Vail EA, Thiele EA (2011) Tuberous sclerosis complex: diagnostic challenges, presenting symptoms, and commonly missed signs. Pediatrics 127:e117–e125

Winterkorn EB, Daouk GH, Anupindi S, Thiele EA (2006) Tuberous sclerosis complex and renal angiomyolipoma: case report and review of the literature. Pediatr Nephrol 21:1189–1193

Case 3: Pediatric Human Immunodeficiency Virus Encephalopathy

Book

Zeichner SL (2005) Textbook of pediatric HIV care. Cambridge University Press, Cambridge. ISBN 0521821533

Web Link

http://www.hivma.org/

Articles

Belman AL (1997) Pediatric neuro-AIDS. Update. Neuroimaging Clin N Am 7:593–613

Boisse L, Gill J, Power C (2008) HIV infection of the central nervous system: clinical features and neuropathogenesis. Neurol Clin 26:799–819

Civitello LA (1991–1992) Neurologic complications of HIV infection in children. Pediatr Neurosurg 17:104–112

de la IMM Sarmiento, Lecumberri Cortés G, Lecumberri Cortés I, Oleaga Zufiria L, Isusi Fontan M, Grande Icaran D (2006) Intracranial calcifications on MRI. Radiologia 48:19–26

Exhenry C, Nadal D (1996) Vertical human immunodeficiency virus-1 infection: involvement of the central nervous system and treatment. Eur J Pediatr 155:839–850

Gavin P, Yogev R (1999) Central nervous system abnormalities in pediatric human immunodeficiency virus infection. Pediatr Neurosurg 31:115–123

Ramos JT, de José MI, Polo R, Fortuny C, Mellado MJ, Muñoz-Fernández MA et al (2005) Recommendations of the CEVIHP/SEIP/AEP/PNS on antiretroviral treatment in HIV-infected children and teenagers. Enferm Infecc Microbiol Clin 23:279–312

Safriel YI, Haller JO, Lefton DR, Obedian R (2000) Imaging of the brain in the HIV-positive child. Pediatr Radiol 30:725–732

Sibtain NA, Chinn RJS (2002) Imaging of the central nervous system in HIV infection. Imaging 14:48–59

States LJ, Zimmerman RA, Rutstein RM (1997) Imaging of pediatric central nervous system HIV infection. Neuroimaging Clin N Am 7:321–339

Case 4: Acute Cerebellitis Secondary to Rotavirus Infection (ACSRI)

Book

Barkovich AJ (2005) Pediatric neuroimaging, 4th ed. Lippincott & Williams and Wilkins, Philadelphia, pp 839–840

Web Link

http://www.slideshare.net/yassermetwally/short-case-postinfectious-cerebellitis-presentation

Articles

Dimova P, Bojinova VS, Milanov IG (2009) Transient mutism and pathologic laughter in the course of cerebellitis. Pediatr Neurol 41:49–52

Fukuda S, Kishi K, Yasuda K et al (2009) Rotavirus-associated encephalopathy with a reversible splenial lesion. Pediatr Neurol 40:131–133

Lynch M, Lee B, Azimi P et al (2001) Rotavirus and central nervous system symptoms: cause or contaminant? Case reports and review. Clin Infect Dis 33:932–938

Mewasingh LD, Kadhim H, Christophe C et al (2003) Nonsurgical cerebellar mutism (anarthria) in two children. Pediatr Neurol 28:59–63

Papavasiliou AS, Kotsalis C, Trakadas S (2004) Transient cerebellar mutism in the course of acute cerebellitis. Pediatr Neurol 30:71–74

Ramig RF (2004) Pathogenesis of intestinal and systemic rotavirus infection. J Virol 78:10213–10220

Shiihara T, Watanabe I, Honma A et al (2007) Rotavirus associated encephalitis/ encephalopathy and concurrent cerebellitis: report of two cases. Brain Dev 29:670–673

Tada H, Takanashi J, Barkovich AJ et al (2004) Clinically mild encephalitis/encephalopathy with a reversible splenial lesion. Neurology 63:1854–1858

Takanashi J (2009) Two newly proposed infectious encephalitis/encephalopathy syndromes. Brain Dev 31:521–528

Case 5: Moyamoya Disease

Book

Barkovich AJ (2005) Pediatric neuroimaging, 4th ed. Lippincott & Williams and Wilkins, Philadelphia

Web Link

http://www.ninds.nih.gov/disorders/moyamoya/moyamoya.htm

Articles

Fujita K, Tamak N, Matsumoto S (1986) Surgical treatment of moyamoya disease in children: which is the more effective procedure, EDAS or EMS? Childs Nerv Syst 2:134–138

Lee SK, Kim DI, Jeong EK, Kim SY, Kim SH, In YK et al (2003) Postoperative evaluation of moyamoya disease with perfusion-weighted MR imaging: initial experience. AJNR Am J Neuroradiol 24:741–747

Lee M, Zaharchuk G, Guzman R, Achrol A, Bell-Stephens T, Steinberg GK (2009) Quantitative hemodynamic studies in moyamoya disease: a review. Neurosurg Focus 26(4):E5

Pandey P, Steinberg GK (2011) Neurosurgical advances in the treatment of moyamoya disease. Stroke 42:3304–3310

Suzuki J, Takaku A (1969) Cerebrovascular "moyamoya" disease: a disease showing abnormal net-like vessels in base of brain. Arch Neurol 20:288–299

Yamada I, Matsushima Y, Suzuki S (1992) Moyamoya disease: diagnosis with three-dimensional time-of-flight MR angiography. Radiology 184:773–778

Yamada I, Suzuki S, Matsushima Y (1995) Moyamoya disease: comparison of assessment with MR angiography and MR imaging versus conventional angiography. Radiology 196:211–218

Yonekawa Y, Goto Y, Ogata N (1986) Moyamoya disease: diagnosis, treatment, and recent achievement. Stroke 1:805–829

Yoon HK, Shin HJ, Lee M, Byun HS, Na DG, Han BK (2000) MR angiography of moyamoya disease before and after encephaloduroarteriosynangiosis. AJR Am J Roentgenol 174:195–200

Yun TJ, Cheon JE, Na DG, Kim WS, Kim IO, Chang KH et al (2009) Childhood moyamoya disease: quantitative evaluation of perfusion MR imaging – correlation with clinical outcome after revascularization surgery. Radiology 251:216–223

Case 6: Pediatric Multiple Sclerosis Revisited

Book

Asenjo García B (2005). Multiple Sclerosis. In: Martínez León MI, Ceres Ruiz L, Gutiérrez J, Learning Pediatric Imaging. Ribes, Luna, Ros (eds)Springer. Berlin, pp 54-55

Web Link

www.mssociety.org.uk

Articles

Filippi M, Agosta F (2007) Magnetization transfer MRI in multiple sclerosis. J Neuroimaging 17(Suppl 1): 22S–26S

Filippi M, Rocca MA (2007) Conventional MRI in multiple sclerosis. J Neuroimaging 17(Suppl 1):3S–9S

Filippi M, Rocca M (2011) MR Imaging of multiple sclerosis. Radiology 259:659–681

Lövblad KO, Anzalone N, Dörfler A et al (2010) MR imaging in multiple sclerosis: review and recommendations for current practice. AJNR Am J Neuroradiol 31:983–989

McDonald WI, Compston A, Edan G, Goodkin D, Hartung HP, Lublin FD et al (2001) Recommended diagnostic criteria for multiple sclerosis: guidelines from the international panel on the diagnosis of multiple sclerosis. Ann Neurol 50:121–127

Okuda DT, Mowry EM, Beheshtian A et al (2009) Incidental MRI anomalies suggestive of multiple sclerosis: the radiologically isolated syndrome. Neurology 72:800–805

Polman CH, Reingold SC, Edan G et al (2005) Diagnostic criteria for multiple sclerosis: 2005 revisions to the "McDonald criteria". Ann Neurol 58:840–846

Simon JH, Li D, Traboulsee A et al (2006) Standardized MR imaging protocol for multiple sclerosis: consortium of MS centers consensus guidelines. AJNR Am J Neuroradiol 27:455–461

Swanton JK, Fernando K, Dalton CM, Miszkiel KA, Thompson AJ, Plant GT et al (2006) Modification of MRI criteria for multiple sclerosis in patients with clinically isolated syndromes. J Neurol Neurosurg Psychiatry 77:830–833

Swanton JK, Rovira A, Tintore M, Altmann DR, Barkhf F, Filippi M et al (2007) MRI criteria for multiple sclerosis in patients presenting with clinically isolated syndromes: a multicentre retrospective study. Lancet Neurol 6:677–686

Case 7: Cystic Craniopharyngioma

Book

Castillo M (2006) Extra-axial tumors. In: Castillo M, Mc Allister L, Baryett K (eds) Neuroradiology companion, 3rd edn. Lippincott Williams & Wilkins, Philadelphia, p 129

Web Link

Wasserman JR, Smirniotopoulos JG. Craniopharyngioma imaging. http://emedicine.medscape.com/article/339424-overview. 2011

Articles

Albright AL, Hadjipanayis CG, Lunsford LD, Kondziolka D, Pollack IF, Adelson PD (2005) Individualized treatment of pediatric Craniopharyngiomas. Childs Nerv Syst 21:649–654

Cáceres A (2005) Intracavitary therapeutic options in the management of cystic craniopharyngioma. Childs Nerv Syst 21:705–718

Curran JG, O'Connor E (2005) Imaging of craniopharyngioma. Childs Nerv Syst 21:635–639

Garnett MR, Puget S, Grill J, Sainte-Rose C (2007) Craniopharyngioma. Review. OJRD 2:1–18

Karavitaki N, Cudlip S, Adams CB, Wass JA (2006) Craniopharyngiomas. Endocr Rev 27:371–397

Molla E, Martí-Bonmatí L, Revert A, Arana E, Menor F, Dosda R et al (2001) Craniopharyngiomas: identification of different semiological patterns with MRI. Eur Radiol 12:1829–1836

Muñoz A, Hinojosa J, Esparza J (2007) Cisternography and ventriculography gadopentate dimeglumine-enhanced MR imaging in pediatric patients: preliminary report. AJNR Am J Neuroradiol 28: 889–894

Rossi A, Cama A, Consales A, Gandolfo C, Garrè ML, Milanaccio C et al (2006) Neuroimaging of pediatric craniopharyngiomas: a pictorial essay. J Pediatr Endocrinol Metab 19:299–319

Vivek BJ, Lakshminarayan R, Ipeson PK, Ari GC (2003) MR ventriculography for the study of CSF flow. AJNR Am J Neuroradiol 24:373–381

Wang KC, Hong SH, Kim SK, Cho BK (2005) Origin of craniopharyngiomas: implication on the growth pattern. Childs Nerv Syst 2:628–634

Case 8: Obstetric Brachial Plexus Injuries and Magnetic Resonance Imaging

Book

Siqueira MG, Malessy MJA (2011) Traumatic brachial plexus lesions: clinical and surgical aspects. In: Siqueira MG, Socolovsky M, Malessy MJA, Devi IB (eds) Treatment of peripheral nerve lesions, vol 10, 1st edn. Prism Books PVT LTD, Bangalore/Chennai/Hyderabad/Kochi/Kolkata, pp 93–110

Web Link

http://www.orthoseek.com/articles/brachialpp.html

Articles

Goetz E (2010) Neonatal spinal cord injury after an uncomplicated vaginal delivery. Pediatr Neurol 42:69–71

Malessy MJA, Pondaag W (2009) Obstetric brachial plexus injuries. Neurosurg Clin N Am 20:1–14

Malessy MJA, Pondaag W, Van Dijk JG (2009) Electromyography, nerve action potential, and compound motor action potentials in obstetric brachial plexus lesions: validation in the absence of a "gold standard". Neurosurgery 65:A153–A159

Mallouhi A, Marik W, Prayer D, Kainberger F, Bodner G, Kasprian G (2011) 3T MR tomography of the brachial plexus: structural and microstructural evaluation. Eur J Radiol doi:10.1016/j.ejrad.2011.05.021

Nath RK, Liu X (2009) Nerve reconstruction in patients with obstetric brachial plexus injury results in worsening of glenohumeral deformity: a case-control study of 75 patients. J Bone Joint Surg Br 91:649–654

Nath RK, Amrani A, Melcher SE, Wentz MJ, Paizi M (2010) Surgical normalization of the shoulder joint in obstetric brachial plexus injury. Ann Plast Surg 65: 4411–4417

Ruchelsman DE, Oetrone S, Price AE, Grossman JÁ (2009) Brachial plexus birth palsy: an overview of early treatment considerations. Bull NYU Hosp Jt Dis 67:83–89

Smith AB, Gupta N, Strober J, Chin C (2008) Magnetic resonance neurography in children with birth-related brachial plexus injuries. Pediatr Radiol 38:159–163

Steens SC, Pondaag W, Malessy MJA, Verbist BM (2011) Obstetric brachial plexus lesions: CT myelography. Radiology 259:508–515

Zafeiriou D, Psychogiou K (2008) Obstetrical brachial plexus palsy. Pediatr Neurol 38:235–242

Case 9: Intradural Lipoma

Book

Tortori-Donati P, Rossi A, Biancheri R (2005) Congenital malformations of the spine and spinal cord. In: Pediatric neuroradiology brain, vol 39. Springer, Berlin/Heidelberg/New York, pp 1551–1608

Web Link

http://seram2010.com/modules.php?name=posters&d_op=diapositivas&file=diapositivas&idpaper=843&forpubli=&idsection=2 Spina bifida: clinical-radiological classification and uncommon forms of presentation (SERAM review)

Articles

Brown E, Mathes JC, Bazan C III, Jinkins JR (1994) Prevalence of incidental intraspinal lipoma of the lumbosacral spine as determined by MRI. Spine 19:833–836

Dick EA, de Bruyn R (2003) Ultrasound of the spinal cord in children: its role. Eur Radiol 13:552–562

Egelhoff J (1999) MR imaging of congenital anomalies of the pediatric spine. Magn Reson Imaging Clin N Am 7:459–479

Korsvik HE (1992) Sonography of occult dysraphism in neonates and infants with MR imaging correlation. Radiographics 12:297–306

Muroi A, Fleming KL, McClomb JG (2010) Split medulla in association with close neural tube defects. Childs Nerv Syst 26:967–971

Rossi A, Biancheri R, Cama A, Piatelli G, Ravegnani M, Tortori-Donati P (2004a) Imaging in spine and spinal cord malformations. Eur J Radiol 50: 177–200

Rossi A, Cama A, Piatelli G, Biancheri R, Tortori-Donati P (2004b) Spinal dysraphism: MR imaging rationale. J Neuroradiol 31:3–24

Rufener S, Ibrahim M, Raybaud CA, Palmar HA (2010) Congenital spine and spinal cord malformations-pictorial review. AJR Am J Roentgenol 194(3 Suppl): S26–S37

Rufener S, Ibrahin M, Parmar HA (2011) Imaging of congenital spine and spinal cord malformations. Neuroimaging Clin N Am 21:659–676

Schijman E (2003) Split spinal cord malformations: report of 22 cases and review of the literature. Childs Nerv Syst 19:96–103

Case 10: Dumbbell Neuroblastoma

Book

Swischuk LE (1997) Chest masses. In: Imaging of the newborn, infant, and young child, 4th edn. Lippincott Williams & Wilkins, Baltimore, pp 143–147

Web Link

http://www.nbglobe.com/

Articles

Angelini P, Plantaz D, De Bernardi B, Passagia JG, Rubie H, Pastore G (2011) Late sequelae of symptomatic epidural compression in children with localized neuroblastoma. Pediatr Blood Cancer 57:473–480

Brisse HJ, Mc Carville MB, Granata C, Drug KB, Wootton-Gorges SL, Kanegawa K et al (2011) Guidelines for imaging and staging of neuroblastic tumors: consensus report from the International Neuroblastoma Risk Group Project. Radiology 261:243–257

Cohn SL, Pearson AD, London WB, Monclair T, Ambros PF, Brodeur GM et al (2009) The International Neuroblastoma Risk Group (INRG) classification system: an INRG Task Force report. J Clin Oncol 27:289–297

De Bernardi B, Balwierz V, Bejent J, Cohn SL, Garre ML, Iehara T et al (2005) Epidural compression in neuroblastoma: diagnostic and therapeutic aspects. Cancer Lett 228:283–299

Maris JM (2010) Recent advances in neuroblastoma. N Engl J Med 362:2202–2211

Maris JM, Hogarty MD, Bagatell R, Cohn SL (2007) Neuroblastoma. Lancet 369:2106–2120

Modak S (2011) Updates in the treatment of neuroblastoma. Clin Adv Hematol Oncol 9:74–76

Monclair T, Brodeur GM, Ambros PF, Brisse HJ, Cecchetto G, Colmes K et al (2009) The International Neuroblastoma Risk Group (INRG) staging system: an INRG Task Force report. J Clin Oncol 27:298–303

Moroz V, Machin D, Faldum A, Hero B, Lehara T, Mosseri V et al (2011) Changes over three decades in outcome and the prognostic influence of age-at-diagnosis in young patients with neuroblastoma: a report from the International Neuroblastoma Risk Group Project. Eur J Cancer 47:561–571

Park JR, Eggert A, Caron H (2008) Neuroblastoma: biology, prognosis, and treatment. Pediatr Clin North Am 55:97–120

Thoracic Imaging

2

María I. Martínez-León

Contents

M.I. Martínez-León et al., *Imaging for Pediatricians*, Imaging for Clinicians,
DOI 10.1007/978-3-642-28629-2_2, © Springer-Verlag Berlin Heidelberg 2012

Case 1: Postinfectious Bronchiolitis Obliterans

Javier Lucaya and Joaquim Piqueras

A 5-year-old boy who, 1 year prior to admission, had suffered adenovirus-induced pneumonia (Fig. 2.1). Since then, he has experienced frequent episodes of cough. Physical examination on admission revealed decreased breath sounds and some crackles in the left hemithorax. Inspiratory and expiratory AP chest X-rays and lung CT were obtained.

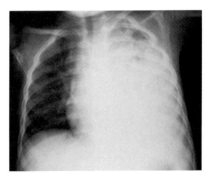

Fig. 2.1

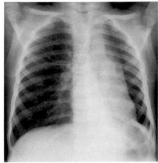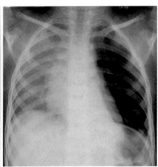

Fig. 2.2

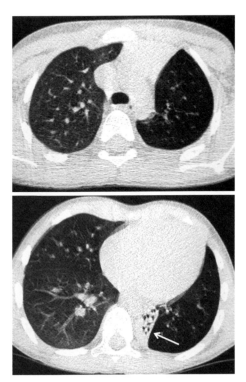

Fig. 2.3

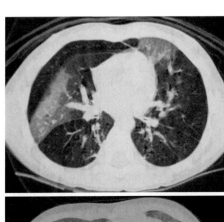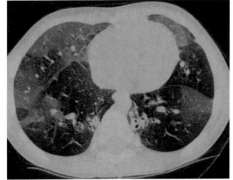

Fig. 2.4

Bronchiolitis obliterans (BO) is an uncommon and severe form of chronic obstructive lung disease in children and adults that results from an insult to the lower respiratory tract. Pathologically, BO is characterized by bronchiectasis of the large airway and obliteration of the small airways. Known etiologies include infection, particularly adenovirus and mycoplasma pneumonia, aspiration, toxic inhalation, lung and bone marrow transplantation, and connective tissue disorders. Presenting signs and symptoms include chronic cough, wheezing, exercise intolerance, tachypnea, and frequent respiratory illnesses. Crackles are a very common finding on auscultation.

A classic manifestation of postinfectious BO is the Swyer-James-MacLeod (SJM) syndrome . First thought to be of congenital origin, SJM is now considered a postinfectious form of BO.

Comments

In children with postinfectious BO, chest X-rays may show five different patterns:

(a) Unilateral hyperlucency of increased volume.
(b) Complete collapse of the affected lobe.
(c) Unilateral hyperlucency of small- or normal-sized lung.
(d) Bilateral hyperlucent lungs.
(e) Mixed pattern of persistent collapse and hyperlucency and peribronchial thickening (Fig. 2.2). When assessing a chest X-ray showing an asymmetrical degree of pulmonary aeration, the lung showing more vascularity is usually the normal one.

Imaging Findings

Chest CT is the imaging technique of choice. Characteristic diagnostic features include pulmonary hyperlucency and vascular attenuation, bronchiectasis, and/or a mosaic attenuation pattern. Lobar collapse, usually associated with bronchiectasis (*arrow*), occurs in 20% of cases (Fig. 2.3). Bilateral involvement (Fig. 2.4) of another patient will be present in 50% of cases. The involved areas on the high-resolution computed tomography correspond to those showing infiltrates on chest X-rays at the time of the initial pneumonia.

In children, the finding of a mosaic pattern of lung attenuation is practically synonymous with peripheral airway obstruction and is most commonly seen in asthma and BO. In our experience, the finding of associated bronchiectasis strongly favors the diagnosis of BO.

Pulmonary function tests (PFT) continue to be an important diagnostic tool in patients with BO. Unlike what occurs in asthma, patients with BO usually fail to respond to bronchodilator therapy. The results of PFTs in patients with BO characteristically show irreversible obstructive lung disease. The diagnosis of BO is usually established by radiologic and PFT findings but may be missed by lung biopsy due to sampling error.

Case 2: Thoracic Rib Invasion from Actinomycosis

Paul Marten and Rodrigo Domínguez

A 38-month-old girl with findings on computed tomography (CT) (Fig. 2.5) of multiple rib periostitis as an otherwise subtle chest wall spread

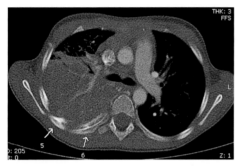
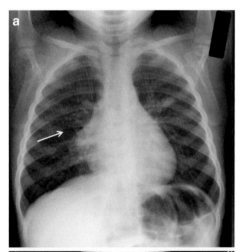

Fig. 2.5

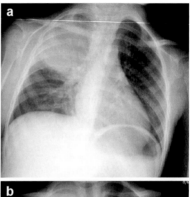
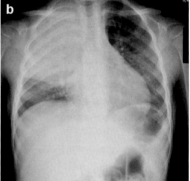

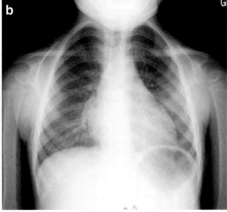

Fig. 2.6

Fig. 2.7

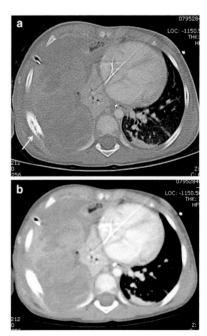

Fig. 2.8

of a presumed pneumonia. Previously, the patient had been treated as an outpatient for pneumonia at age 20 months. Subsequently, the findings became more widespread and in the very same location at 34 months, and kept worsening despite treatment, which prompted her admission.

Comments

Actinomycosis is an uncommon lower respiratory tract infection with aggressive features known to invade the chest wall and is associated with periostitis. Other aggressive pathogens which may be associated with chest wall invasion include tuberculosis or *Nocardia*. Particularly, if associated with empyema necessitans, other infections such as fungal (*Aspergillosis, Mucormycosis, Cryptococcosis*, etc.), *Staphylococcus aureus* (most common cause of pediatric osteomyelitis), *Streptococcus pyogenes*, etc.

Given the chronicity and resistance to treatment, two major differential categories should be considered: resistant infection with probable immune deficiency or tumor. Tumors considered are: Langerhans cell histiocytosis, Askin/PNET, primary bone tumor (Ewing more than osteosarcoma), rhabdomyosarcoma/other sarcomas, desmoid, lymphoma, or leukemia – often disseminated. Pleuropulmonary blastoma or metastatic tumors would be rare.

In our case, this patient tested negative for HIV with normal immunity but was prone to repeat infections from an undiagnosed non-cystic, non-cystic (solid) congenital cystic adenomatoid malformation. *Actinomyces israelii*, a slow-growing Gram-positive bacterium, often affects the gastrointestinal tract and head and neck. Pathologically, *Actinomycosis* and *Nocardia* behave similar to fungal infections causing solid peripheral mass, with *Actinomycosis* more prone to cause periostitis (like tuberculosis). Diagnosis is by biopsy and anaerobic culture.

Common imaging findings in Actinomyces infection are:

- Peripheral dense consolidation (non-segmental, often in the lower lobes) or mediastinal mass.
- Solid and slow progression consolidation. Cavitation and even fibrosis if left untreated.
- If the consolidation is untreated, it dissects along tissue planes with cutaneous sinus tracts with yellow thick pustulent drainage (with sulfur granules) and pleuritis with chest wall abscess.
- Pleural effusions and/or pericardial effusion.
- Multiple rib periostitis, +/− rib destruction, and severe rib eburnation.

Imaging Findings

(Fig. 2.5). Contrast-enhanced CT with solid parenchymal mass with subtle wall extension with posterior rib periostitis (*arrows*). Initial pneumonia at age 20 months (*arrow*) (Fig. 2.6a) appears resolved by age 29 months (Fig. 2.6b). (Fig. 2.7). Recurrence age 34 months (Fig. 2.7a), worsening and not responsive to antibiotics 38 months (Fig. 2.7b). Comparison with case of Ewing's sarcoma: note periostitis is confined to one rib (*arrow*) with more heterogeneous pleural mass and atelectasis right lung. No significant effusion (Fig. 2.8a, b).

Case 3: Non-Cystic Fibrosis Bronchiectasis

Estela Pérez Ruiz and Pilar Caro Aguilera

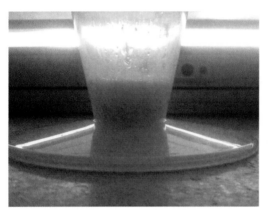

Fig. 2.9

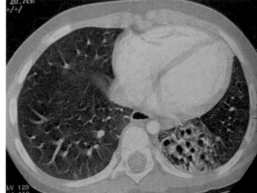

Fig. 2.10

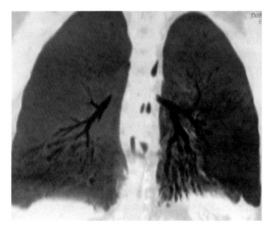

Fig. 2.11

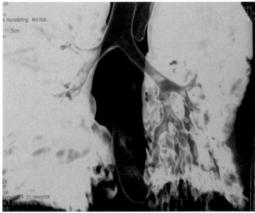

Fig. 2.12

An 8-year-old girl from the north of Africa presented with copious daily production of mucopurulent sputum. She had a history of previous pneumonia at the age of 2 years and recurrent respiratory tract infections since then.

Nowadays, an increase in the frequency of diagnosing non-cystic fibrosis bronchiectasis (NCFB) in children has been observed due probably to both heightened awareness of the disease and the wider availability of high-resolution computed tomography (HRCT). Moreover, NCFB remains an important cause of chronic suppurative lung disease in the developing world. Bronchiectasis is characterized by chronic airway inflammation that is driven by persistent infection and defined by the presence of permanent abnormally dilated medium-sized airways, with progressive destruction of the bronchial walls. Underlying causes have been described in 50–60% of NCFB. The most common underlying conditions include previous pneumonic illness, congenital and acquired immunodeficiency, primary ciliary dyskinesia, mechanical obstruction (inhaled foreign body, extrinsic compression, slow-growing tumor), and chronic aspiration. Fifty percent of cases keep without diagnosis. Postinfectious bronchial damage, particularly following adenovirus infection, still accounts for the majority of cases in childhood.

NCFB may be classified as a localized (one lobe) or generalized disease (multilobular) and also according to the pathological or radiographic appearance of the airways: *cylindrical,* dilated bronchi alone; *varicose,* focal constrictive areas between the dilated airways caused by defects in the bronchial wall; and *cystic,* airways ending in large cyst, saccules, or grape-like clusters.

In recent years, other terms have been proposed: *pre-bronchiectasis* (bronchial wall thickening on the HRCT scan, which may resolve entirely or progress), *HRCT bronchiectasis* (bronchial dilatation which may persist, resolve, or progress), and *established bronchiectasis* (the HRCT findings persist after 2 years, probably as an irreversible condition).

(Fig. 2.9). Copious daily mucopurulent sputum expectorated by the patient. (Fig. 2.10). HRCT (lung window setting): established bronchiectasis: mucous impaction, bronchial dilatation, and thickening with smaller adjacent pulmonary vessel (signet ring sign) in left lower lobe. (Fig. 2.11). Coronal reconstruction HRCT, mini-maximum intensity projection (miniMIP) reconstruction technique and (Fig. 2.12) tridimensional reconstruction HRCT provide a good depiction of established varicose bronchiectasis: bronchial dilatation (tram lines) and focal constrictive areas between the dilated airways caused by defects in the bronchial wall.

Case 4: Congenital Unilateral Pulmonary Vein Atresia

Estela Pérez Ruiz and Pilar Caro Aguilera

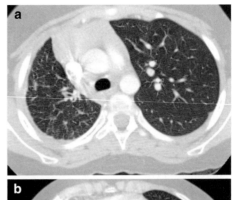

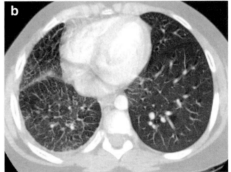

Fig. 2.14

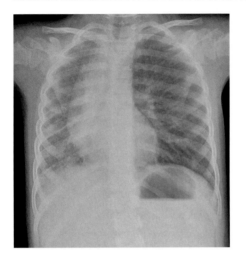

Fig. 2.13

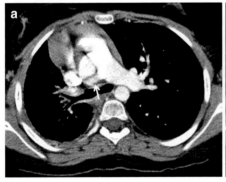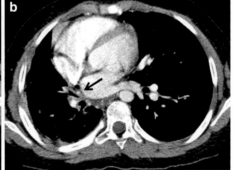

Fig. 2.15

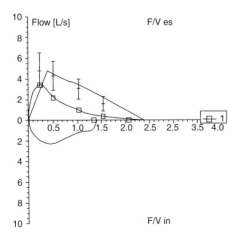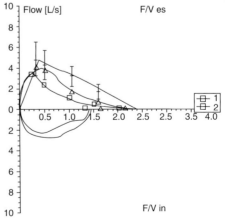

Fig. 2.16

A 3-year-old girl presents with history of both recurrent bronchitis and pneumonia since the age of 3 months. An asymmetric right hypoventilation was noted on thorax auscultation. She did not have a history of congenital heart disease nor evidence of bronchial obstruction at bronchoscopy. Clinical evolution has consisted of bronchial hyperresponsiveness, asthma-like symptoms, until the age of 11 years.

Comment

Unilateral pulmonary vein atresia without anomalous connection is a rare congenital abnormality that is usually present in infants, although some cases have been reported in adult patients. It results from failure of incorporation of the common pulmonary vein into the left atrium. It may occur in either lung, with no right- or left-side predominance. Pulmonary artery and parenchymal abnormalities are also present. Ipsilateral hypoplasia of the pulmonary artery is likely because of preferential pulmonary artery perfusion to the contralateral side and would account for the arterial systemic-to-pulmonary collateral vessels. Parenchymal manifestations include interlobular septal thickening, bronchial wall thickening, and ground-glass opacities, probably reflected in both pulmonary vein hypertension and engorged lymphatics. The most frequent presenting symptoms include recurrent infections in the hypoplastic lung, exercise intolerance, and hemoptysis due to the systemic collateral supply to the affected lung. Other associated congenital heart defects are found in approximately 50% of patients. Pulmonary artery hypertension may also be associated.

Imaging Findings

(Fig. 2.13). Anteroposterior chest radiograph reveals small right hemithorax with ipsilateral mediastinical shift and right diffuse interstitial infiltrate. (Fig. 2.14). CT scan (lung window setting): upper field section (a), lower field section (b). Septal pattern throughout right parenchyma with diffuse ground-glass attenuation and smooth thickening of the interlobular septa and bronchovascular bundles. The small right hemithorax is confirmed. (Fig. 2.15). Contrast-enhanced CT scan (artery phase): (a) Small right pulmonary artery (*white arrow*). (b) Absence of right pulmonary venous connection into left atrium, revealing a left atrial margin completely smooth at expected location of right pulmonary veins (*black arrow*). (Fig. 2.16). Flow volume curve with moderate degree of airway obstruction. The shape of the loop shows an intrathoracic obstructive ventilatory pattern (loop 1) with reversibility to bronchodilator test (loop 2). Bronchial hyperresponsiveness.

Case 5: Late Complications of Congenital Esophageal Atresia and Tracheoesophageal Fistula

Francisco Javier Pérez-Frías and Estela Pérez Ruiz

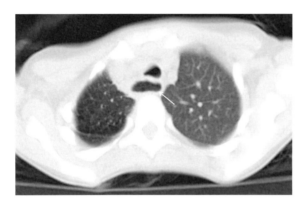

Fig. 2.17

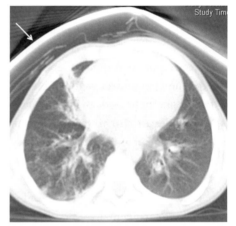

Fig. 2.18

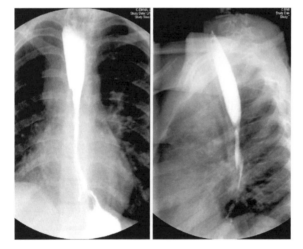

Fig. 2.19

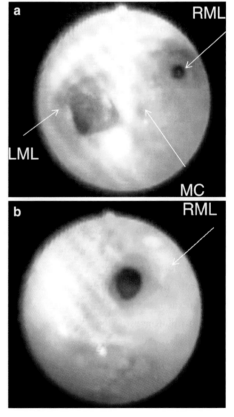

Fig. 2.20

An 8-year-old girl presents with recurrent bronchitis and pneumonia. She had a history of operated esophageal atresia (EA) with distal tracheoesophageal fistula (TEF).

Following EA and/or TEF surgery, patients have several long-term respiratory and esophageal symptoms during childhood, with a reported prevalence in up to 40% of cases which may persist life-long. In fact, "doctor-diagnosed asthma" has been described in 20% of cases. Late complications include tracheomalacia, a recurrence of the TEF, esophageal stricture, and gastroesophageal reflux (GR). Recurrent retrograde pulmonary aspiration can be due to either esophageal stricture or GR. Anastomotic stricture is especially common after repairing a gap of more than 2.5 cm, as an anastomosis under tension appears to increase the incidence of this complication, especially if a GR is present. The diagnosis of esophageal stenosis in the anatomosis site needs to be confirmed by esophagography or esophageal endoscopy. The esophageal stricture associated to GR origins recurrent airways aspiration which has been suggested to contribute to a persistent inflammation that may lead to several pulmonary diseases and other conditions, including chronic coughing, chronic hoarseness, posterior laryngitis, nocturnal choking, airway hyperreactivity (asthma), and recurrent pneumonitis, which may progress to obstructive and restrictive ventilatory defects. In cases of recurrent pneumonia, a bronchoscopy may evidence bronchial edema and hyperemia associated to a variable degree of bronchial stenosis, especially in the right bronchial tree. Performing a bronchoalveolar lavage also helps to investigate possible markers for GR disease and their relation to oxidation and inflammation and to correlate these with endobronchial biopsy findings. In conclusion, aspiration should be excluded in children and adults with a history of EA/TEF who present with respiratory symptoms and/or recurrent lower respiratory infections to prevent chronic pulmonary disease.

(Fig. 2.17). Axial thorax CT, lung window. Air entrapment in right upper lobe. Dilatation of proximal portion of the esophagus (*arrow*). (Fig. 2.18). Axial thorax CT, lung window. Bilateral diffuse bronchiectasis, predominantly in right lower lobe. Segmental atelectasis and bronchiectasis in middle lobe. Thorax protection with bismuth (*arrow*). (Fig. 2.19). Anteroposterior and lateral projection of esophagogram with oral contrast. Dilatation of proximal portion of the esophagus with straight stenosis in middle portion (at the anastomosis site). (Fig. 2.20). Flexible bronchoscopy: view of trachea at main-stem carina (MC). (a) Stenotic right main-stem bronchus (RML) compares to normal left main-stem bronchus (LML). (b) Hyperemia, inflammation, and stenosis of RMB secondary to recurrent pulmonary aspiration.

Case 6: Congenital Tracheal Stenosis with Tracheoesophageal Fistula

Pilar Caro Aguilera and Estela Pérez Ruiz

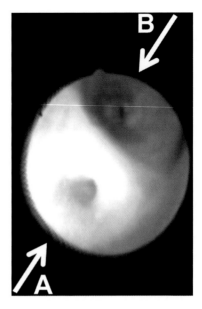

Fig. 2.23

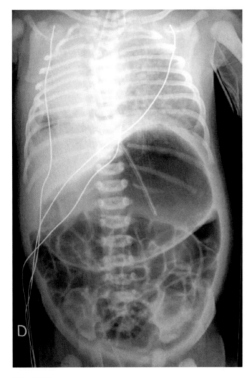

Fig. 2.21

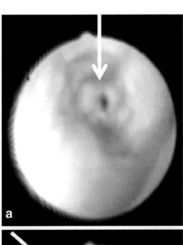

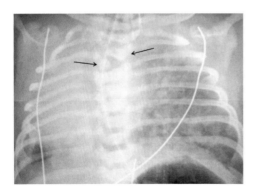

Fig. 2.22

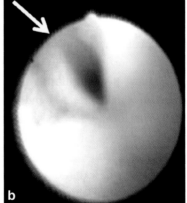

Fig. 2.24

An 8-day-old female newborn was admitted to the neonatal intensive care unit as she suffered from an acute respiratory insufficiency at birth. She needed endotracheal intubation and mechanical ventilation with severe ventilation problems.

Congenital tracheal stenosis (CTS) may be the result of an abnormality of the trachea itself or the effect of external forces compressing the airway. However, the common characteristic is narrowing of the trachea producing airway obstruction. Severe CTS and atresia of the trachea are rare malformations occurring with an estimated rate of two per 100,000 live births. Severe CTS, resulting in functional tracheal atresia, is frequently combined with other anomalies such as vertebral anomalies, anal atresia, cardiovascular anomalies, tracheoesophageal fistula (TEF), esophageal atresia, renal/radial anomalies, and limb defects (VACTERL association). Affected neonates present with severe respiratory distress immediately after birth. Without TEF, severe CTS is fatal and usually results in death within the first minutes of life. Survival is only possible with either a small tracheal lumen remaining, large enough for spontaneous breathing, or an emergency tracheotomy.

Prenatal magnetic resonance imaging (MRI) may provide a definitive diagnosis. Postnatal diagnosis is based on recognition of clinical signs in the newborn. The diagnostic should begin with thorax X-rays which may show unusual air distribution, deviation of the heart and mediastinum, and evidence of tracheal compression. Other diagnostic imaging studies may be used, including contrast esophagography, tracheobronchography, echocardiography, bronchoscopy (BC), and cardiac catheterization. Spiral sequencing or 3-dimensional reformatting CT scans and virtual BC are used to reconstruct the trachea and proximal bronchi. BC coupled with bronchography is a simple procedure that has excellent spatial and temporal resolution. Despite progress in surgical interventions, mortality remains high.

(Fig. 2.21). Thorax and abdomen X-ray. Central alveolar pattern, more evident in the left lung. Heart deviation to the right. Great gastric distension with bowel luminogram. Devices: endotracheal tube in D2, nasogastric tube in stomach. (Fig. 2.22). Detail of the thorax X-ray. Dorsal vertebral malformations (*arrows*) and dextrocardia. (Fig. 2.23) BC. TEF in a proximal and posterior position (*arrow* "A") and the CTS distally (*arrow* "B"). (Fig. 2.24) BC. (a) Severe CTS in the middle/distal tracheal third with a punctate lumen (*arrow*). (b) Tracheal lumen at maximal obstruction (*arrow*); the small size of the trachea did not allow the pass of the 2.5-mm-diameter bronchoscope.

Case 7: Multidetector CT of the Central Airways in Children: 3D Imaging and Virtual Bonchoscopy

Isabel Gordillo Gutiérrez

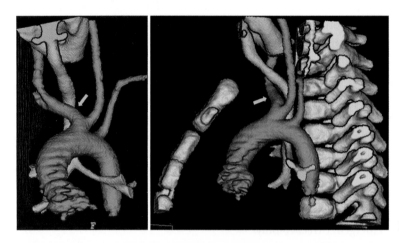

Fig. 2.25

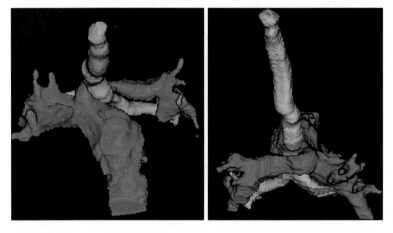

Fig. 2.26

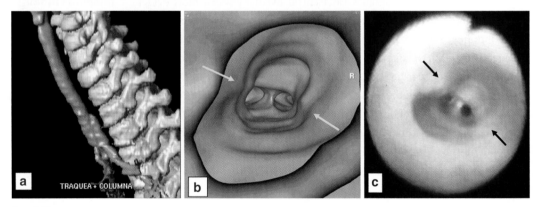

Fig. 2.27

Recent advances in multidetector computed tomography (MDCT) have revolutionized the noninvasive imaging evaluation of the central airways in pediatric patients.

Fiberoptic bronchoscopy (FOB) is the gold standard for diagnosis of tracheobronchial abnormalities. However, it remains an uncomfortable procedure and is of limited use in patients with severe stenosis of the bronchial lumen. MDCT-3D airway and mediastinal vascular reconstruction and virtual bronchospocpy (VB) is a good diagnostic tool in the evaluation of the large airways in children and presents information that renders abnormalities more obvious than they are on axial images.

Comments

Several limitations are associated with axial CT images: limited ability to detect subtle airway stenosis, underestimation of the craniocaudal extent of disease, difficulty displaying 3D relationships of the airways, and inadequate representation of the airways that are oriented obliquely to the axial plane.

Accurate identification and measurement of airway diseases are of paramount importance for assigning the appropriate diagnosis and planning the surgical procedures: this can be obtained with MDCT-3D and VB.

Advantages of this MDCT technology are:

1. Noninvasive procedure.
2. The creation of 3D reconstruction can help overcome the limitations of axial images.
3. Provides endoluminal, extraluminal, and extra-airway information that facilitates evaluation of spatial relationships.
4. VB is able to visualize areas beyond even high-grade stenosis.
5. It can give 3D road maps to surgeons and help in endobronchial treatments.
6. Can replace more invasive examinations such as FOB in selected cases (patients with no tolerance, high-risk patients and children).

Disadvantages are (1) it is not dynamic and is unable to show information such as pulsation from external pressure indicating vascular compression; (2) it does not evaluate mucosal surface; (3) motion artifacts, mucous plugs, or secretions inside the lumen can create false positives; (4) and it cannot provide samples for histological analysis.

MDCT-3D Imaging. VB and FOB are complementary techniques. Clinical applications of MDCT technology include assisting with diagnosis, helping in surgical planning treatments, and replacing invasive examinations such as FOB in selected cases.

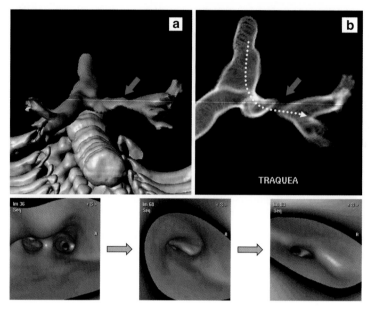

Fig. 2.28

MDCT-3D reconstruction in a girl with tracheal compression by an innominate artery (*arrow*) (Fig. 2.25) and in a boy with airway compression by a pulmonary sling (Fig. 2.26). Postsurgery exploration, 3D airway reconstruction (a), VB (b), and FOB (c) in a 2-year-old boy with tracheoplasty (*arrows*) (Fig. 2.27). 3D imaging (Fig. 2.28a) and VB (Fig. 2.28b) in a boy with left main bronchus stenosis (*red arrow*). FOB was not possible, but VB is able to visualize areas beyond even high-grade stenosis (Fig. 2.28). (Discontinuous line in b and gray arrows show the endoscopic way).

Imaging Findings

Case 8: Recurrent Spontaneous Pneumothorax

Pilar Caro Aguilera and
Francisco Javier Pérez-Frías

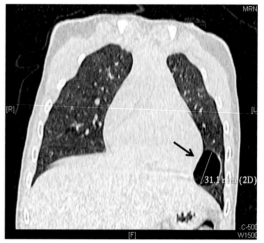

Fig. 2.31

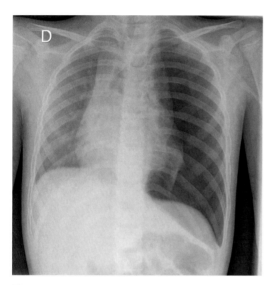

Fig. 2.29

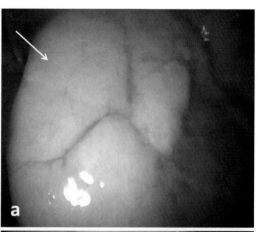

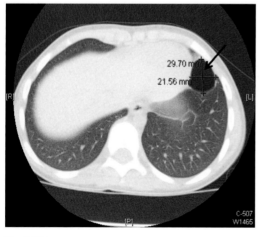

Fig. 2.30

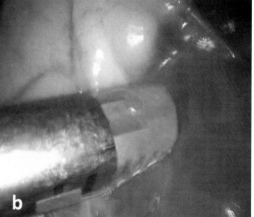

Fig. 2.32

An 8-year-old boy who suffered from recurrent spontaneous pneumothorax (SPT) at the ages of 5 and 7 years. He was admitted to the hospital as he had a severe chest pain. The auscultation showed hypoventilation in the left hemithorax.

Comments

Primary SPT is defined as a pneumothorax occurring in the absence of underlying lung disease and with no apparent pathology. SPT is a relatively rare condition in the pediatric population. The peak age of occurrence in this age group is bimodal, with most cases occurring either in the neonatal period or in late adolescence.

The risk of recurrent pneumothorax after a single episode of SPT with conservatory therapy ranges from 16% to 52%, whereas following surgical management of SPT, it is less than 5%. The mechanism involved in this predisposition is thought to be related to the presence of blebs or bullae in the most apical portions of the lungs. In children, SPT is thought to be related to rupture of these apical subpleural blebs or bullae. The typical symptoms of pneumothorax, such as chest pain and dyspnoea, may be relatively minor or even absent in SPT so that a high degree of initial diagnostic suspicion is required. When the patient presents severe symptoms or signs of cardiorespiratory distress, tension pneumothorax must be considered. The diagnosis of SPT is usually confirmed by imaging techniques. Thorax X-ray must be the first step in the diagnosis of PST, although it has limitations, such as the difficulty in accurately quantifying pneumothorax size. Computed tomography (CT) is useful in the detection of small pneumothoraces and in size estimation. It allows identifying the presence of surgical emphysema and bullous lung disease or additional lung pathology.

Therapeutic management ranges from a conservative attitude in mild cases receiving supplemental oxygen, to active intervention – needle aspiration and chest drain insertion – or surgical intervention. It may include removal of underlying cysts or bullae thought to be responsible for the occurrence or persistence of the pneumothorax. Open thoracotomy or limited axillary thoracotomy and pleurectomy remain the procedures with the lowest recurrence rate, but video-assisted thoracoscopic surgery (VATS) with pleurectomy and pleural abrasion has good results as well and is better tolerated.

Imaging Findings

(Fig. 2.29). Thorax X-ray: left SPT.

(Figs. 2.30 and 2.31). CT image, axial and coronal reconstructions: large bullae (29.7 × 21.56 × 31.1 mm) on the left lower lobe (*arrows*).

(Fig. 2.32). VATS photographs: (a) Bullae as white structure (*arrow*) in the region of the left lower lobe. (b) Photograph during the resection of the bullae.

Case 9: Bronchotracheal Foreign Body

Pilar Caro Aguilera and Francisco Javier Pérez-Frías

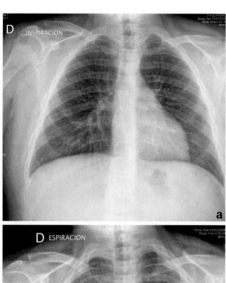

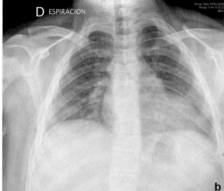

Fig. 2.33

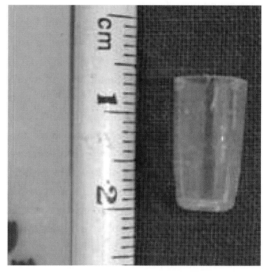

Fig. 2.35

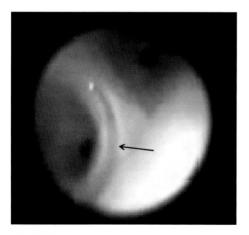

Fig. 2.34

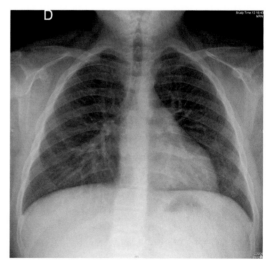

Fig. 2.36

A 13-year-old boy was referred from another center with a clinical history of foreign body aspiration and two negative flexible bronchoscopes. The child was without respiratory distress and non-pathologic signs during the exploration, except for moderate auscultatory signs of left hemithorax hypoventilation.

Foreign body (FB) aspiration is one of most frequent episodes in child respiratory pathologies. FB aspiration is a significant cause of morbidity and mortality in childhood.

Comments

The severity of the acute obstruction of the upper airway and the complications that FB creates in the lower airway require early diagnosis and treatment. Classically, the FB was previously removed by surgeons with a rigid bronchoscope under general anesthesia.

Nowadays, there are publications on removing FB with flexible bronchoscopy. At present, the discussion is which instrument is the best, a rigid or flexible bronchoscope. Flexible bronchoscopy is a minimal invasive procedure that allows making the diagnosis and locating the FB, which can only be removed in selected cases. Therefore, authors believe that FB removal is more effective with rigid bronchoscopy. It guarantees patient safety and the success of the procedure.

However, flexible and rigid bronchoscopes are complementary, so their combined use is the most appropriate choice. We report the management of this case of FB in pediatric patients with a combined procedure using flexible and rigid bronchoscopes.

Normal thorax X-ray in inspirations (Fig. 2.33a) and signs of air entrapment in the left lower lobe at the expiratory thorax X-ray (Fig. 2.33b).

Imaging Findings

Bronchoscope vision with rigid bronchoscope before extraction. The pen cap is in the left lower lobe bronchus and it seems a bronchial stenosis (*arrow*) (Fig. 2.34).

Plastic pen cap of a mechanical pencil (Fig. 2.35).

Final normal chest X-ray (Fig. 2.36).

Case 10: Endobronchial Lymphoma

María I. Martínez-León and
Antonio Martínez-Valverde

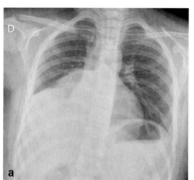
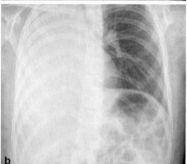
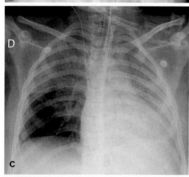
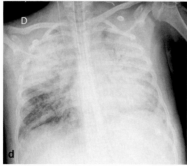

Fig. 2.37

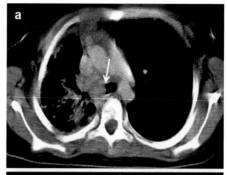
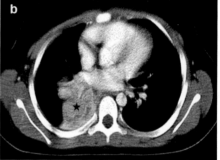

Fig. 2.38

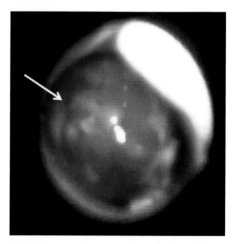

Fig. 2.39

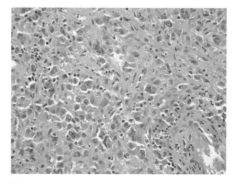

Fig. 2.40

A 10-year-old male patient was sent to the Traumatology Service of our hospital with a history of progressive right ankle pain with no response to treatment. No other symptoms were referred. A gammagraphy was performed, showing areas of hypercaptation in tibia and basal right lung. The bronchial lymphoma was diagnosed by chance while he was being investigated for a benign bone disease, due to the initial absence of respiratory symptoms.

This is a presentation of CD30+ anaplastic large-cell lymphoma (ALCL) with an unusual endobronchial polypoid mass. ALCL is a very rare disorder in childhood. The most common localization of this lymphoma is in the lymph node and skin, with endobronchial involvement being extremely rare among the pediatric population. **Comments**

Clinical findings in the few reported cases of ALCL are nonspecific, including cough, dyspnea, hemoptysis, fever, shortness of breath, etc. Radiographic features include nodules, mass, air space consolidation, pleural effusion, cavitations, and cystic lesions, which are indistinguishable from a broad spectrum of disorders. All these reasons, together with the malignancy of the process, make an early diagnosis necessary in order to begin treatment as soon as possible.

This case illustrates that ALCL should be included in the differential diagnosis of endobronchial mass lesions.

(Fig. 2.37). (a) Initial chest X-ray shows right hiliar mass with middle and inferior lobe atelectasis. (b) Chest X-ray 25 days later: white right lung with collapse and homolateral mediastinal deviation. (c) Chest X-ray after chemotherapy: there is no hiliar mass, but now there is a white left lung. (d) Follow-up chest X-ray indicates an alveolo-interstitial pulmonary bilateral pattern with the need of intubation. It is compatible with acute adult respiratory distress syndrome. **Imaging Findings**

(Fig. 2.38). A thorax CT without contrast (a) and enhanced (b) revealed a right hilum mass protruding into the carina (*arrow*) and a secondary collapse of the right lung (*asterisk*).

(Fig. 2.39). Flexible fiberoptic bronchoscopy revealed an endobronchial polypoid mass (*arrow*), with high vascularization, completely filling the lumen. This mass reached the lower third of the trachea, with its origin in the main right bronchus; partial resection with LASER was made, obtaining a tissue sample which gave the diagnosis.

(Fig. 2.40). Endobronchial ALCL pathology, Hematoxilin-Eosin.

Even though chemotherapy was started, the patient's outcome was unfavorable, and he died 18 days later.

Further Reading

Case 1: Postinfectious Bronchiolitis Obliterans

Book

Lucaya J, Le Pointe HD (2008) High-resolution CT of the lung in children. In: Lucaya J, Strife JL (eds) Pediatric chest imaging. Chest imaging in infants and children, 2nd edn. Springer, Berlin/Heidelberg, pp 103–104

Web Link

Wikipedia contributors (2006). Bronchiolitis obliterans [Internet]. Wikipedia, the free encyclopedia; Available from: http://en.wikipedia.org/wiki/Bronchiolitis_obliterans

Articles

Chang AB, Masel JP, Masters B (1998) Post-infectious bronchiolitis obliterans: clinical, radiological and pulmonary function sequelae. Pediatr Radiol 28:23–29

Colom AJ, Teper AM, Vollmer WM, Diette GB (2006) Risk factors for the development of bronchiolitis obliterans in children with bronchiolitis. Thorax 61:503–506

Dillman JR, Sanchez R, Ladino-Torres MF, Yarram SG, Strouse PJ, Lucaya J (2011) Expanding upon the unilateral hyperlucent hemithorax in children. Radiographics 31:723–741

Franquet T (2011) Imaging of pulmonary viral pneumonia. Radiology 260:18–39

Kim CK, Kim SW, Kim JS et al (2001) Bronchiolitis obliterans in the 1990s in Korea and the United States. Chest 120:1101–1106

Lucaya J, Gartner S, García-Peña P, Cobos N, Roca I, Liñan S (1998) Spectrum of manifestations of Swyer-James-MacLeod syndrome. J Comput Assist Tomogr 22:592–597

MacLeod WM (1954) Abnormal transradiancy of one lung. Thorax 9:147–153

Murtagh P, Giubergia V, Viale D, Bauer G, Pena HG (2009) Lower respiratory infections by adenovirus in children. Clinical features and risk factors for bronchiolitis obliterans and mortality. Pediatr Pulmonol 44:450–456

Smith KJ, Fan LL (2006) Insights into post-infectious bronchiolitis obliterans in children. Thorax 61:462–463

Swyer PR, James GCW (1953) A case of unilateral pulmonary emphysema. Thorax 8:133–136

Case 2: Thoracic Rib Invasion from Actinomycosis

Book

Ellis ME (1998) Infectious diseases of the respiratory tract. Cambridge University Press, Cambridge. ISBN 9780521405546

Web Link

http://www.learningradiology.com/notes/chestnotes/ACTINOMYCOSIS.htm

Articles

Benammar S, Herlardot P, Sapin E, Adamsbaum C, Raymond J (1995) Childhood actinomycosis: report of 2 cases. Eur J Pediatr Surg 5:180–183

Frank P, Strickland B (1974) Pulmonary actinomycosis. Br J Radiol 47:373–378

Jeung MY, Afshin G, Bernard G, Cornelia V, Gilbert M, Wihlm JM et al (1999) Imaging of chest wall disorders. Radiographics 19:617–637

Kuo TY, Gutman E (1974) Lesion of the lungs, chest wall, and ribs. JAMA 230:1051–1052

Lee JP, Rudoy R (2003) Pediatric thoracic actinomycosis. Hawaii Med J 62:30–32

Pinarly FG, Mutlu B, Celenk C, Yildiz L, Elli M, Dagdemir A et al (2005) Pulmonary actinomycosis mimicking chest wall tumor in a child. Jpn J Infect Dis 58:247–249

Thompson J, Carty H (1979) Pulmonary actinomycosis in children. Pediatr Radiol 8:7–9

Webb R, Sagel SS (1982) Actinomycosis involving the chest wall: CT findings. AJR Am J Roentgenol 139:1007–1009

Wilson DC, Redmond AO (1990) An unusual case of thoracic mass. Arch Dis Child 65:991–992

Young JK (1908) Actinomycosis of the ribs and vertebrae. JBJS s2–6:252–255

Case 3: Non-Cystic Fibrosis Bronchiectasis

Book

Andrés Martín A, Valverde Molina J (2010) Manual de Neumología Pediátrica. Sociedad Española de Neumología Pediátrica (SENP), 1st ed. Ed Médica Panamericana

Web Link

www.separ.es

Articles

Bilton D (2008) Update on non-cystic fibrosis bronchiectasis. Curr Opin Pulm Med 14:595–599

Douros K, Alexopoulou E, Nicopoulou A, Anthracopoulos MB, Fretzayas A, Yiallouros P et al (2011) Bronchoscopic and high-resolution CT scan findings in children with chronic wet cough. Chest 140:317–323

Eastham KM, Fall AJ, Mitchell L, Spencer DA (2004) The need to redefine non-cystic fibrosis bronchiectasis in childhood. Thorax 59:324–327

Javidan-Nejad C, Sanjeev Bhalla S (2009) Bronchiectasis. Radiol Clin North Am 47:289–306

Kapur N, Masters IB, Chang AB (2009) Exacerbations in noncystic fibrosis bronchiectasis: clinical features and investigations. Respir Med 103:1681–1687

King P (2011) Pathogenesis of bronchiectasis. Paediatr Respir Rev 12:104–110

Oili GC, Khong PL, Chan-Leung M, Ho JCM, Lee JCK, Lam WK et al (2002) Resolution CT quantification of bronchiectasis: clinical and functional correlation. Radiology 3:663–672

Redding GJ (2009) Bronchiectasis in children. Pediatr Clin North Am 56:157–171

Stafler P, Carr S (2010) Non-cystic fibrosis bronchiectasis: its diagnosis and management. Arch Dis Child Educ Pract Ed 95:73–82

Vendrell M, de Gracia J, Olveira Cl, Martínez MA, Girón R, de Máiz L et al (2008) Diagnóstico y tratamiento de las bronquiectasias. Arch Bronconeumol 44: 629–640

Cabrera A, Alcibar J (2002) Atresia bilateral de venas pulmonares. Rev Esp Cardiol 55:671–672

Heyneman LE, Nolan RL, Harrison JK, McAdams HP (2001) Congenital unilateral pulmonary vein atresia: radiologic findings in three adult patients. AJR Am J Roentgenol 177:681–685

Hsing-Yuan L, Betau H, Pi-Chang L (2008) Congenital atresia of unilateral pulmonary veins associated with a single ventricle. A rare case report and literature review. Circ J 72:1544–1546

Kim Y, Yoo IR, Ahn MI, Han DH (2011) Asymptomatic adults with isolated, unilateral right pulmonary vein atresia: multidetector CT findings. Br J Radiol 84:e109–e113

Mataciunas M, Gumbiene L, Cibiras S, Tarutis V, Tamosiunas AE (2009) CT Angiography of mildly symptomatic, isolated, unilateral right pulmonary vein atresia. Pediatr Radiol 39:1087–1090

Nam Lee H, Tong Kim Y, Sik S (2011) Individual pulmonary vein atresia in adults: report of two cases. Korean J Radiol 12:395–399

Pourmoghadam KK, Moore JW, Khan M, Geary EM, Madan N, Wolfson BJ et al (2003) Congenital unilateral pulmonary venous atresia: definitive diagnosis and treatment. Pediatr Cardiol 24:73–79

Shuhaiber J, Rehman M, Jenkins K, Fynn-Thompson F, Bacha F (2011) The role of surgical therapy for pulmonary vein atresia in childhood. Pediatr Cardiol 32:639–645

Tissot C, Corbelli R, Aggoum Y, Beghetti M, Da Cruz E (2008) Bronchoscopic diagnosis of asymptomatic unilateral pulmonary vein atresia in an infant. Pediatr Cardiol 29:976–979

Case 4: Congenital Unilateral Pulmonary Vein Atresia

Book

Allen HD, Driscoll DJ, Shaddy RE, Feltes TF (2008) Moss and Adams' heart disease in infants, children, and adolescents: including the fetus and young adult, 7th edn. Lippincott Williams & Wilkins, Philadelphia

Web Link

http://www.mendeley.com/research/congenital-unilateral-pulmonary-vein-atresia-radiologic-findings-three-adult-patients/

Articles

Artero Muñoz I, Serrano Puche F, Padín Martín MI, Serrano Ramos F (2008) Atresia congénita unilateral de las venas pulmonares: hallazgos radiológicos. Radiologia 50:82–85

Case 5: Late Complications of Congenital Esophageal Atresia and Tracheoesophageal Fistula

Book

Cobos N, Pérez Yarza EG (2009) Tratado de Neumología Infantil, 1st edn. Ergon, Madrid

Web Link

http://www.neumoped.org

Articles

Castilloux J, Noble AJ, Faure C (2010) Risk factors for short- and long-term morbidity in children with esophageal atresia. J Pediatr 156:755–760

Jadcherla SR, Hogan WJ, Shaker R (2010) Physiology and pathophysiology of glottic reflexes and pulmonary aspiration: from neonates to adults. Semin Respir Crit Care Med 31:554–560

Koivusalo A, Pakarinen MP, Rintala RJ (2007) The cumulative incidence of significant gastrooesophageal reflux in patients with oesophageal atresia with a distal fistula–a systematic clinical, pH-metric, and endoscopic follow-up study. J Pediatr Surg 42:370–374

Kovesi K, Rubin S (2004) Long-term complications of congenital esophageal atresia and/or tracheoesophageal fistula. Chest 126:915–925

Lacher M, Froehlich S, von Schweinitz D, Dietz HG (2010) Early and long term outcome in children with esophageal atresia treated over the last 22 years. Klin Padiatr 222:296–301

Malmström K, Lohi J, Lindahl H, Pelkonen A, Kajosaari M, Sarna S, Malmberg LP, Mäkelä MJ (2008) Longitudinal follow-up of bronchial inflammation, respiratory symptoms, and pulmonary function in adolescents after repair of esophageal atresia with tracheoesophageal fistula. J Pediatr 153:396–401

Nasr A, Ein SH, Gerstle JT (2005) Infants with repaired esophageal atresia and distal tracheoesophageal fistula with severe respiratory distress: is it tracheomalacia, reflux, or both? J Pediatr Surg 40:901–903

Sistonen SJ, Pakarinen MP, Rintala RJ (2011) Long-term results of esophageal atresia: Helsinki experience and review of literature. Pediatr Surg Int 27:1141–1149

Starosta V, Kitz R, Hartl D, Marcos V, Reinhardt D, Griese M (2007) Bronchoalveolar pepsin, bile acids, oxidation, and inflammation in children with gastroesophageal reflux disease. Chest 132:1557–1564

Touloukian RJ, Seashore JH (2004) Thirty-five-year institutional experience with end-to-side repair for esophageal atresia. Arch Surg 139:371–374

Bercker S, Kornak U, Bührer C, Henrich W, Kerner T (2006) Tracheal atresia as part of an exceptional combination of malformations. Int J Pediatr Otorhinolaryngol 70:1137–1139

De Groot-van der Mooren MD, Haak MC, Lakeman P, Cohen-Overbeek TE, Van der Voorn JP, Bretschneider JH et al (2012) Tracheal agenesis: approach towards this severe diagnosis. Case report and review of the literature. Eur J Pediatr 171(3):425–431. doi:10.1007/s00431-011-1563-x

Fuchimoto Y, Mori M, Takasato F, Tomita H, Yamamoto Y, Shimojima N et al (2011) A long-term survival case of tracheal agenesis: management for tracheoesophageal fistula and esophageal reconstruction. Pediatr Surg Int 27:103–106

Gunlemez A, Anik Y, Elemen L, Tugay M, Gökalp AS (2009) H-type tracheoesophageal fistula in an extremely low birth weight premature neonate: appearance on magnetic resonance imaging. J Perinatol 29:393–395

Heimann K, Bartz C, Naami A, Peschgens T, Merz U, Hörnchen H (2007) Three new cases of congenital agenesis of the trachea. Eur J Pediatr 166:79–82

Krause U, Rödel RM, Paul T (2011) Isolated congenital tracheal stenosis in a preterm newborn. Eur J Pediatr 170:1217–1221

Mong A, Johnson AM, Kramer SS, Coleman BG, Hedrick HL, Kreiger P et al (2008) Congenital high airway obstruction syndrome: MR/US findings, effect on management, and outcome. Pediatr Radiol 38:1171–1179

Phipps LM, Raymond JA, Angeletti TM (2006) Congenital tracheal stenosis. Crit Care Nurse 26:60–69

Russell HM, Backer CL (2010) Pediatric thoracic problems: patent ductus arteriosus, vascular rings, congenital tracheal stenosis, and pectus deformities. Surg Clin North Am 90:1091–1113

Case 6: Congenital Tracheal Stenosis with Tracheoesophageal Fistula

Book

Pérez Ruiz E, Martínez León MI, Caro Aguilera P (2009) Anomalías congénitas de las vías aéreas. In: Cobos N, Pérez-Yarza EG (eds) Tratado de Neumología Infantil, 2nd edn. Ergon, Madrid, pp 223–248

Web Link

Neumoped. The official site of SENP (Sociedad Española de Neumología Pediátrica). http://www.neumoped.org/

Articles

Antón-Pacheco JL, López M, Moreno C, Bustos G (2011) Congenital tracheal stenosis caused by a new tracheal ring malformation. J Thorac Cardiovasc Surg 14:e39–e40

Case 7: Multidetector CT of the Central Airways in Children: 3D Imaging and Virtual Bonchoscopy

Book

Lee EY, Siegel MJ (2008) Pediatric airways disorders: large airways. In: Lynch DA, Boiselle PM (eds) CT of the airways. The Humana Press, Totowa, pp 351–380

Web Link

D'Alessandro DM, D'Alessandro MP. Virtual pediatric hospital. A digital library of pediatric information: http://www.virtualpediatrichospital.org/providers/ElectricAirway/Text/IntroEduObjectives.shtml(1992-2012)

Articles

Beigelman-Aubry C, Brillet PY, Grenier PA (2009) MDCT of the airways: technique and normal results. Radiol Clin North Am 47:185–201

Berrocal T, Madrid C, Novo S, Gutiérrez J, Arjonilla A, Gómez-León N (2004) Congenital anomalies of the tracheobronchial tree, lung and mediastinum: embryology, radiology, and pathology. Radiographics 24:e17, http://radiographics.rsna.org/content/24/1/e17.full

Boiselle PM, Reynolds KF, Ernst A (2002) Multiplanar and three-dimensional imaging of the central airways with multidetector CT. Am J Roentgenol 179:301–308

Choo KS, Lee HD, Ban JE, Sung SC, Chang YH, Kim ChW et al (2006) Evaluation of obstructive airway lesions in complex congenital heart disease using composite volume-rendered images from multislice CT. Pediatr Radiol 36:219–223

Lee EY (2008) Advancing CT and MR imaging of the lungs and airways in children: imaging into practice. Pediatr Radiol 38(Suppl 2):S208–S212

Lee EY, Siegel MJ, Hildebolt CF, Gutiérrez FR, Bhalla S, Fallah JH (2004) MDCT evaluation of thoracic aortic anomalies in pediatric patients and young adults: comparison of axial, multiplanar, and 3D images. Am J Roentgenol 182:777–784

Lee EY, Greenberg SB, Boiselle PM (2011) Multidetector computed tomography of pediatric large airway diseases: state of the art. Radiol Clin North Am 49:869–893

Papaioannou G, Young C, Owens CM (2007) Multidetector row CT for imaging the paediatric tracheobronchial tree. Pediatr Radiol 37:515–529

Siegel M (2003) Multiplanar and three-dimensional multi-detector row CT of thoracic vessels and airways in the pediatric population. Radiology 229:641–650

Yedururi S, Guillerman RP, Chung T, Braverman RM, Dishop MK, Giannoni CM, Krishnamurthy R (2008) Multimodality imaging of tracheobronchial disorders in children. Radiographics 28:e29, http://radiographics.rsna.org/content/28/3/e29.full.pdf+html

pneumothorax in children: is there an optimal technique? J Pediatr Surg 43:2151–2155

Butterworth SA, Blair GK, LeBlanc JG, Skarsgard ED (2007) An open and shut case for early VATS treatment of primary spontaneous pneumothorax in children. Can J Surg 50:171–174

Ganesalingam R, O'Neil RA, Shadbolt B, Tharion J (2010) Radiological predictors of recurrent primary spontaneous pneumothorax following non-surgical management. Heart Lung Circ 19:606–610

Guimaraes CV, Donnelly LF, Warner BW (2007) CT findings for blebs and bullae in children with spontaneous pneumothorax and comparison with findings in normal age-matched controls. Pediatr Radiol 37:879–884

Kim DH (2011) The feasibility of axial and coronal combined imaging using multi-detector row computed tomography for the diagnosis and treatment of a primary spontaneous pneumothorax. J Cardiothorac Surg 6:71

Laituri CA, Valusek PA, Rivard DC, Garey CL, Ostlie DJ, Snyder CL et al (2011) The utility of computed tomography in the management of patients with spontaneous pneumothorax. J Pediatr Surg 46:1523–1525

MacDuff A, Arnold A, Harvey J (2010) BTS pleural disease guideline group. Management of spontaneous pneumothorax: British thoracic society pleural disease guideline 2010. Thorax 65(Suppl 2):ii18–ii31

O'Lone E, Elphick HE, Robinson PJ (2008) Spontaneous pneumothorax in children: when is invasive treatment indicated? Pediatr Pulmonol 43:41–46

Robinson PD, Cooper P, Ranganathan SC (2009) Evidence-based management of paediatric primary spontaneous pneumothorax. Paediatr Respir Rev 10:110–117

Shih CH, Yu HW, Tseng YC, Chang YT, Liu CM, Hsu JW (2011) Clinical manifestations of primary spontaneous pneumothorax in pediatric patients: an analysis of 78 patients. Pediatr Neonatol 52:150–154

Case 8: Recurrent Spontaneous Pneumothorax

Book

Schaarschmidt K, Uschinshy K (2008) The thoracoscopic approach to pneumothorax in children. In: Bax KM, Georgeson KE, Rothenberg S, Valla JS, Yeung CK (eds) Endoscopic surgery in infants and children. Part 2. Springer, Berlin/Heidelberg, pp 111–116. doi:10.1007/978-3-540-49910-7_14

Web Link

http://www.uptodate.com/contents/spontaneous-pneumothorax-in-children

Articles

Bialas RC, Weiner TM, Phillips JD (2008) Video-assisted thoracic surgery for primary spontaneous

Case 9: Bronchotracheal Foreign Body

Book

Pérez-Frías J, Pérez-Ruiz E, Cordón A (2010a) Broncoscopia Pediátrica, 2nd edn. Ergon, Madrid

Web Link

Neumoped. The official site of SENP (Sociedad Española de Neumología Pediátrica). http://www.neumoped.org/

Articles

Cutrone C, Pedruzzi B, Tava G, Emanuelli E, Barion U, Fischetto D et al (2011) The complimentary role of diagnostic and therapeutic endoscopy in foreign body aspiration in children. Int J Pediatr Otorhinolaryngol 75:1481–1485

D'Agostino J (2010) Pediatric airway nightmares. Emerg Med Clin North Am 28:119–126

Fidkowski CW, Zheng H, Firth PG (2010) The anesthetic considerations of tracheobronchial foreign bodies in children: a literature review of 12,979 cases. Anesth Analg 111:1016–1025

Guanà R, Gesmundo R, Maiullari E, Bianco ER, Vinardi S, Cortese MG et al (2009) The value of lung scintigraphy in the management of airways foreign bodies in children. Minerva Pediatr 61:477–482

Pérez-Frías J, Caro-Aguilera P, Pérez-Ruiz E, Moreno-Requena L (2010b) Manejo del cuerpo extraño intra-bronquial. Broncoscopia combinada. An Pediatr (Barc) 72:67–71

Pérez-Frías J, Moreno Galdó A, Pérez Ruiz E, Barrio Gómez De Agüero MI, Escribano Montaner A, Caro Aguilera P (2011) Normativa SEPAR de Broncoscopia Pediátrica. Pediatric bronchoscopy guidelines. Arch Bronconeumol 47:350–360

Rodrigues AJ, Scussiatto EA, Jacomelli M, Scordamaglio PR, Gregório MG, Palomino AL et al (2012) Bronchoscopic techniques for removal of foreign bodies in children's airways. Pediatr Pulmonol 47(1):59–62. doi:10.1002/ppul.21516, Epub 2011 Aug 9

Shah RK, Patel A, Lander L, Choi SS (2010) Management of foreign bodies obstructing the airway in children. Arch Otolaryngol Head Neck Surg 136:373–379

Shlizerman L, Mazzawi S, Rakover Y, Ashkenazi D (2010) Foreign body aspiration in children: the effects of delayed diagnosis. Am J Otolaryngol 31:320–324

Sternberg TG, Thompson JW, Schoumacher RA, Lew DB (2010) Recurrent stridor in a 9-year-old child after a choking and aspiration event. Allergy Asthma Proc 31:154–157

Case 10: Endobronchial Lymphoma

Book

Warnke RA, Weiss LM, Chan JKC, Dorfman RF (1995) Anaplastic large cell lymphoma: tumors of the lymph nodes and spleen. In: Rosai J (ed) Atlas of tumor pathology, vol fasc 14, Third series. Armed Forces Institute of Pathology, Washington, pp 187–198

Web Link

Pérez Frías J, Pérez Ruiz E, Cordón Martínez A, Spitaleri G. Broncoscopia Pediátrica. 2nd edn. http://www.neumoped.org/docs/broncoscopia2.pdf

Articles

Al-Qahtani AR, Di Lorenzo M, Yazbeck S (2003) Endobronchial tumors in children: institutional experience and literature review. J Pediatr Surg 38:773–776

Bhalla R, McCluree S (2003) Pathologic quiz case: a 17 year old adolescent girl with a short history of dyspnea. Arch Pathol Lab Med 127:e430–e431

Erbaycu AE, Karasu I, Ozdemirkirian FG, Yücel N, Ozsöz A, Bilgir O (2004) Endobronchial low-grade MALT lymphoma causing unilateral hypertranslucency. Monaldi Arch Chest Dis 61:237–240

Greer JP, Kinney MC, Collins RD, Salhany KE, Wolff SN, Hainsworth JD et al (1991) Clinical features of 31 patients with Ki-1 anaplastic large cell lymphoma. J Clin Oncol 9:539–547

Guerra J, Echevarria-Escudero M, Barrios N, Velez-Rosario R (2006) Primary endobronchial anaplastia large cell lymphoma in a pediatric patient. PRHSJ 25:159–161

Kim DH, Ko YH, Lee MH, Ree HJ (1998) Anaplastic large cell lymphoma presenting as an endobronchial polypoid mass. Respiration 65:156–158

Le Deley MC, Reiter A, Williams D et al (2008) Prognostic factors in childhood anaplastia large cell lymphoma: results of a large European intergroup study. Blood 111:1560–1566

Massimino M, Gasparini M, Giardini R (1995) Ki-1 (CD30) anaplastic large cell lymphoma in children. Ann Oncol 6:915–920

Rose RM, Grigas D, Strattemeir E, Harris NL, Linggood RM (1986) Endobronquial involvement with non-Hodgkin's Lymphoma. Cancer 57:1750–1755

Scott KJ, Greinwald JH, Darrow D, Smith R (2001) Endobronchial tumors in children: an uncommon clinical entity. Ann Otol Rhinol Laryngol 110:63–69

Contents

M.I. Martínez-León et al., *Imaging for Pediatricians*, Imaging for Clinicians,
DOI 10.1007/978-3-642-28629-2_3, © Springer-Verlag Berlin Heidelberg 2012

Case 1: Atrial Septal Defect Ostium Secundum Type

Sofía Granja and
Constancio Medrano

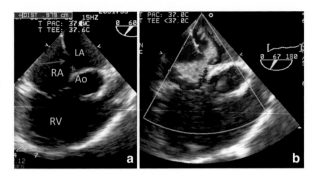

Fig. 3.1

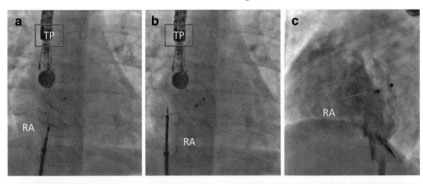

Fig. 3.2

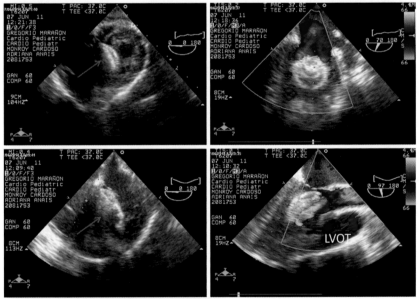

Fig. 3.3

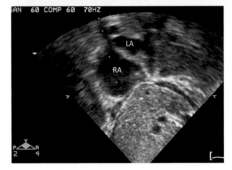

Fig. 3.4

A 3-year-old girl evaluated because of a cardiac murmur and low weight gain. A large secundum atrial septal defect (ASD OS) was diagnosed, and percutaneous closure of the defect was performed. The procedure was complicated by left ventricular migration of the device, leading to urgent cardiac surgery.

Comments

ASDs may be detected from early age through late adulthood and represent 6–10% of all cardiac anomalies. The most common type is *secundum* ASD, the result of a deficiency in the *septum primum*. A significant number of ASDs are small and close spontaneously. In the setting of large defects, they are usually asymptomatic throughout early childhood, and recurrent lower respiratory tract infections or poor growth are very rare. Progressively, the chronic left-to-right shunt imposes a volume overload on the right cardiac chambers, with consequent enlargement of the right atrium and ventricle. Precordial examination shows a wide and fixed splitting of the second heart sound associated with a systolic ejection murmur at the second left intercostal space and an early/mid-diastolic murmur, heard at the lower left sternal border. Chest radiography presents increased cardiothoracic ratio with intensification of pulmonary vascular markings. Echocardiography is the gold standard diagnostic method: it sizes and locates the defect, determines its margins, excludes associated lesions, and clarifies its relevance in the hemodynamic status of the patient (magnitude of the shunting, effects on right heart volume, and cardiac function). Compared to a transthoracic echo, transesophageal echocardiography (TEE) adds accuracy and precision to the measurements. The lesser invasiveness of the transcatheter occlusion technique associated with the development of new and successful percutaneous occluding devices has favored the nonsurgical treatment. Complications associated with percutaneous closure include residual shunts, fractures of the hardware, device embolization, obstruction of the pulmonary veins or coronary sinus, atrioventricular (AV) valve dysfunction, and AV block.

Imaging Findings

(Fig. 3.1a). TEE-transversal plane image showing a moderate-sized secundum ASD (*arrow*). (b) Color Doppler flow mapping showing a left-to-right shunting at the atria level. LA – left atrium; RA – right atrium; RV – right ventricle; Ao – aorta. (Fig. 3.2a). Percutaneous closure of the ASD was done. Images report the implantation and delivery of the device (*arrows*) (3.2b, c) and the angiographic control in the RA showing no residual shunting. TEE probe can be seen (TP). (Fig. 3.3). 24 h after percutaneous intervention, control echocardiogram shows LV migration of the device. TEE shows the device (*arrow*) moving freely in the LV cavity, protruding into the LV outflow tract (LVOT). (Fig. 3.4). After urgent surgery, the device was removed and surgical closure of the ASD was performed. TTE bicaval view after surgery shows no residual shunt across the atrial septum.

Case 2: Mitral Valve Endocarditis

Sofía Granja and Enrique Maroto

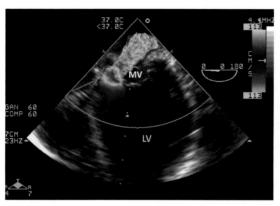

FIG. 3.5

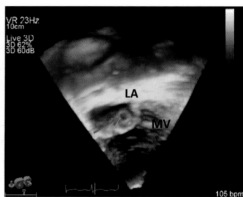

Fig. 3.6

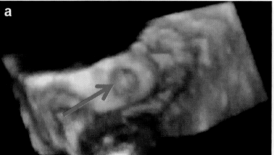

Fig. 3.7

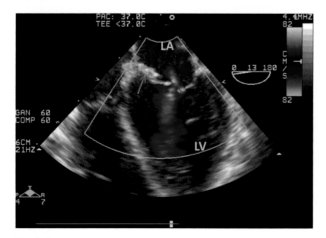

Fig. 3.8

A 2-year-old girl presenting cardiac murmur and recent history of amigdalitis, hip arthritis, and thromboembolic obstruction of a femoral artery. Cardiac ultrasound showed severe mitral insufficiency due to perforation of the anterior mitral leaflet, suggesting an infective origin. The patient underwent surgical treatment with good outcome.

Comments

Infective endocarditis (IE) is a relatively rare disease among the pediatric population, affecting 0.8–3.3/1,000 hospital admissions. It is defined as a subacute infection of the heart and surrounding vessels that usually develops in patients with underlying structural heart malformations, associated with a significant morbimortality. Some cases of IE affecting normal hearts have been reported, mostly in adults, with previous history of instrumentation and use of indwelling catheters, drug abuse, or pacemaker placement (in these cases, with IE lesions affecting the right cardiac structures). Literature is scarce with respect to small children with normal heart and mitral valve infective endocarditis. The clinical presentation is usually subtle, and the diagnosis demands a high level of suspicion. Patients with mild mitral lesion are asymptomatic. As the degree of severity increases, patient can develop symptoms of heart failure. When mitral regurgitation is moderate to severe, chest radiography can demonstrate a straight left heart border (left chambers enlargement "cephalization"), cardiomegaly and prominent pulmonary venous pattern. Cardiac ultrasound provides a complete structural and functional cardiac evaluation, clarifies the mitral valve anatomy (valve apparatus, annulus, leaflets, chordae, papillary muscles, and associated lesions), and grades the severity of the lesion and its hemodynamic significance (size of the left atrium (LA) and left ventricle (LV), ventricular function). When the suspicion of IE is high but TTE does not confirm the diagnosis, transesophageal echocardiography (TEE) should be performed without delay.

Imaging Findings

(Fig. 3.5). 2D TEE (apical view) shows a defect of the anterior leaflet of the mitral valve (MV), causing a significant regurgitant jet (*arrow*), left ventricle (LV).

(Fig. 3.6). 3D echocardiogram (apical view): round defect (*arrow*) of the anterior leaflet of the MV, left atrium (LA).

(Fig. 3.7). MV viewed from the ventricular (*arrow*) (a) and atrial (*arrow*) (b) aspects. Optimal anatomical orientation is obtained by rotation of the 3D dataset and cropping away intervening structures. Combination of clinical and imaging findings must at least raise the hypothesis of an infective aggression and perforation of the mitral anterior leaflet.

(Fig. 3.8). TEE 4 chamber view after surgical repair shows a well-positioned patch (*arrow*), with no residual shunts. Mild central mitral regurgitation is observed, left ventricle (LV), left atrium (LA).

Case 3: Sinus Venosus Defect and Partial Anomalous Pulmonary Venous Connection

Sofía Granja and Carlos Marín

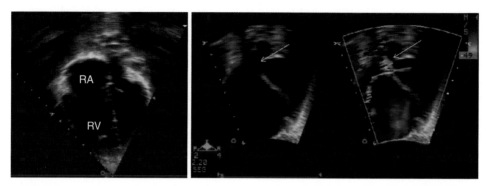

Fig. 3.9

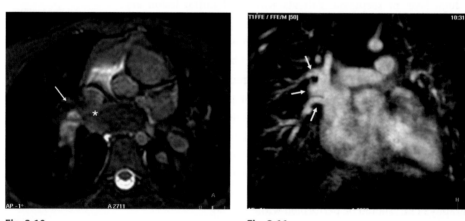

Fig. 3.10   Fig. 3.11

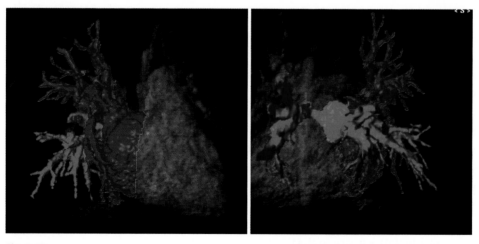

Fig. 3.12

A 6-year-old girl evaluated for low weight gain. Cardiac imaging performed showed partial anomalous pulmonary venous connection (PAPVC) and an atrial sinus venosus defect (SVD). She underwent cardiac surgery with good results.

Comments

Anomalous connections of pulmonary veins occur when one or more pulmonary veins drain into the right cardiac structures, namely, to the superior vena cava, right atrium, or inferior vena cava. Frequently, they are associated with SVD (5–10% of all atrial septal defects (ASDs)), located posterior and superiorly to the fossa ovalis. Depending on the number of veins anomaly connected, the condition may be symptomatic or go undetected until later in life. Growth failure, recurrent lower respiratory tract infections, or heart failure are uncommon. The chronic volume overload imposed on the right side cardiac chambers determines enlargement of both right atrium and right ventricle. At the pulmonary level, there is also dilation of the pulmonary vascular bed. The auscultatory features are a fixed and widely splitting of the second heart sound, a systolic ejection murmur, and a mid-diastolic murmur at the left lower sternal border. As regards images, radiological evaluation may show some degree of cardiomegaly and increased pulmonary vascular markings, but the diagnosis is established by echocardiography. Transthoracic echocardiogram first draws one's attention because of the dilated right cardiac chambers, but a careful evaluation demonstrates the SVD and the PAPVC. Transesophageal echocardiogram (TEE) imaging gives accuracy to the diagnosis, being particularly useful in the pre- and postoperative assessment. Surgical correction implies the construction of a tunnel redirecting the anomalous pulmonary vein to the left atrium through the ASD. Sometimes the pulmonary venous drainage is not clearly defined by ultrasound, and other cardiac imaging techniques may be required (as cardiac magnetic resonance, cardiac computed tomography, or even cardiac catheterization).

Imaging Findings

Transthoracic echocardiogram shows dilated right atrium (RA) and right ventricle (RV) on the apical view and a sinus venosus type atrial defect (*arrow*) with left-to-right shunt (red flow) on the subcostal view (Fig. 3.9). Whole heart 3D image (Fig. 3.10) shows sinus venosus septal defect (*asterisk*) and an abnormal pulmonary vein reaching the superior vena cava (*arrow*). Magnetic resonance (MR) angiographic images (Fig. 3.11) demonstrate the right upper lobe and middle lobe veins draining into the superior vena cava (*arrows*). Volume-rendered images (Fig. 3.12) from the MR angiography nicely depict the pulmonary venous connections to the right atrium (*blue*) and left atrium (*red*).

Case 4: Double Aortic Arch

Mariano del Valle Diéguez and Carlos Marín

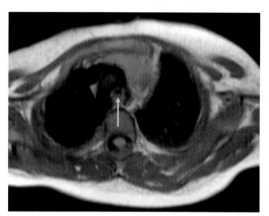

Fig. 3.13

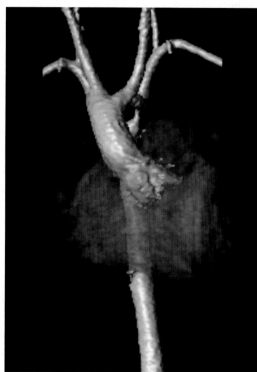

Fig. 3.15

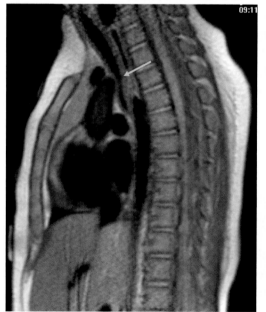

Fig. 3.14

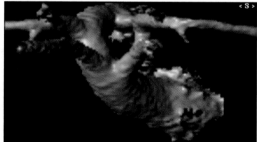

Fig. 3.16

Ten-month-old girl with stridor. Vascular ring is suspected in transthoracic ultrasound.

The most common vascular rings are double aortic arch and right aortic arch with aberrant subclavian artery. Vascular rings represent 1% of congenital vascular malformations and manifest at an early age (typically the first weeks of life). Respiratory symptoms are the most common clinical presentation, followed by dysphagia, emesis, and choking. Double aortic arch usually occurs without associated malformations. There are several forms of double aortic arch: both arches may be patent or one may be atretic. The right arch is dominant in 75% of cases. Each arch passes over the ipsilateral mainstem bronchus, gives rise to the ipsilateral carotid and subclavian arteries, and fuses into the descending aorta, which is usually located at the left of the spine. Typically, there is a marked narrowing of the tracheal lumen at the level of the arches.

Since patients present mostly with respiratory symptoms, imaging evaluation usually starts with chest radiographs. In some cases, tracheal compression by the aortic arches can be seen. Although barium esophagogram is a reliable technique for the detection of vascular rings, the specific type cannot be confidently determined. Posterior esophageal impression on the lateral projection is the most common finding. US allows a correct definition of the anatomy and prenatal diagnosis of vascular rings but is limited by its poor capacity to determine tracheal compression and to provide a large field of view for surgical orientation. CT and MRI are the imaging modalities of choice for the diagnosis and characterization of vascular rings: both allow 3D and multiplanar evaluation of the double arch and its adjacent structures, providing an adequate surgical map. CT is currently more reliable than MRI for the evaluation of lung parenchyma and the airways. In addition, the short scanning times of modern CTs allow imaging without sedation. MRI avoids radiation and the use of intravenous iodinated contrast and provides additional information on ventricular function and blood flow. On the other hand, it has longer imaging times requiring sedation in most pediatric patients. The choice between these two imaging modalities depends on their availability, medical expertise, and the patient's individual needs.

MRI T1 TSE sequences, axial (Fig. 3.13) and sagittal (Fig. 3.14) views, show a double aortic arch with right dominance and hypoplasia of the left arch. There is a significant tracheal stenosis secondary to the ring (*arrows*). Volume-rendered contrast-enhanced MR angiogram, anterior (Fig. 3.15) and superior views (Fig. 3.16), show the permeability of the aortic arches, each giving rise to the respective common carotid and subclavian arteries.

Case 5: Tetralogy of Fallot

Sofía Granja and José Luis Zunzunegui

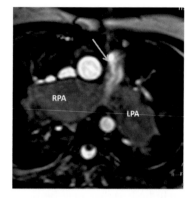

Fig. 3.19

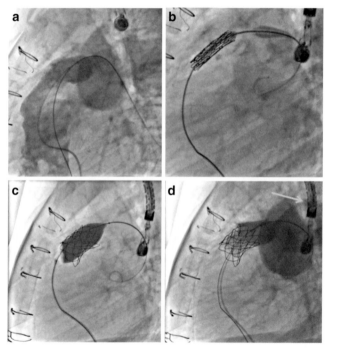

Fig. 3.17

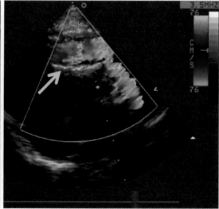

Fig. 3.20

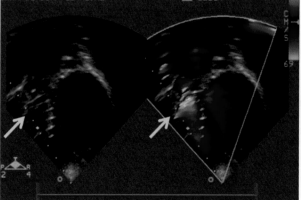

Fig. 3.18

A 16-year-old female with tetralogy of Fallot (TOF) and absent pulmonary valve. She underwent surgical correction at 3 years of age, and at six, the calcified pulmonary conduit was replaced. Due to severe dysfunction of the pulmonary conduit, a transcatheter pulmonary valve was successfully implanted at the age of 12.

Comments

TOF is the most common cyanotic defect affecting 32.6 per 100,000 live births. Despite the heterogeneity of the morphological phenotype presentation, it is characterized by a common anatomical picture: (1) large conoventricular ventricular septal defect (VSD), (2) overriding of the aorta over the VSD, (3) right ventricle outflow tract (RVOT) obstruction, and (4) RV hypertrophy. The age and severity of symptoms are closely related with the anatomy, reflecting the degree of RVOT obstruction. In respect to imaging, echocardiographic findings are elucidative and diagnostic for TOF in infants and young children; a complete and careful study may obviate the diagnostic angiography in the routine preoperative assessment. Depending on the complexity of the case, radiography, cardiac magnetic resonance imaging (cMRI), and angiography may add important data to the anatomical clarification (coronary artery distribution, peripheral pulmonary circulation). During the last few years, progress in the surgical techniques and perioperative care has significantly improved the quality of life of these patients; nevertheless, reinterventions over the course of a lifetime are frequent. Percutaneous alternatives to the surgical treatment of RVOT dysfunction (transcatheter pulmonary valves) have emerged, with good results. The imaging follow-up of these patients includes echocardiographic and cMRI evaluation. Cardiac ultrasound evaluates residual RVOT obstruction and branch pulmonary arteries, ventricular or atrial septal defects, atrioventricular valve regurgitation, aortic root dilation or regurgitation, ventricular size and function. On the other hand, cMRI provides a quantitative assessment of cardiac output, right and left ventricular function, determination of the severity of the pulmonary insufficiency, and evaluation of branch pulmonary arteries.

Imaging Findings

Cardiac catheterization (Fig. 3.17) evidences RVOT anatomy and severe pulmonary regurgitation (a). Positioning of the Ensemble balloon catheter delivery system with the premounted Melody transcatheter pulmonary valve can be seen (b). Inflation of the endoprosthesis was performed (c), with good results and no regurgitation. Transesophageal probe (*arrow*) (d). Figure 3.18 shows the Melody transcatheter pulmonary valve implanted in the RVOT (*arrow*) seen by 2D imaging (a) and by color Doppler (b) from the anteriorly angled apical view and in the long axis view (c). Magnetic resonance 3D whole heart images (Fig. 3.19) and volume-rendering MR angiographic images (Fig. 3.20) show the large bilateral pulmonary artery aneurisms (left pulmonary artery (LPA) and right pumonary artery (RPA)), as well as the pulmonary valve conduit (*arrow*).

Case 6: Transposition of the Great Arteries (TGA)

Sofía Granja and Carlos Marín

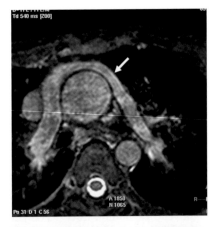

Fig. 3.21

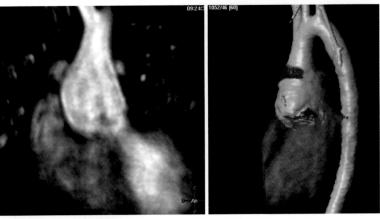

Fig. 3.22

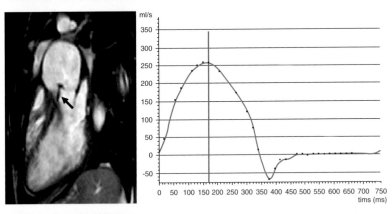

Fig. 3.23

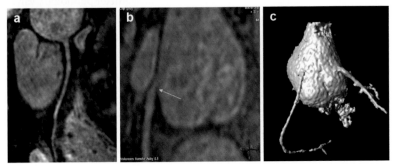

Fig. 3.24

A 11-year-old male followed at the Paediatric Cardiology outpatient clinic because of dextro-TGA (D-TGA), treated by Jatene surgery in the neonatal period.

Comments

TGA results from an abnormal development of the fetal heart during the first 8 weeks of pregnancy. The most common form is D-TGA, in which the aorta becomes connected to the right ventricle and the pulmonary artery to the left ventricle, the opposite of a normal heart anatomy. This condition can be associated with other anatomical lesions, the most common being a ventricular septal defect and left ventricular outflow tract obstruction.

Clinical presentation is determined by the anatomical picture. Nevertheless, cyanosis is the rule, being noted in the first hours of life in about half of the infants with TGA, and within the first days of life in 90% of cases. The immediate newborn's survival depends on adequate blood mixing, assured by a nonrestrictive foramen ovale and a persistent ductus arteriosus. With this objective, an atrial septostomy may have to be performed.

Chest X-ray supports the diagnosis of transposition by showing an oval heart with narrow superior mediastinum, cardiomegaly, and an increase of pulmonary vascularization. However, the final diagnosis is established by echocardiography. Ultrasound confirms the diagnosis and offers a full assessment of cardiac anatomy, including the adequacy of intracardiac and ductal mixing, and the likely ability of the left ventricle to support the systemic circulation. Cardiac catheterization is no longer routinely performed. Within the first weeks of life, TGA is surgically repaired. Prior to the early 1990s, TGA was generally treated surgically with a Mustard or a Senning procedure (atrial switch). These procedures created a tunnel, or baffle, in the atria to correct blood flow. Later, in the 1980s, the Jatene operation procedure (arterial switch) was introduced, "switching" the aorta and pulmonary artery to the proper locations. After TGA repair, child follow-up is scheduled on a regular basis, checking the development of arrhythmias, valvular dysfunction, stenosis at vessel connection site(s), and narrowing of the coronary arteries at their switch connection site. In the long-term follow-up, magnetic resonance imaging gains relevance, proving an excellent assessment of the reconstructed arterial trunks and origins of the reimplanted coronary arteries (in the arterial switch), ventricular function, or venous vessel connections (in atrial switch).

Imaging Findings

Whole heart 3D (WH3D) image shows mild stenosis of the left pulmonary artery (*arrow*) (Fig. 3.21). Magnetic resonance angiography (Fig. 3.22) depicts moderate dilatation of the aortic root. Aortic incompetence jet is shown (*arrow*) (Fig. 3.23a). Flow curve in the aortic root was obtained with phase contrast MR imaging (Fig. 3.23b). Mild aortic regurgitation was confirmed, with a regurgitant fraction of 10%. WH3D images of the coronary arteries (Fig. 3.24) show normal left coronary artery (a) and moderate stenosis of right coronary artery (*arrow*) (b). Volume-rendered image (c) of WH3D depicts coronary artery anatomy.

Case 7: Hypoplastic Left Heart Syndrome

Carlos Marín and Mariano del Valle Diéguez

A 3-year-old patient with hypoplastic left heart syndrome (HLHS). Postsurgical evolution is shown.

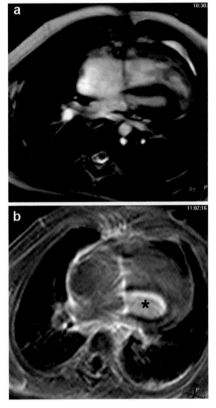

Fig. 3.25

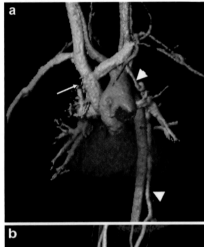

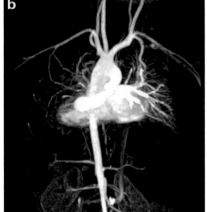

Fig. 3.27

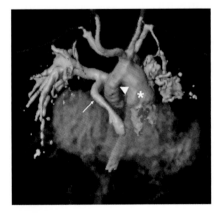

Fig. 3.26

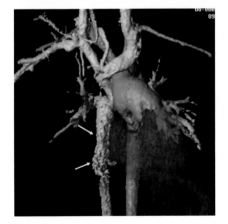

Fig. 3.28

HLHS has a reported prevalence between 0.21% and 0.28%. Until recent advances in surgery and postnatal care, HLHS was an invariably lethal cardiac malformation. In fact, it is the most common cause of cardiac deaths in infants. The left ventricle is small and there is some degree of mitral or aortic atresia, stenosis, or both. With an atretic aortic valve, survival depends on a patent ductus arteriosus.

Ultrasound (US) in the 22nd week of gestation is accurate for prenatal diagnosis. Postnatal US usually suffices for prenatal diagnosis confirmation and surgical planning. In the 1980s, Norwood described a three-stage palliative surgical procedure. The first stage (Norwood I) consists in the construction of a neoaorta from the pulmonary trunk and aortic arch, converting the right ventricle into a systemic ventricle. Ductus arteriosus and atrial septum are excised. Pulmonary arterial flow is obtained by means of a systemic-pulmonary fistula (modified Blalock-Taussig) or a right ventricle-pulmonary artery conduit (Sano procedure). Which of these procedures is better in the long term is currently under debate. The second surgical stage (Norwood II) consists in the creation of a bidirectional cavopulmonary shunt, a termino-lateral connection between superior vena cava and right pulmonary artery (modified Glenn procedure). It is performed at the age of 4–6 months, when pulmonary resistance decreases. The third stage is the modified Fontan procedure. A total separation of systemic and pulmonary circulation is achieved by connecting the inferior vena cava with the pulmonary artery. This step is usually performed at 4–6 years of age. The goal of imaging follow-up in these patients is to assess the hemodynamic status and to diagnose complications as early as possible. The presence of thrombi and malfunction of the AV valve is adequately detected by US. To evaluate pulmonary resistance, especially prior to the Norwood II procedure, cardiac catheterization is generally performed. Cardiac MRI is a reliable technique for the follow-up of anastomoses and pulmonary artery stenoses, aortic recoarctation, arterial or venous collaterals, ventricular function, and the presence of myocardial infarction.

Comments

A small left ventricle is shown in a four-chamber gradient echo image (Fig. 3.25a). Late enhancement of left ventricular myocardium represents endocardial fibroelastosis (*asterisk*) (Fig. 3.25b). In the Norwood I stage, volume-rendered MR angiogram (Fig. 3.26) shows the neoaorta (*asterisk*), the primitive aorta (*arrowhead*), and the Sano conduit (*arrow*). Same patient at the age of five (Fig. 3.27), volume rendered (a) and maximum intensity projection (b) MR angiogram. Bidirectional Glenn shunt shows normal caliber (*arrow*). A venous systemic collateral vein from the hemiazygos vein to the inferior vena cava is shown (*arrowheads*). Multiple arterial to pulmonary collateral arteries from the aortic arch and abdominal aorta are demonstrated in the MIP image. Third stage (modified Fontan procedure) is shown in a 9-year-old boy (Fig. 3.28, different patient). Extracardiac Fontan conduit from the inferior vena cava to the right pulmonary artery is shown (*arrows*).

Imaging Findings

Case 8: Cavopulmonary Thrombosis in Bidirectional Glenn

Fermín Sáez Garmendia

A 2-year-old female with VACTERL (vertebral, anorectal, cardiac anomalies, tracheoesophageal atresia, renal malformations, and limb defects), whose cardiac anomalies consisted of tricuspid atresia and other complex heart defects, underwent a bidirectional Glenn (connection of the superior vena cava to the right pulmonary artery which diverts this blood flow from the heart

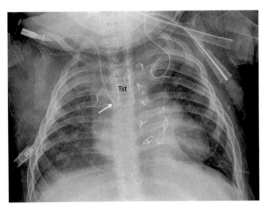

Fig. 3.29

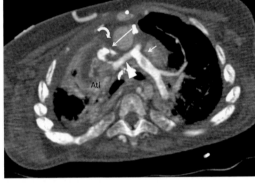

Fig. 3.30

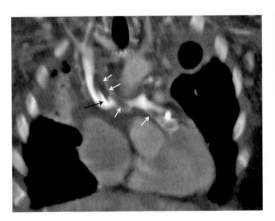

Fig. 3.31

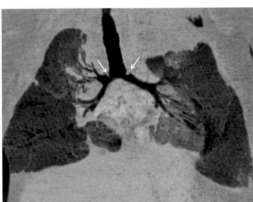

Fig. 3.32

directly to the lungs) when she was 13 months old. Previously, she had required the insertion of a tracheal stent to treat a severe tracheomalacy. After 2 months at the intensive care unit, her clinical situation worsened with increasing tachypnea and cyanosis (61% O_2 sat.).

Comments

Major early complications after bidirectional Glenn include transient superior vena cava syndrome, hematoma, abscess, and persistent pleural or pericardial effusion. Delayed complications include stenosis of the cavopulmonary anastomosis, thrombosis, development of systemic venous to pulmonary venous collateral vessels, arrhythmias, obstructed venous pathways, and protein-losing enteropathy.

Low-dose multidetector CT angiography (MDCTA) is the imaging modality of choice for the study of the thoracic vessels and lung parenchyma. No sedation is required and the examination is performed in a few seconds. MDCTA allows the visualization of the patency and caliber of the cavopulmonary anastomosis and pulmonary arteries, and it is of great help in the diagnostic work-up of these patients.

In this case, chest X-ray (Fig. 3.29) showed mild pulmonary edema and segmental bilateral atelectasis, but these findings did not explain the patient's severe symptoms. A chest CT angiography (CTA) (Figs. 3.30, 3.31, and 3.32) led to the diagnosis of partial thrombosis of the superior vena cava, cavopulmonary anastomosis, and pulmonary arteries. The central venous line was then removed from the superior vena cava, and after adequate medical treatment, the thrombus disappeared with subsequent clinical improvement.

Imaging Findings

(Fig. 3.29). Chest X-ray showed the tracheal stent (Tst), the tracheal tube, and a central venous catheter (inserted 2 months ago) with the tip at the cavopulmonary junction (*arrow*). A pleural tube in the left upper quadrant is draining a localized pleural effusion. A prosthesis obliterates the right ventricular outflow tract. Mild edema and bilateral segmental atelectasis are also demonstrated. (Fig. 3.30) CTA. Oblique subvolume reconstruction. Several filling defects (thrombus) are visualized in the cavopulmonary anastomosis (*long arrow*) and the left pulmonary artery (*short arrow*). The lower end of the tracheal stent (*arrowhead*), the tip of the central venous catheter (*curved arrow*), and the right upper lobe atelectasis (Atl) are also shown. (Fig. 3.31) CTA. Coronal oblique reconstruction. The superior vena cava and the right and left pulmonary arteries are partially filled with thrombi (*white arrows*). The tip of the central venous catheter is demonstrated at the level of the cavopulmonary anastomosis (*black arrow*). Hydropneumothorax in the upper left. Atelectasis of the right upper lobe. (Fig. 3.32) CTA. Coronal subvolume reconstruction, minimal intensity projection, the best method to visualize the airway. The tips of the tracheal stent (*arrows*) protrude slightly into both the right and left main bronchi. The rest of the airway is unremarkable.

Case 9: Single Coronary Artery

Pilar García-Peña
and Cristian Quezada Jorquera

A 6-year-old boy with Noonan syndrome. Cardiac US shows hypertrophic septal cardiomyopathy and a prominent left coronary artery. A coronary CT angiography (CTA) was performed posteriorly.

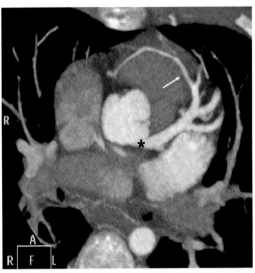

Fig. 3.33

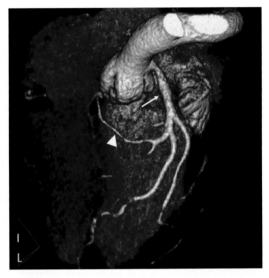

Fig. 3.34

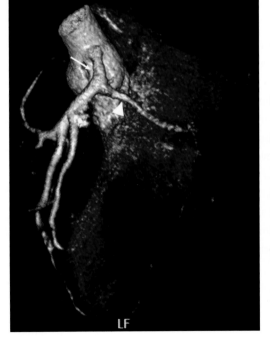

Fig. 3.35

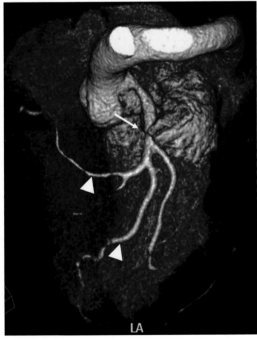

Fig. 3.36

Congenital coronary anomalies are uncommon, and the vast majority are diagnosed incidentally during coronary angiography or necropsy. The prevalence of these anomalies has been estimated in 1–2% of the general population. Types of coronary artery anomalies include a coronary artery originating from the wrong aortic sinus, a single coronary ostium, the left coronary artery originating from the pulmonary trunk, a high takeoff coronary ostium from the aortic wall, and a stenosis of the coronary ostium. Most coronary anomalies are usually of little or no clinical significance. However, several types can result in an increased incidence of symptoms including angina pectoris, myocardial infarction, syncope, and sudden death.

In this case, there is a single coronary ostium in the left sinus of Valsalva, from which the left main coronary artery originates, which later has two branches supplying the right ventricle. The left anterior descendent artery has a normal course. There is no ostium for the right coronary artery.

A single coronary ostium is a rare anomaly seen in only 0.024–0.044% of the population. In this condition, the left main coronary artery and the right coronary artery arise from a common ostium situated on the left, right, or posterior sinus.

The coronary artery involved may have an anomalous course and run interarterially between the aortic root and the pulmonary trunk. This can have an adverse clinical outcome with an increased risk of sudden death.

Today, echocardiography remains the examination of choice in studying patients with suspected cardiac abnormalities. However, the study of the coronary arteries has traditionally required the use of conventional angiography. The development of MDCT has allowed the noninvasive study of the coronary arteries. In children, the use of this method requires employing dose reduction strategies to minimize their effects. Cardiac MRI is another technique that can depict the proximal coronary arteries. However, it is not as widely available as MDCT and is limited in the evaluation of the course and the distal area of the coronary arteries.

Comments

(Fig. 3.33). Axial maximum intensity projection CT image shows a single coronary ostium (*asterisk*) from which the prominent left main coronary artery originates. There is no ostium for the right coronary artery. One of the coronary branches runs toward the right ventricle (*arrow*). (Fig. 3.34). Volume-rendered CT image shows a single left coronary artery (*arrow*) from which the left descending artery originates and then reaches the right ventricular apex and the first diagonal branch. The other coronary branch runs to the right (*arrowhead*). (Fig. 3.35). Volume-rendered CT image shows the left coronary artery (*arrow*) from which the circumflex artery originates and then travels in the left atrioventricular groove (*arrowhead*). The left descendent artery and its branches are visualized to the right of the image. (Fig. 3.36). Volume-rendered CT image shows the left descendent artery (*arrow*) and one of its branches supplying the apex and the right ventricle (*arrowheads*).

Imaging Findings

Case 10: Hypertrophic Cardiomyopathy (HCM)

Sofía Granja and Carlos Marín

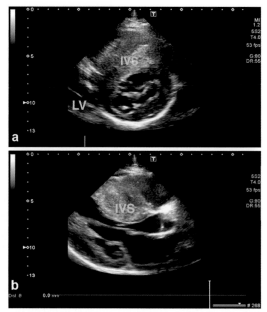

Fig. 3.37

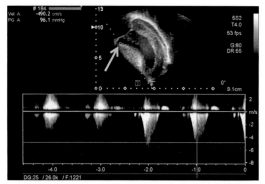

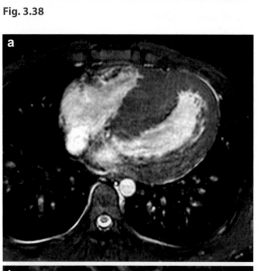

Fig. 3.38

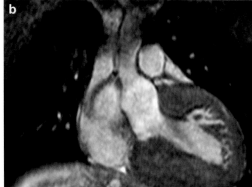

Fig. 3.39

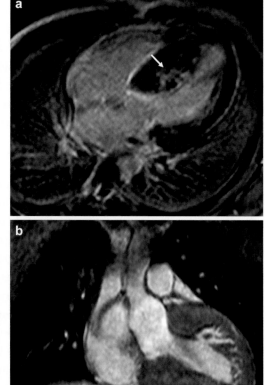

Fig. 3.40

An 8-year-old male diagnosed with obstructive asymmetric ventricular septal HCM after a cardiac murmur evaluation. At 14 years of age suffers first syncope. Genetic test was positive for a sarcomeric protein gene mutation, and cardiac MR (CMR) showed areas of myocardial fibrosis. An implantable cardiac defibrillator (ICD) was implanted.

Comments

HCM is a complex entity with unique physiopathologic characteristics and marked genotypic, phenotypic, and clinical heterogeneity. It can be defined as myocardial hypertrophy in the absence of a causative condition, with an estimated prevalence of 10–100 cases per 100,000 people. Multiple mutations in myocyte contractile proteins have been implicated in the development of HCM. Ventricular septal hypertrophy is the most frequent form of hypertrophy, with mid-ventricular and apical types being far less common. The onset of symptoms typically occurs in early adulthood, with patients reporting chest pain, palpitations, dyspnea, or syncope. Sudden death may be the presenting symptom (HCM is the most common cause of sudden death among young athletes). HCM is generally diagnosed during cardiac evaluation for murmurs, symptoms, electrocardiographic abnormalities, and screening of offspring of affected adults. The echocardiogram provides definitive noninvasive assessment of ventricular size, wall thickness, systolic and diastolic function, outflow obstruction, and valvular insufficiency in nearly all children. Complementing the echocardiographic study, delayed hyperenhancement on MRI has been identified as a sensitive imaging technique for myocardial scar, correlating with histologically proven myocardial fibrosis, a known risk factor for ventricular arrhythmias. Avoidance of high-intensity physical activity is usually recommended, but medical therapies are initiated only in symptomatic patients. In this last group, procedures like alcohol septal ablation, surgical myectomy, pacemaker, or ICD implantation may be indicated. The overall mortality is less than 1% per year. However, a subgroup of patients is at high risk of sudden death, primarily as a result of ventricular arrhythmias.

Imaging Findings

Transthoracic echocardiogram (TTE), short axis view (Fig. 3.37a) and long axis view (Fig. 3.37b), shows severe septal hypertrophy (IVS, interventricular septum). Reverse curvature septum HCM shows a predominant mid-septal convexity toward the left ventricular (LV) cavity, with the cavity itself often having an overall crescent shape. Continuous wave Doppler spectra from the apex (Fig. 3.38) demonstrate dynamic subaortic obstruction (*arrow*). A typical late-peaking configuration similar to a dagger is noted; peak velocity is 4.9 m/s, corresponding to a peak gradient of 96 mmHg. Whole heart 3D images (Fig. 3.39) show septal hypertrophy, affecting the subvalvular left ventricular outflow tract. Ejection fraction was 67%. Late enhancement MR images in four chamber and short axis views (Fig. 3.40) show enhancing nodules in the IV septum (*arrows*).

Further Reading

Case 1: Atrial Septal Defect Ostium Secundum Type

Book

Geva T (2009) Anomalies of the atrial septum. In: Lai W, Mertens L, Cohen M, Geva T (eds) Echocardiography in pediatric and congenital heart disease: from fetus to adult, 1st edn. Wiley-Blackwell, Hoboken, pp 158–174

Web Link

Abdulla R et al (2011) Heart diseases in children information center – pediatric cardiology for medical professionals. The University of Chicago Website. http://pediatriccardiology.uchicago.edu/MP/CHD/ASD/asd.htm. Accessed 26 Oct 2011

Articles

Arrington CB, Tani LY, Minich LL, Bradley DJ (2007) An assessment of the electrocardiogram as a screening test for large atrial septal defects in children. J Electrocardiol 40:484–488

Azhari N, Shihata MS, Al-Fatani A (2004) Spontaneous closure of atrial septal defects within the oval fossa. Cardiol Young 14:148–155

Butera G, Carminati M, Chessa M et al (2006) Percutaneous versus surgical closure of secundum atrial septal defect: comparison of early results and complications. Am Heart J 151:228–234

Hanslik A, Pospisil U, Salzer-Muhar U, Greber-Platzer S, Male C (2006) Predictors of spontaneous closure of isolated secundum atrial septal defect in children: a longitudinal study. Pediatrics 118(4):1560–1565

McMahon CJ, Feltes TF, Fraley JK, Bricker DJ, Grifka RG, Tortoriello TA et al (2002) Natural history of growth of secundum atrial septal defects and implications for transcatheter closure. Heart 87:256–259

Post MC, Suttorp MJ, Jaarsma W, Plokker HW (2006) Comparison of outcome and complications using different types of devices for percutaneous closure of a secundum atrial septal defect in adults: a single-center experience. Catheter Cardiovasc Interv 67:438–443

Saxena A, Divekar A, Soni NR (2005) Natural history of secundum atrial septal defect revisited in the era of transcatheter closure. Indian Heart J 57:35–38

Spence M, Qureshi S (2005) Complications of transcatheter closure of atrial septal defects. Heart 91:1512–1514

Vaidyanathan B, Simpson JM, Kumar RK (2009) Transesophageal echocardiography for device closure of atrial septal defects – case selection, planning, and procedural guidance. JACC Cardiovasc Imaging 2:1238–1242

Vida VL, Barnoya J, O'Connell M, Leon-Wyss J, Larrazabal LA, Castañeda AR (2006) Surgical versus percutaneous occlusion of ostium secundum atrial septal defects: results and cost-effective considerations in a low-income country. J Am Coll Cardiol 47:326–331

Case 2: Mitral Valve Endocarditis

Book

Vogt MO (2009) Infective endocarditis. In: Lai W, Mertens L, Cohen M, Geva T (eds) Echocardiography in pediatric and congenital heart disease: from fetus to adult, 1st edn. Wiley-Blackwell, Hoboken, pp 657–668

Web Link

Brusch J et al (2011) Infective endocarditis. In Medscape reference site. http://emedicine.medscape.com/article/216650-overview. Updated July 27, 2011. Accessed November 6, 2011

Articles

Casella F, Rana B, Casazza G, Bhan A, Kapetanakis S, Omigie J et al (2009) The potential impact of contemporary transthoracic echocardiography on the management of patients with native valve endocarditis: a comparison with transesophageal echocardiography. Echocardiography 26(8):900–906

Castro S, Cartoni D, d'Amati G, Beni S, Yao J, Fiorelli M et al (2000) Diagnostic accuracy of transthoracic and multiplane transesophageal echocardiography for valvular perforation in acute infective endocarditis. Clin Infect Dis 30:825–826

Chatzis AC, Saroglou G, Giannopoulos NM, Sarris GE (2005) Subtle infective endocarditis and congenital cardiac disease. Cardiol Young 15:617–620

Di Filippo S, Delahaye F, Semiond B et al (2006) Current patterns of infective endocarditis in congenital heart disease. Heart 92:1490–1495

Ferrieri P, Gewitz MH, Gerber MA et al (2002) From the committee on rheumatic fever, endocarditis, and Kawasaki disease of the American heart association council on cardiovascular disease in the young. Unique features of infective endocarditis in childhood. Circulation 105:2115–2126

Holmes AA, Hung T, Human DG, Campbell AI (2011) Kingella kingae endocarditis: a rare case of mitral valve perforation. Ann Pediatr Cardiol 4:210–212

Penk JS, Webb CL, Shulman ST, Anderson EJ (2011) Echocardiography in pediatric infective endocarditis. Pediatr Infect Dis J 30:1109–1111

Simpson JM, Miller O (2011) Three-dimensional echocardiography in congenital heart disease. Arch Cardiovasc Dis 104:45–56

Wilson W, Taubert KA, Gewitz M et al (2007) Prevention of infective endocarditis: guidelines from the American heart association: a guideline from the American Heart Association Rheumatic Fever, Endocarditis, and Kawasaki Disease Committee, Council on Cardiovascular Disease in the Young, and the Council on Clinical Cardiology, Council on Cardiovascular Surgery and Anesthesia, and the Quality of Care and Outcomes Research Interdisciplinary Working Group. Circulation 116:1736–1754

Youssef D, Henaine R, Di Filippo S (2010) Subtle bacterial endocarditis due to Kingella kingae in an infant: a case report. Cardiol Young 20:448–450

Case 3: Sinus Venosus Defect and Partial Anomalous Pulmonary Venous Connection

Book

Allen HD, Driscoll DJ, Shaddy RE, Feltes TF (eds) (2008) Moss and Adams' heart disease in infants, children, and adolescents: including the fetus and young adult, 7th edn. Lippincott Williams and Wilkins, Philadelphia

Web Link

Congenital heart disease – sinus venosus atrial septal defect. Yale University School of Medicine Website. http://www.yale.edu/imaging/chd/e_asd_sinus_venos/. Accessed October 26, 2011

Articles

Alsoufi B, Cai S, Van Arsdell GS, Williams WG, Caldarone CA, Coles JG (2007) Outcomes after surgical treatment of children with partial anomalous pulmonary venous connection. Ann Thorac Surg 84:2020–2026

Ammash NM, Seward JB, Warnes CA, Connolly HM, O'Leary PW, Danielson GK (1997) Partial anomalous pulmonary venous connection: diagnosis by transesophageal echocardiography. J Am Coll Cardiol 29:1351–1358

Campbell M (1970) Natural history of atrial septal defect. Br Heart J 32:820–826

Davia JE, Cheitlin MD, Bedynek JL (1973) Sinus venosus atrial septal defect: analysis of fifty cases. Am Heart J 85:177–185

Festa P, Ait-Ali L, Cerillo AG, De Marchi D, Murzi B (2006) Magnetic resonance imaging is the diagnostic tool of choice in the preoperative evaluation of patients with partial anomalous pulmonary venous return. Int J Cardiovasc Imaging 22:685–693

Li J, Al Zaghal AM, Anderson RH (1998) The nature of the superior sinus venosus defect. Clin Anat 11:349–352

Riesenkampff EM, Schmitt B, Schnackenburg B, Huebler M, Alexi-Meskishvili V, Hetzer R et al (2009) Partial anomalous pulmonary venous drainage in young pediatric patients: the role of magnetic resonance imaging. Pediatr Cardiol 30:458–464

Sachweh JS, Daebritz SH, Hermanns B et al (2006) Hypertensive pulmonary vascular disease in adults with secundum or sinus venosus atrial septal defect. Ann Thorac Surg 81:207–213

Van Praagh S, Carrera ME, Sanders S, Mayer JE Jr, Van Praagh R (1995) Partial or total direct pulmonary venous drainage to right atrium due to malposition of septum primum. Anatomic and echocardiographic findings and surgical treatment: a study based on 36 cases. Chest 107:1488–1498

Vida VL, Padalino MA, Boccuzzo G, Tarja E, Berggren H, Carrel T et al (2010) Scimitar syndrome: a European Congenital Heart Surgeons Association (ECHSA) multicentric study. Circulation 122:1159–1166

Case 4: Double Aortic Arch

Book

Powell AJ, Mandell VS (2006) Vascular rings. In: Keane JF, Lock JE, Fyler CF (eds) NADAS' pediatric cardiology, 2nd edn. Elsevier, Philadelphia, pp 811–825

Web Link

McElhinney DB, Wernovsky G, Berger S (2009) Vascular ring, double aortic arch. Medscape reference. http://emedicine.medscape.com/article/899609-overview. Updated Oct 29, 2009. Accessed August 2, 2011

Articles

Browne LP (2009) What is the optimal imaging for vascular rings and slings? Pediatr Radiol 39(Suppl 2):S191–S195

Hernanz-Schulman M (2005) Vascular rings: a practical approach to imaging diagnosis. Pediatr Radiol 35:961–979

Jaffe RB (1991) Radiographic manifestations of congenital anomalies of the aortic arch. Radiol Clin North Am 29:319–334

Kellenberg CJ (2010) Aortic arch malformations. Pediatr Radiol 40:876–884

Lee EY, Siegel MJ, Hildebolt CF, Gutierrez FR, Bhalla S, Fallah JH (2004) MDCT evaluation of thoracic aortic anomalies in pediatric patients and young adults: comparison of axial, multiplanar and 3D images. AJR Am J Roentgenol 182:777–784

Oddone M, Granata C, Vercellino N, Bava E, Tomá P (2005) Multi-modality evaluation of the abnormalities of the aortic arches in children: techniques and imaging spectrum with emphasis on MRI. Pediatr Radiol 35:947–960

Pickhardt P, Siegel M, Gutierrez F (1997) Vascular rings in symptomatic children: frequency of chest radiographic findings. Radiology 203:423–426

Turner A, Gavel G, Coutts J (2005) Vascular rings presentation, investigation and outcome. Eur J Pediatr 164:266–270

Weinberg PM (2006) Aortic arch anomalies. J Cardiovasc Magn Reson 8:633–643

Yoo SJ, Min JY, Lee YH, Roman YK, Jaeggi E, Smallhorn J (2003) Fetal sonographic diagnosis of aortic arch anomalies. Ultrasound Obstet Gynecol 22:535–546

Case 5: Tetralogy of Fallot

Book

Srivastava S, Parness IA (2009) Tetralogy of fallot. In: Lay WW, Mertens LL, Cohen MS, Geva T (eds) Echocardiography in pediatric and congenital heart disease from fetus to adult, 1st edn. Blackwell Publishing Ltd, Oxford, pp 362–384

Web Link

MedlinePlus (2009) Tetralogy of Fallot. MedlinePlus®, the National Library of Medicine's consumer health web site. http://www.nlm.nih.gov/medlineplus/ency/article/001567.htm. Updated December 1, 2011

Articles

Aboulhosn J, Child JS (2006) Management after childhood repair of tetralogy of fallot. Curr Treat Options Cardiovasc Med 8:474–483

Anderson RH, Weinberg PM (2005) The clinical anatomy of tetralogy of fallot. Cardiol Young 15(Suppl 1):38–47

Boechat MI, Ratib O, Williams PL, Gomes AS, Child JS, Allada V (2005) Cardiac MR imaging and MR angiography for assessment of complex tetralogy of Fallot and pulmonary atresia. Radiographics 25:1535–1546

Duro RP, Moura C, Leite-Moreira A (2010) Anatomophysiologic basis of tetralogy of fallot and its clinical implications. Rev Port Cardiol 29:591–630

Kanter KR, Kogon BE, Kirshbom PM, Carlock PR (2010) Symptomatic neonatal tetralogy of fallot: repair or shunt? Ann Thorac Surg 89:858–863

Park CS, Lee JR, Lim HG, Kim WH, Kim YJ (2010) The long-term result of total repair for tetralogy of fallot. Eur J Cardiothorac Surg 38:311–317

Redington AN (2006) Determinants and assessment of pulmonary regurgitation in tetralogy of fallot: practice and pitfalls. Cardiol Clin 24:631–639, vii

Starr JP (2010) Tetralogy of fallot: yesterday and today. World J Surg 34:658–668

Tsang FH, Li X, Cheung YF, Chau KT, Cheng LC (2010) Pulmonary valve replacement after surgical repair of tetralogy of fallot. Hong Kong Med J 16:26–30

Zahn E, Hellenbrand W, Lock J, McElhinney D, Zahn E, Hellenbrand W, Lock J, McElhinney D (2009) Implantation of the melody transcatheter pulmonary valve in patients with a dysfunctional right ventricular outflow tract conduit: early results from the U.S. Clinical trial. J Am Coll Cardiol 54:1722–1729

Case 6: Transposition of the Great Arteries (TGA)

Book

Paul MH, Wernovsky G (1998) Transposition of the great arteries. In: Moss and Adams heart disease in infants, children, and adolescents, vol 2. Williams & Wilkins, Baltimore, pp 1154–1224

Web Link

Transposition of the Great Arteries (TGA). Children's heart federation web site: http://www.chfed.org.uk/information/heart_conditions/transposition_of_the_great_arteries_tga. Accessed October 28, 2011

Articles

Aseervatham R, Pohlner P (1998) A clinical comparison of arterial and atrial repairs for transposition of the great arteries: early and midterm survival and functional results. Aust N Z J Surg 68:206–208

Jatene AD, Fontes VF, Paulista PP, Souza LC, Neger F, Galantier M et al (1976) Anatomic correction of transposition of the great vessels. J Thorac Cardiovasc Surg 72:364–370

Lissin LW, Li W, Murphy DJ, Hornung T, Swan L, Mullen M et al (2004) Comparison of transthoracic echocardiography versus cardiovascular magnetic resonance imaging for the assessment of ventricular function in adults after atrial switch procedures for complete transposition of the great arteries. Am J Cardiol 93:654–657

Losay J, Touchot A, Capderou A, Piot JD, Belli E, Planché C et al (2006) Aortic valve regurgitation after arterial switch operation for transposition of the great arteries incidence, risk factors, and outcome. J Am Coll Cardiol 47:2057–2062

Qamar ZA, Goldberg CS, Devaney EJ, Bove EL, Ohye RG (2007) Current risk factors and outcomes for the arterial switch operation. Ann Thorac Surg 84:871–878

Rao PS (2009) Diagnosis and management of cyanotic congenital heart disease: part I. Indian J Pediatr 76(1):57–70

Rashkind WJ, Miller WW (1966) Creation of an atrial septal defect without thoracotomy: a palliative approach to complete transposition of the great arteries. JAMA 196:991–992

Rodríguez E, Soler R, Fernández R, Raposo I (2007) Postoperative imaging in cyanotic congenital heart disease. Part 1. Normal findings. AJR Am J Roentgenol 189:1353–1360

Salehian O, Schwerzmann M, Merchant N, Webb GD, Siu SC, Therrien J (2004) Assessment of systemic right ventricular function in patients with transposition of the great arteries using the myocardial performance index: comparison with cardiac magnetic resonance imaging. Circulation 110:3229–3233

Soongswang J, Adatia I, Newman C, Smallhorn JF, Williams WG, Freedom RM (1998) Mortality in potential arterial switch candidates with transposition of the great arteries. J Am Coll Cardiol 32(3):753–757

Case 7: Hypoplastic Left Heart Syndrome

Book

Lang P, Fyler CF (2006) Hypoplastic left heart syndrome. In: Keane JF, Lock JE, Fyler CF (eds) NADAS' pediatric cardiology, 2nd edn. Elsevier, Philadelphia, pp 715–728

Web Link

Ohye RG, Mosca RS, Bove EL (2010) Pediatric hypoplastic left heart syndrome and the staged norwood procedure. Medscape Reference. http://emedicine.medscape.com/article/904137-overview. Updated Jul 9, 2010. Accessed September 28, 2011

Articles

Andrews RE, Tulloh RM, Anderson DR, Lucas SB (2004) Acute myocardial infarction as a cause of death in palliated hypoplastic left heart syndrome. Heart 90:e17

Bardo DM, Frankel DG, Applegate KE, Murphy DJ, Saneto RP (2001) Hypoplastic left heart syndrome. Radiographics 21:705–717

Dillman JR, Dorfman AL, Attili AK, Agarwal PP, Bell A, Mueller GC, Hernandez RJ (2010) Cardiovascular magnetic resonance imaging of hypoplastic left heart syndrome in children. Pediatr Radiol 40:261–274

Fiore AC, Tobin C, Jureidini S, Rahimi M, Kim ES, Schowengerdt K (2011) A comparison of the modified Blalock-Taussig shunt with the right ventricle-to-pulmonary artery conduit. Ann Thorac Surg 91:1479–1484

Hughes ML, Tsang VT, Kostolny M, Giardini A, Muthurangu V, Taylor AM, Brown K (2011) Lessons

from inter-stage cardiac magnetic resonance imaging in predicting survival for patients with hypoplastic left heart syndrome. Cardiol Young 31:1–8

Khairy P, Fernandes SM, Mayer JE Jr, Triedman JK, Walsh EP, Lock JE, Landzberg MJ (2008) Long-term survival, modes of death, and predictors of mortality in patients with Fontan surgery. Circulation 117:85–92

Mery CM, Lapar DJ, Seckeler MD, Chamberlain RS, Gangemi JJ, Kron IL, Peeler BB (2011) Pulmonary artery and conduit reintervention rates after norwood using a right ventricle to pulmonary artery conduit. Ann Thorac Surg 92:1483–1489

Muthurangu V, Taylor AM, Hegde SR, Johnson R, Tulloh R, Simpson JM, Qureshi S, Rosenthal E, Baker E, Anderson D, Razavi R (2005) Cardiac magnetic resonance imaging after stage I Norwood operation for hypoplastic left heart syndrome. Circulation 22(112):3256–3263

Norwood WI, Lang P, Casteneda AR, Campbell DN (1981) Experience with operations for hypoplastic left heart syndrome. J Thorac Cardiovasc Surg 82:511–519

Sano S, Ishino K, Kawada M et al (2003) Right ventricle-pulmonary artery shunt in first-stage palliation of hypoplastic left heart syndrome. J Thorac Cardiovasc Surg 126:504–509

Case 8: Cavopulmonary Thrombosis in Bidirectional Glenn

Book

Thelen M, Kreitner KF, Erbel R, Barkhausen J (2009) Cardiac imaging: a multimodality approach. Thieme, Stuttgart

Web Link

http://www.learningradiology.com/toc/tocorgansystems/toccardiac.htm

Articles

Dillman JR, Hernandez RJ (2009) Role of CT in the evaluation of congenital cardiovascular disease in children. AJR Am J Roentgenol 192:1219–1231

Eichhorn JG, Jourdan C, Hill SL, Raman SV, Cheatham JP, Long FR (2008) CT of pediatric vascular stents used to treat congenital heart disease. AJR Am J Roentgenol 190:1241–1246

Gaca AM, Jaggers JJ, Dudley LT, Bisset GS 3rd (2008a) Repair of congenital heart disease: a primer. Part 1. Radiology 247:617–631

Gaca AM, Jaggers JJ, Dudley LT, Bisset GS 3rd (2008b) Repair of congenital heart disease: a primer. Part 2. Radiology 248:44–60

Goo HW (2011) Haemodynamic findings on cardiac CT in children with congenital heart disease. Pediatr Radiol 41:250–261

Haramati LB, Glickstein JS, Issenberg HJ, Haramati N, Crooke GA (2002) MR imaging and CT of vascular anomalies and connections in patients with congenital heart disease: significance in surgical planning. Radiographics 22:337–347

Hlavacek MA (2010) Imaging of congenital cardiovascular disease: the case for computed tomography. J Thorac Imaging 25:247–255

Leschka S, Oechslin E, Husmann L, Desbiolles L, Marincek B, Genoni M et al (2007) Pre- and postoperative evaluation of congenital heart disease in children and adults with 64-section CT. Radiographics 27:829–846

Spevak PJ, Johnson PT, Fishman EK (2008) Surgically corrected congenital heart disease: utility of 64-MDCT. AJR Am J Roentgenol 191:854–861

Taylor AM (2008) Cardiac imaging: MR or CT? Which to use when. Pediatr Radiol 38(Suppl 3):S433–S438

Kim SY, Seo JB, Do K-H, Heo J-N, Lee JS, Song J-W et al (2006) Coronary artery anomalies: classification and ECG-gated multi-detector Row CT findings with angiographic correlation. Radiographics 26:317–333

Ko ar P, Ergun E, Oztürk C, Ko ar U (2009) Anatomic variations and anomalies of the coronary arteries: 64-slice CT angiographic appearance. Diagn Interv Radiol 15:275–283

Solanki P, Gerula C, Randhawa P, Benz M, Maher J, Haider B et al (2010) Right coronary artery anatomical variants: where and how? J Invasive Cardiol 22:103–106

Young PM, Gerber TC, Williamson EE, Julsrud PR, Herfkens RJ (2011) Cardiac imaging: part 2, normal, variant, and anomalous configurations of the coronary vasculature. AJR Am J Roentgenol 197:816–826

Zeina AR, Blinder J, Sharif D, Rosenschein U, Barmeir E (2009) Congenital coronary artery anomalies in adults: non-invasive assessment with multidetector CT. Br J Radiol 82:254–261

Case 9: Single Coronary Artery

Book

Sena L, Krishnamurthy R, Chung T (2008) Pediatric cardiac CT. In: Lucaya J, Strife JL (eds) Pediatric chest imaging, 2nd edn. Springer, Berlin/Heidelberg, pp 361–395

Web Link

http://www.appliedradiology.com/Issues/2011/06/Articles/AR_06-11_Agarwal/Coronary-artery-anomalies-on-CT-angiography.aspx

Articles

Bastarrika Alemañ G, Alonso Burgos A, Azcárate Agüero PM, Castaño Rodríguez S, Pueyo Villoslada JC, Alegría Ezquerra E (2008) Normal anatomy, anatomical variants, and anomalies of the origin and course of the coronary arteries on multislice CT. Radiologia 50:197–206

Cademartiri F, La Grutta L, Malagò R, Alberghina F, Meijboom WB, Pugliese F et al (2008) Prevalence of anatomical variants and coronary anomalies in 543 consecutive patients studied with 64-slice CT coronary angiography. Eur Radiol 18:781–791

Castorina S, Privitera G, Luca T, Panebianco M, Tolaro S, Patanè L et al (2009) Detection of coronary artery anomalies and coronary aneurysms by multislice computed tomography coronary angiography. Ital J Anat Embryol 114:77–86

Goo HW, Park I-S, Ko JK, Kim YH, Seo D-M, Yun T-J et al (2005) Visibility of the origin and proximal course of coronary arteries on non-ECG-gated heart CT in patients with congenital heart disease. Pediatr Radiol 35:792–798

Joshi SD, Joshi SS, Athavale SA (2010) Origins of the coronary arteries and their significance. Clinics (Sao Paulo) 65:79–84

Case 10: Hypertrophic Cardiomyopathy (HCM)

Book

Maron BJ (2009) Hypertrophic cardiomyopathy. In: Lai W, Mertens L, Cohen M, Geva T (eds) Echocardiography in pediatric and congenital heart disease: from fetus to adult, 1st edn. Wiley-Blackwell, Hoboken, pp 1172–1195

Web Link

Sander G (2011) Hypertrophic cardiomyopathy. http://emedicine.medscape.com/article/152913-overview. Updated Sep 29, 2011. Accessed October 24, 2011

Articles

Bos JM, Towbin JA, Ackerman MJ (2009) Diagnostic, prognostic, and therapeutic implications of genetic testing for hypertrophic cardiomyopathy. J Am Coll Cardiol 54:201–211

Colan SD (2010) Hypertrophic cardiomyopathy in childhood. Heart Fail Clin 6:433–444, vii–iii

Colan SD, Lipshultz SE, Lowe AM, Sleeper LA, Messere J, Cox GF, Lurie PR, Orav EJ, Towbin JA (2007) Epidemiology and cause-specific outcome of hypertrophic cardiomyopathy in children: findings from the pediatric cardiomyopathy registry. Circulation 115:773–781

Kwon DH, Smedira NG, Rodriguez ER, Tan C, Setser R, Thamilarasan M et al (2009) Cardiac magnetic resonance detection of myocardial scarring in hypertrophic cardiomyopathy: correlation with histopathology and prevalence of ventricular tachycardia. J Am Coll Cardiol 54:242–249

Maron BJ, McKenna WJ, Danielson GK, Kappenberger LJ, Kuhn HJ, Seidman CE et al (2003) American college of cardiology/European society of cardiology clinical expert consensus document on hypertrophic cardiomyopathy. A report of the American college of cardiology foundation task force on clinical expert consensus documents and the European society of cardiology committee for practice guidelines. J Am Coll Cardiol 42:1687–1713

Maron BJ, Spirito P, Shen WK, Haas TS, Formisano F, Link MS et al (2007) Implantable cardioverter-defibrillators and prevention of sudden cardiac death in hypertrophic cardiomyopathy. J Am Med Assoc 298:405–412

Ostman-Smith I, Wettrell G, Keeton B, Riesenfeld T, Holmgren D, Ergander U (2005) Echocardiographic and electrocardiographic identification of those children with hypertrophic cardiomyopathy who should be considered at high-risk of dying suddenly. Cardiol Young 15:632–642

Pelliccia A, Zipes DP, Maron BJ (2008) Bethesda conference #36 and the European society of cardiology consensus recommendations revisited a comparison of U.S. and European criteria for eligibility and disqualification of competitive athletes with cardiovascular abnormalities. J Am Coll Cardiol 52: 1990–1996

Spirito P, Autore C, Rapezzi C, Bernabò P, Badagliacca R, Maron MS et al (2009) Syncope and risk of sudden death in hypertrophic cardiomyopathy. Circulation 119:1703–1710

Syed IS, Ommen SR, Breen JF, Tajik AJ (2008) Hypertrophic cardiomyopathy: identification of morphological subtypes by echocardiography and cardiac magnetic resonance imaging. JACC Cardiovasc Imaging 1:377–379

Abdominal Imaging

CINTA SANGÜESA NEBOT

Contents

M.I. Martínez-León et al., *Imaging for Pediatricians*, Imaging for Clinicians,
DOI 10.1007/978-3-642-28629-2_4, © Springer-Verlag Berlin Heidelberg 2012

Case 1: Choledochal Cyst

Sara Desamparados Picó Aliaga

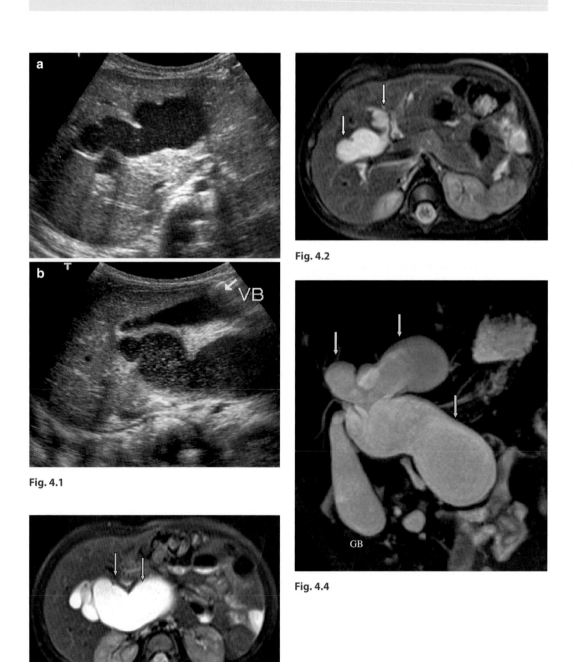

Fig. 4.1

Fig. 4.2

Fig. 4.3

Fig. 4.4

A 10-month-old girl presents jaundice and abdominal pain for 3 days and clinical picture of gastroenteritis the previous week. On examination, there was moderate hepatomegaly. Laboratory test shows signs of cholestasis.

Choledochal cysts are characterized by a cystic dilatation of a segment of the biliary ductal system with a female predilection (4:1). It is an infrequent cause of neonatal jaundice and usually is diagnosed in childhood or in the adult age. The choledochal cyst in the neonate may be a separate entity from the choledochal cyst that presents in childhood and adolescence. The pathogenesis in these two groups differs; in the neonate, the choledochal cyst is congenital and may be associated with atresia of the distal common bile duct, whereas in the older child, it may be acquired in association with an anomalous pancreaticobiliary union.

Five types of biliary cysts based on the Todani classification system have been described. The majority of cysts are type 1, which is diffuse involvement of the choledochal biliary duct (CBD) and common hepatic duct. In type 2, the choledochal cyst is a diverticulum of the extrahepatic bile duct. Type 3, a choledochocele, emerges from the intraduodenal portion of the CBD. In type 4, multiple cystic dilatations involve intra- and extrahepatic ducts (type 4A) or are limited to extrahepatic ducts (type 4B). Type 5 is known as Caroli's disease, an autosomal recessive disorder that results from the arrest of or a derangement in the normal embryologic remodeling of ducts, causing varying degrees of destructive inflammation and nonobstructive cystic segmental dilatation of the intrahepatic ducts.

Abdominal pain, jaundice, and an abdominal mass are the classic triad of signs and symptoms, but they are present in less than one third of cases, and the diagnosis should be suspected in children with any one or combination of these features.

US is an effective, noninvasive procedure that should be used in all patients with cholestatic jaundice. A cystic or fusiform mass in the porta hepatis separate from the gallbladder, with bile ducts leading into or out of it, is diagnostic of a choledochal cyst. Its relationship to the pancreas and intrahepatic biliary tree should be ascertained. The central dot sign is considered suggestive of Caroli disease. Biliary origin can be confirmed by MR cholangiopancreatography or with radionuclide imaging. Surgical resection is necessary to prevent complications that include purulent cholangitis, progressive biliary obstruction, and eventual hepatic cirrhosis with portal hypertension. Spontaneous or traumatic rupture with biliary peritonitis may also occur.

(Fig. 4.1a, b). US shows a cystic structure in the porta hepatis, separate from the gallbladder (*arrow*) (VB), representing type IVA choledochal cyst with severe biliary dilatations. (Figs. 4.2 and 4.3). Axial T2-weighted TSE shows marked cystic dilatation of the common bile duct and of the intrahepatic biliary tree (*arrows*), which is well demonstrated on the coronal reconstruction image (*arrows*) (Fig. 4.4) GB (*gall bladder*).

Case 2: Gastric Duplication Cyst

Cinta Sangüesa Nebot

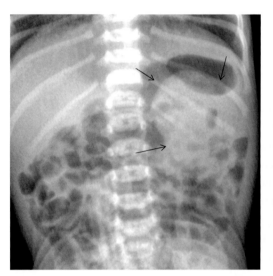

Fig. 4.5

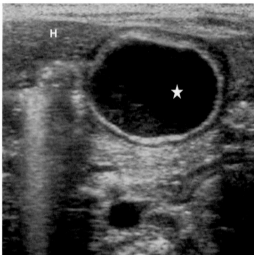

Fig. 4.6

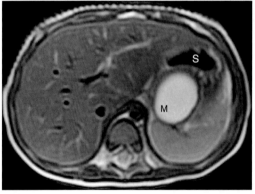

Fig. 4.7

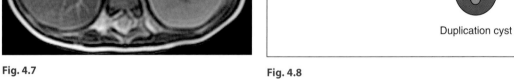

Epithelial plug   Vacuolization

Recanalization

Duplication cyst

Fig. 4.8

A 3-year-old girl presents with a 10-day history of abdominal pain. Physical exploration reveals an abdominal mass.

Gastrointestinal (GI) duplication cysts constitute a rare congenital anomaly that may occur anywhere along the mesenteric side of the GI tract. A duplication cyst is most common in the distal ileum, followed by the esophagus, colon, jejunum, stomach, and duodenum. It is usually attached to the GI tract, has smooth muscle in its wall, and is lined with GI epithelium. The cause remains unclear, the most accepted theory being the abnormal recanalization of vacuoles in the lumen of the gut tube; another possible cause is an intrauterine vascular accident during early fetal development.

They are two types of GI duplication cysts: cystic duplication (80% of cases), spherical in shape without any communication with the bowel lumen, and tubular duplication (20% cases), which communicates with the bowel lumen. Most GI cysts manifest during the first year of life as an abdominal distension, vomiting, bleeding, pain, and abdominal mass. Complications are rare but may include obstruction by volvulus or intussusception, bleeding, infection, and perforation. GI bleeding may occur as a result of peptic ulcers in the presence of heterotopic gastric mucosa. Surgical excision is the treatment of choice.

The characteristic US appearance consists of an echogenic inner mucosa surrounded by a hypoechoic outer muscular layer, a finding known as the "double wall" or "muscular rim" sign. CT is only performed to evaluate a duplication cyst in case of suspected complications. In this case, the CT appearance is a fluid-filled cyst mass with an area of high attenuation inside due to hemorrhage or proteinaceous material. A thick enhancing wall or septa and surrounding inflammation may indicate a duplication cyst complicated by infection. On MR, most duplications have low signal intensity on T1 images and very high signal intensity on T2-weighted images.

Radiography of the abdomen shows a soft-tissue mass in the left upper quadrant (*arrows*) (Fig. 4.5).

Ultrasound reveals an echogenic thick-wall cystic mass (*asterisk*) at the posterior aspect of the left hepatic lobe (H). Stomach is collapsed (Fig. 4.6).

On the T2-weighted axial MR image, the lesion (M) appears hyperintense and it is behind the stomach (S) (Fig. 4.7).

The diagram shows the normal and abnormal development of the gastrointestinal lumen with the abnormal recanalization of vacuoles in the lumen of the gut tube (Fig. 4.8).

Case 3: Meckel's Diverticulum

Cinta Sangüesa Nebot

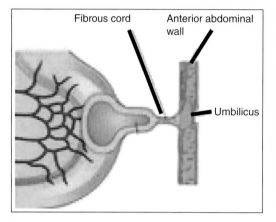

Fig. 4.9

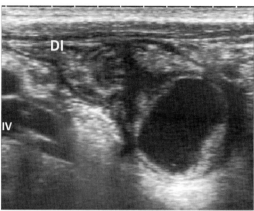

Fig. 4.10

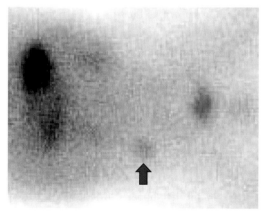

Fig. 4.11

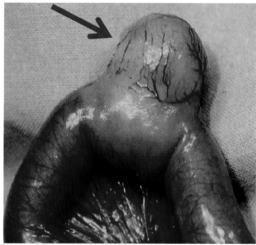

Fig. 4.12

A 6-year-old girl presents to the emergency department with abdominal pain, vomiting, and acute intestinal bleeding.

Meckel's diverticulum (MD) is the most common congenital gastrointestinal anomaly in children. Embryologically, it is caused by failure of obliteration of the omphalomesenteric duct. MD arises from the antimesenteric border of the distal small bowel, typically 40–100 cm from the ileocecal valve.

Most patients with MD are asymptomatic. However, when MD is symptomatic, it has varied clinical manifestations and entails a diagnostic challenge for pediatricians. About 50% of diverticula contain ectopic gastric mucosa. Gastric mucosal secretions can cause peptic ulceration resulting in pain, bleeding, and perforation.

High-resolution ultrasound shows a fluid-filled structure in the right lower quadrant having the appearance of a blind-ending thick-walled loop of bowel and a connection to a normal small-bowel loop. Complicated MD can appear as a thick irregular wall lacking gut signature, concentric rings, or double target sign simulating intussusception in an inverted Meckel. CT imagings vary according to the complication, but the most frequent is a dilated loop with a thick wall and inflammatory change in the surrounding mesentery. Technetium-99m ((99m) Tc) pertechnetate scintigraphy is helpful in diagnosing ectopic gastric mucosa.

(Fig. 4.9). Embryological scheme: The omphalomesenteric duct obliterates during the seventh week. If it fails, its proximal part persists as a diverticulum from the small intestine. It can be attached to the abdominal wall by a fibrous cord at the umbilicus (*Source*: http://cuefllash.com/decks/Development of the GI System. Lane Anatomy Block II. Unit II).

(Fig. 4.10). Abdominal ultrasound reveals a cystic lesion in the antimesenteric border of the distal ileum (DI), iliac vein (IV).

(Fig. 4.11). Technetium-99m scintigraphy demonstrates hypercaptation in the right lower paraumbilical region (*arrow*) highly suggestive of Meckel's diverticulum.

(Fig. 4.12). Surgery piece showing Meckel's diverticulum along the antimesenteric border of the intestine (*arrow*).

Case 4: Severe Acute Pancreatitis

Dolores Muro Velilla

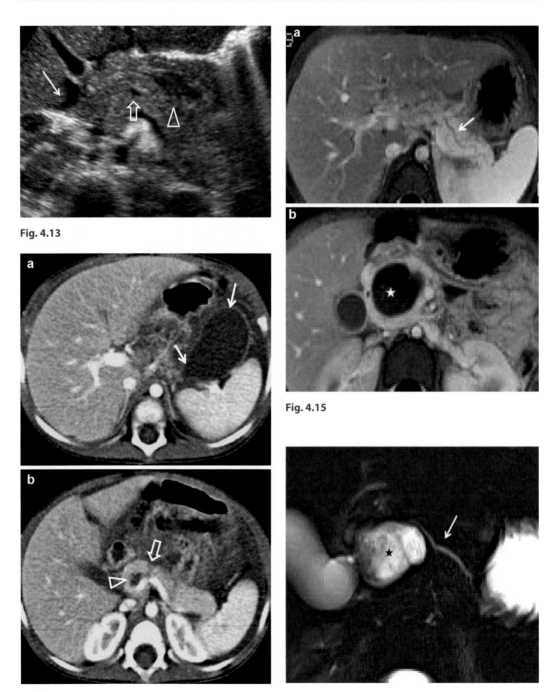

Fig. 4.13

Fig. 4.14

Fig. 4.15

Fig. 4.16

An 8-month-old girl presented with a history of abdominal pain, fever, and vomiting. Tenderness to palpation with guarding was noted on physical examination. Ultrasound was performed.

Acute pancreatitis is an acute inflammatory process of the pancreas with variable involvement of adjacent tissues and organs. Acute pancreatitis is characterized by sudden-onset abdominal pain and a rise in pancreatic enzymes with ultimate complete structural and functional restitution. Acute pancreatitis is idiopathic in 23% of patients, traumatic (22%), caused by structural anomalies (15%), multisystem diseases (14%), drugs and toxins (12%), and viral infections (10%).

Acute pancreatitis is further classified as mild or severe based on histologic and clinical findings. Mild acute pancreatitis is usually a self-limited disease with a rapid response to conservative medical therapy. Severe acute pancreatitis is associated with major organ failure and local complications, such as pseudocyst formation, pancreatic abscess, necrosis, and vascular complications.

Ultrasound (US) is the primary imaging modality for the detection of pancreatic abnormalities and is used to exclude extrapancreatic disease. On computer tomography (CT), the imaging features include swelling of the pancreas, blurring of the contours, inhomogeneous enhancement, inflammatory changes in the peripancreatic fat, intra- or retroperitoneal fluid collections, and thickening of facial planes.

In this case, the initial US shows no pancreatic abnormality. Evolution was torpid, with many complications during several months. Finally, the patient developed a pancreatic pseudocyst that required a cystojejunostomy. One year later, the patient is fine.

Imaging Findings

US obtained a few days after the acute onset (Fig. 4.13) shows a markedly enlarged and ill-defined pancreas, with pancreatic inflammatory changes (*arrowhead*), peripancreatic fluid (*arrow*), and pancreatic duct dilatation (*open arrow*), findings that are consistent with a diagnosis of acute pancreatitis. Several weeks later (Fig. 4.14a, b), CT scan shows a pseudocysts in the head and pancreatic body (*arrowhead*), a vertically oriented linear area of low density at the anterior aspect of the pancreatic body (*open arrow*), peripancreatic fluid, inflammatory stranding in the peripancreatic fat, and a large pseudocyst in the yuxtasplenic area (*arrows*). (Fig. 4.15a, b). Axial T1 FS + Gd, and some weeks later (Fig. 4.16), MRCP MIP shows a marked increase in diameter of the pseudocystic formation (*) and pancreatic duct dilatation (*arrow*).

Case 5: Chronic Pancreatitis

Dolores Muro Velilla

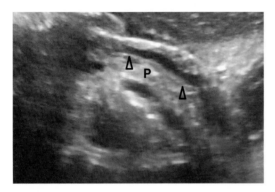

Fig. 4.17

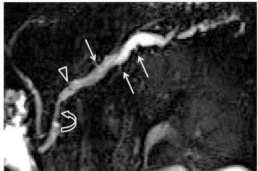

Fig. 4.19

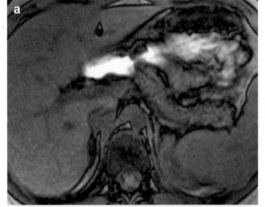

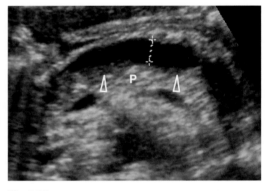

Fig. 4.20

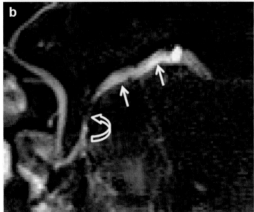

Fig. 4.18

A 7-year-old girl presented with recurrent episodes of acute pancreatitis, consistent with abdominal pain that fluctuated during the course of the disease. The pain was typically epigastric, often radiating to the back.

Chronic pancreatitis is a progressive inflammatory disease of the pancreas. It is characterized by irreversible structural changes that result in irreversible exocrine and/or endocrine pancreatic insufficiency. The structural changes include irregular sclerotic and diffuse or focal destruction, acinar cell loss, islet cell loss, inflammatory cell filtrate, and pancreatic duct abnormalities. Intraductal obstruction may be caused by protein plugs and/or calculi.

Pediatric patient data on the incidence and prevalence of chronic pancreatitis is limited. Most chronic pancreatitis in children is associated with hereditary pancreatitis and pancreaticobiliary ductal anomalies. Less common causes are cystic fibrosis, malnutrition, and hyperparathyroidism. Other rarer causes are idiopathic fibrosing pancreatitis and autoimmune pancreatitis. About 10–20% of children with acute pancreatitis develop recurrent or chronic pancreatitis. Idiopathic pancreatitis is considered to be the most common cause of chronic pancreatitis in children.

Abdominal pain can be intense. In later stages, steatorrhea and weight loss will manifest. The complications of chronic pancreatitis include pancreatic pseudocyst, pseudoaneurysm, splenic vein thrombosis, pancreatic fistula, common bile duct, and duodenal obstructions.

In chronic pancreatitis, imaging features on US and CT include tissue loss, irregular contours, ductal dilatation, and ductal and parenchymal calcifications. MRI with pre- and postcontrast sequences, including MR cholangiopancreatography, may be considered the next possible imaging technique after US.

A 7-year-old girl with chronic pancreatitis with unknown underlying predisposing factor (Fig. 4.17). Transverse US image shows significant atrophy of the pancreatic parenchyma (P) and dilated and tortuous main pancreatic duct in the body and tail of the pancreas (*arrowheads*). (Fig. 4.18a). Axial T1-OUT MR shows pancreatic atrophy and (Fig. 4.18b) coronal T2 MRCP image shows dilatation of the main pancreatic duct (*arrows*) with narrowing in the neck of the gland (*curved arrow*). (Fig. 4.19). Coronal T2 MRCP image taken several months later shows marked dilatation of the main pancreatic duct (*curved arrow*) with intraductal stone appearing as hypointense filling defect (*arrowhead*), with dilated side branches (*straight arrows*). (Fig. 4.20). Follow-up US obtained several months later shows an increased diameter of the pancreatic duct (*arrowheads*) and more pancreatic atrophy (P).

Case 6: Pediatric Crohn's Disease

María I. Martínez-León
and Víctor Navas López

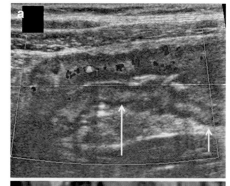

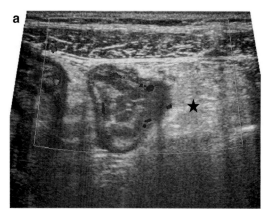

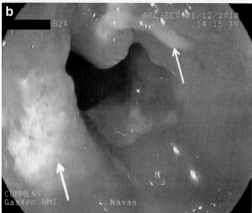

Fig. 4.21

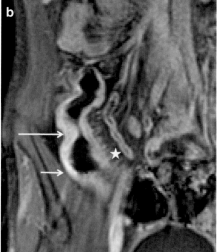

Fig. 4.23

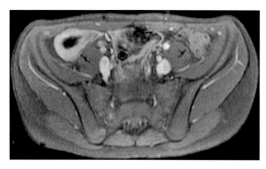

Fig. 4.22

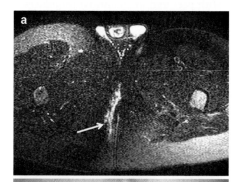

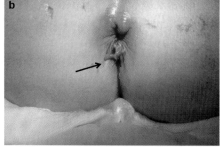

Fig. 4.24

Patient 1: A 13-year-old girl with short height, anemia, diarrhea, and secondary amenorrhea. She was diagnosed with Crohn's disease (CD) (A1b, L3, B1, G1). Patient 2: Fibrostenosing Crohn's disease in activity (A1b, L2, B2B3). Patient 3: A 11-year-old girl with colonic Crohn's disease, proctitis, and perianal disease (A1b, L1, B1p).

Comments

Radiological nonradiating studies such as ultrasound (US) and magnetic resonance (MR) are key to the diagnosis and follow-up of CD. For this complex illness, radiologists must be integrated in a multidisciplinary group that includes pediatricians and surgeons.

There are some radiological signs in each technique that help to establish an early diagnosis and periodic reevaluation:

US findings: Intestinal mural thickening is the main sign, as well as loss of the normal gut layer stratification, hyperemia, and evaluation of the complications. MR findings (colono-MR and entero-MR): Wall thickening, changed mural signal, mural enhancement, bowel rigidity, transmural affectation (fistula, fatty proliferation, adenopathy, abscess), and perianal disease.

The last revision of the CD classification (Paris classification) tries to integrate clinical and radiological findings:

1. Age at diagnosis: A1a, below 10 years; A1b, 10–17 years; A2, 17–40 years; A3, above 40 years.
2. Location: L1, distal third of the ileum +/− limited cecal disease; L2, colonic; L3, ileocolonic; L4a, upper disease proximal to Treitz; L4b, upper disease distal to Treitz and proximal to distal third of the ileum.
3. Behavior: B1, nonstructuring nonpenetrating; B2, structuring; B3, penetrating; B2B3, both penetrating and structuring disease, either at the same or different times; p, perianal disease modifier.
4. Growth: G0, no evidence of growth delay; G1, growth delay.

Imaging Findings

Patient 1: Color Doppler ultrasound (CDUS) and colonoscopic correlation. Thickening of the terminal ileum with loss of the mural stratification; there is also increased mural vascularization and transmural infiltration with echogenic and thickened mesenteric surrounding fat (*asterisk*) (Fig. 4.21a). Colonoscopic correlation, inflamed mucosa of terminal ileum, and ileocecal valve with marked friability and ulceration (*arrows*). (Fig. 4.21b). Colono-MR, axial T1-weighted fat suppression (FS) and contrast. Thick, homogeneous, and marked enhanced cecal base and part of the terminal ileum (Fig. 4.22). Patient 2: (Fig. 4.23) CDUS (a) and MR, coronal localized T1-weighted FS with contrast (b), stenosis (*long arrow*), prestenotic segment (*short arrow*), and "comb sign" (*asterisk*). Patient 3: Perianal MR, axial plane, simple intersphincteric fistula (*white arrow*) (Fig. 4.24a) and Seton* placement (*black arrow*) (Fig. 4.24b).

Case 7: Hepatocellular Adenoma

Sara Desamparados Picó Aliaga

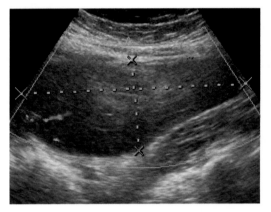

Fig. 4.25

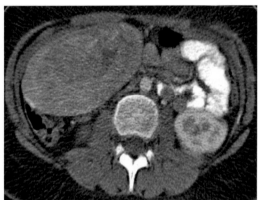

Fig. 4.26

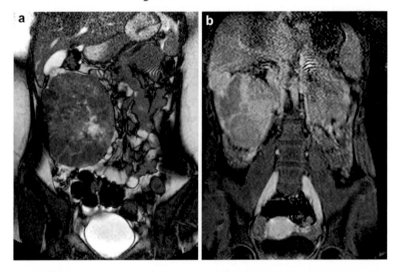

Fig. 4.27

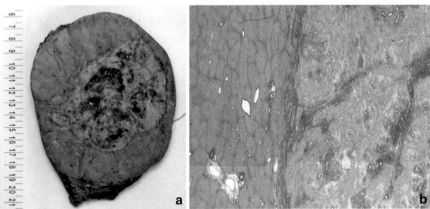

Fig. 4.28

An obese girl, 13 years and 10 months old, described having vague abdominal pain not associated with nausea, vomiting, diarrhea, or weight loss. She had a history of irregular menses. Examination reveals a palpable abdominal mass.

We present the case of a biopsy-proven pedunculated hepatocellular adenoma in a girl without risk factors. No ovarian or adrenal tumor was seen at imaging. The commonly seen benign liver tumors in children are infantile hemangioma, mesenchymal hamartoma, and focal nodular hyperplasia. Rare benign tumors are hepatic adenoma, occasionally seen in teenage girls, and teratoma. Hepatocellular adenomas account for approximately 2–4% of all pediatric liver tumors and approximately 7.5% of all benign hepatic tumors. Liver adenomas vary in size from 1 to 30 cm but typically measure between 8 and 15 cm. There is a marked female preponderance with a female-to-male ratio of 11:1.

The pathogenesis of HA remains uncertain. In children, most patients are diagnosed before the age of 5. Oral contraceptives, glycogen storage disease, diabetes mellitus, and tyrosinemia have all been causally proved. Exogenous androgens, most commonly used in aplastic anemias as well as in many other conditions, such as endocrine abnormalities, hereditary angioedema, immune thrombocytopenia, and body building, have been associated with HA. This evidence supports the role of hormonal regulation in HA development. Presentation usually consists of localized upper abdominal pain because of hemorrhage, enlargement, or compression of local viscera. The risk of hemorrhage is highest in symptomatic patients, ranging from 25% to 40%. Malignant transformation varies from 6% to 13%, and the causes remain unclear. Surgical excision is the treatment of choice for hepatic adenomas measuring in excess of 4 cm. Liver transplantation is recommended for treatment of large central tumors. Furthermore, some researchers have incorporated other approaches, such as radiofrequency ablation (RFA) and transcatheter-arterial embolization (TAE), as potential alternatives to surgical resection with some success. Recurrence of liver adenoma after resection is not reported.

(Fig. 4.25). On US, the lesions may be hypo-, iso-, or hyperechoic. (Fig. 4.26). On CT, HCA is typically a discrete, hypodense lesion that shows arterial-phase enhancement and may become isoattenuating on delayed images. This study revealed the presence of a $14 \times 12 \times 6$-cm pedunculated hepatic mass. (Fig. 4.27a). On T2WI, the lesions are isointense to slightly hyperintense. (b) On fat saturated with gadolinium, T1WI the enhancement is maximal during the arterial phase, with rapid fading in the venous phase. (Fig. 4.28a). Cross section gross image through the liver cell adenoma. (b) Histologically, it is composed of cells larger than normal hepatocytes that do not follow a defined cord architecture. The portal tracts and bile ducts are absent.

Case 8: Gastrointestinal Stromal Tumor (GIST) of Stomach in a Pediatric Patient

Cinta Sangüesa Nebot

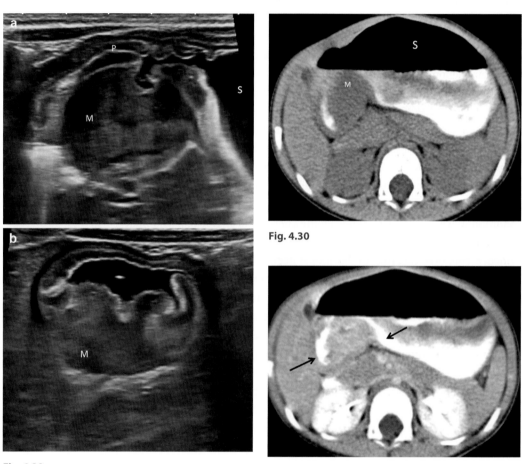

Fig. 4.29

Fig. 4.30

Fig. 4.31

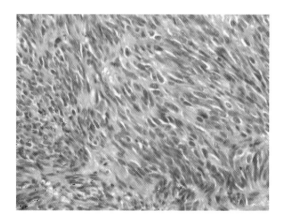

Fig. 4.32

A 3-year-old girl with a 1-month history of daily vomitings and weight loss of 4 kg.

Gastrointestinal stromal tumor (GIST) is a mesenchymal tumor extremely rare in children. It may be familial and has an association with neurofibromatosis (NF1), urticaria pigmentosa, and Carney's triad (pulmonary chondroma, extra-adrenal paraganglioma, and gastric smooth-muscle tumor in young females). GIST can occur anywhere along the gastrointestinal tract, stomach (70%), small intestine (20–30%), anorectum (7%), colon, and esophagus.

Comments

Clinical presentation depends on the site and size of the mass and can include abdominal pain, vomiting, gastrointestinal bleeding, and anemia.

Radiologically, GIST appears as a well-defined solid or partially cystic mass that may be accompanied by areas of hemorrhage or necrosis. On CT, GISTs vary from small and well-defined homogeneous soft-tissue masses to large necrotic heterogeneous masses with variable contrast enhancement. MR imaging features of gastric stromal tumors have been described as a mass with variable T1 and T2 signals because of necrosis and hemorrhage and enhanced with gadolinium.

The main radiological differential diagnoses include other mesenchymal tumors (leiomyoma, leiomyosarcoma), other submucosal gastrointestinal lesions (ectopic pancreas, carcinoid), and lymphoma.

It arises from the muscularis mucosa of the bowel wall. Microscopy analysis reveals a hypercellular neoplasm that contains numerous spindle cells. The major diagnostic criterion for GIST is CD117 antigen positive. Its importance lies in its malignant potential. Complete surgical resection of the lesion is the treatment of choice. Predictions of malignancy in GIST are tumors with higher mitotic counts and size of more than 5 cm.

Axial US view through the upper abdomen reveals a well-defined submucosal mass (M) in the pyloric (P) posterior wall (Fig. 4.29a, b).

Imaging Findings

Nonintravenous contrast axial CT confirms the origin of the mass (M) in the pyloric wall with secondary gastric dilatation (S) (Fig. 4.30).

Contrast CT shows an eccentric and heterogeneous mass (*arrows*) (Fig. 4.31).

The histological sample shows a typical morphologic GIST pattern: spindle cell GIST stained with hematoxylin and eosin (Fig. 4.32).

Case 9: Pancreatic Acinar Cell Carcinoma

Dolores Muro Velilla

PANCREATIC TUMORS IN CHILDREN
1. Epithelial tumors
a. Exocrine tumors
Ductal cell origin
Ductal adenocarcinoma (exceedingly rare)
Acinar cell origin
Pancreatoblastoma
Acinar cell carcinoma
Uncertain origin
Solid-pseudopapillary tumor
b. Endocrine cell origin
2. Nonepithelial tumors (exceedingly rare)
Lymphoma, particularly Burkitt
Sarcomas, particularly rhabdomyosarcoma
Dermoid cyst
Source: Jaffe R. The pancreas. In: Stocker J, Dehner L, eds. Pediatric pathology. 2nd ed. Philadelphia, Pa: Lippincott Williams & Wilkins, 2002;797-834.

Fig. 4.33

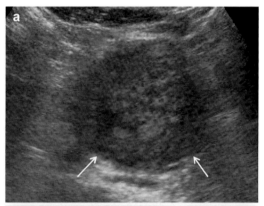
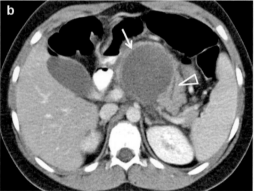

Fig. 4.34

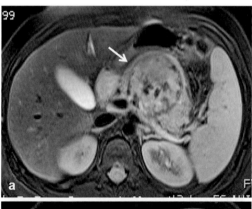
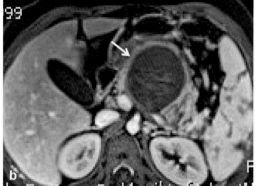

Fig. 4.35

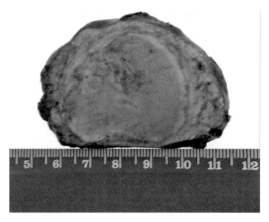

Fig. 4.36

An 11-year-old boy presented to the emergency department with a history of mild abdominal pain and vomiting for a few days. Ultrasound and a contrast-enhanced abdominal CT were performed.

Comments

Pancreatic tumors are uncommon in children, accounting for 0.2% of all pediatric tumors (Fig. 4.33, Jaffe 2002). Acinar cell carcinoma represents 1–2% of pancreatic exocrine tumors, but a small number of cases have been reported in children. Acinar cell carcinoma occurs throughout the pancreas with no preferential location. Symptoms are related to local tumor expansion and metastasis at presentation. The most common complaint is abdominal pain.

At CT, the tumor is almost always well demarcated, and most show a well-defined, partial, or complete capsule. Most tumors show a central hypodense area, often large, which represents tumoral necrosis. The tumor usually enhances, but less than the normal pancreas. Magnetic resonance (MR) imaging shows a well-delineated, homogeneous, and slightly LESION hypointense on T1-weighted images and hypointense on T2-weighted images relative to the normal pancreas. Central necrosis may result in high signal intensity on T2-weighted images and low signal intensity on T1-weighted images. Enhancement of this mass is homogeneous and less than that of the surrounding parenchyma. The imaging appearance of acinar cell carcinoma is reminiscent of that of solid-pseudopapillary tumor and pancreatoblastoma. The age of the patient may help differentiate tumors. Pancreatoblastoma occurs in children less than 10 years of age, while one third of solid-pseudopapillary tumors occur in adolescents, and acinar cell carcinomas are quite rare in children and are almost exclusively seen in older patients.

In this case, the patient underwent subtotal pancreatectomy for complete excision of the neoplasm and cystojejunostomy via a Roux limb of yeyunum. Microscopy showed the typical features of acinar cell carcinoma. The patient remains well 2 years later.

Imaging Findings

(Fig. 4.34a). Transverse sonogram of the upper abdomen shows a well-defined, predominantly hypoechoic mass in the body of the pancreas (*arrows*). (Fig. 4.34b). The enhanced CT scan shows a well-defined, fairly homogeneous, predominantly hypoattenuating mass arising in the body of the pancreas (*arrow*). Note the dilated intrahepatic ducts (*arrowhead*). (Fig. 4.35a). Axial T2-W MR image shows a heterogeneous mass with a hypointense rim (*arrow*). (Fig. 4.35b). Axial post-Gd T1 MR image shows marked enhancement of only the capsule of the mass (*arrow*). (Fig. 4.36). Photograph of the cut surface of the resected gross specimen shows the encapsulated solid mass involving the body of the pancreas.

Case 10: Omental Infarction in Children

Cinta Sangüesa Nebot

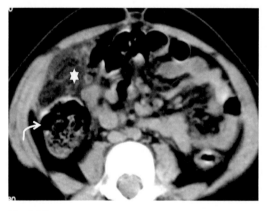

Fig. 4.37

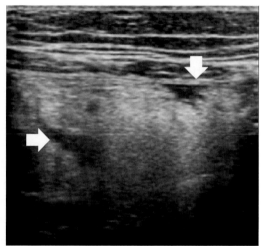

Fig. 4.38

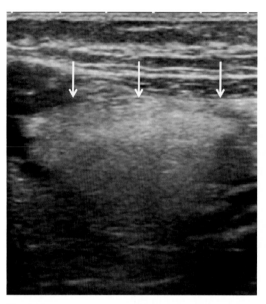

Fig. 4.39

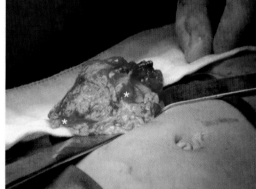

Fig. 4.40

An 8-year-old girl with abdominal pain to the right of the umbilicus.

Comments

Omental infarction is rare. Of all cases described, 15% of the patients are children.

Clinically, omental infarction often mimics acute appendicitis because patients usually present with acute onset of right lower quadrant pain, and approximately 50% report nausea, vomiting, bowel disorders, dysuria, and fever.

Its pathogenesis is still unknown and it occurs with or without torsion. Idiopathic omental infarction is associated with predisposing factors, such as kinking of veins caused by the patient's position or vascular congestion, which may lead to thrombosis and infarction of the omentum. In omental torsion, the omentum twists gradually, resulting in omental infarction and necrosis. Omental torsion may be primary or secondary. Predisposing factors to primary torsion are bifid omentum and obesity. Secondary torsion may be caused by attachment of part of the omentum to acquired lesions (hernias, previous surgical scars, cysts, etc.). Omental infarction typically occurs on the right side, but it may be seen on the left side. The predilection has been attributed to a congenital variant blood supply of the right portion of the greater omentum that predisposes it to venous thrombosis.

Imaging is required to achieve an accurate diagnosis and to avoid unnecessary laparoscopy or laparotomy and antibiotic therapy.

The most frequent ultrasonographic appearance is an ovoid or cake-like hyperechoic mass adherent to the peritoneum and located in the umbilical region or anterolaterally to the right half of the colon. It corresponds to preserved omental tissue with edema and vascular congestion. When some poorly defined nodular or linear hypoechoic areas appear inside the mass, torsion omental infarction is most probable. Visualizing an artery around the tubular structure to define the mechanism of infarction is very rare.

The typical CT features of omental infarction include a solitary, well-circumscribed, triangular or oval heterogeneous fatty mass, sometimes with a whorled pattern of concentric linear fat stranding.

Approximately 0.1% of children undergo laparotomy for suspected appendicitis that later is diagnosed surgically as omental infarction associated with torsion.

(Fig. 4.37). Transverse grayscale sonogram shows a cake-like hyperechoic mass next to anterior abdominal wall (*arrows*) in right lower quadrant that corresponds to the patient's point of maximal tenderness on physical examination. The lesion contains (Fig. 4.38) hypoechoic areas (*short arrows*) inside and around the lesion. (Fig. 4.39). Axial CT image demonstrates an oval lesion with heterogeneous and fatty attenuation (*star*) well separated from colon (*curved arrow*) in the right lower quadrant. Intraoperative surgical finding (Fig. 4.40) presents an omental infarction with torsion. Hemorrhage areas can be seen inside (*asterisk*).

Imaging Findings

Further Reading

Case 1: Choledochal Cyst

Book

Siegel MJ, Babyn PS, Lee EY (2008) Liver and biliary tract. Pediatric body CT, 2nd edn. Wolters Kluwer/Lippincott Williams & Wilkins, Philadelphia, pp 209–211

Web Link

http://www.springerlink.com/index/y68463042w126r31. pdf. Accessed 6 Sept 2011

Articles

Anupindi SA (2008) Pancreatic and biliary anomalies: imaging in 2008. Pediatr Radiol Suppl 2:S267–S271

Karrer FM, Bensard DD (2000) Neonatal cholestasis. Semin Pediatr Surg 9:166–169

Kim OH, Chung HJ, Choi BG (1995) Imaging of the choledochal cyst. Radiographics 15:69–88

Kim WS, Kim IO, Yeon KM, Park KW, Seo JK, Kim CJ (1998) Choledochal cyst with or without biliary atresia in neonates and young infants: US differentiation. Radiology 209:465–469

Meyers RL, Scaife ER (2000) Benign liver and biliary tract masses in infants and toddlers. Semin Pediatr Surg 9:146–155

Rozel C, Garel L, Rypens F, Viremouneix L, Lapierre C, Décaire JC et al (2011) Imaging of biliary disorders in children. Pediatr Radiol 41:208–220

Tani C, Nosaka S, Masaki H, Kuroda T, Honna T (2009) Spontaneous perforation of choledochal cyst: a case with unusual distribution of fluid in the retroperitoneal space. Pediatr Radiol 39:629–631

Torrisi JM, Haller JO, Velcek FT (1990) Choledochal cyst and biliary atresia in the neonate: imaging findings in five cases. AJR Am J Roentgenol 155:1273–1276

Veigel MC, Prescott-Focht J, Rodriguez MG, Zinati R, Shao L, Moore C, Lowe L (2009) Fibropolycystic liver disease in children. Pediatr Radiol 39:317–327

Wootton-Gorges S, Thomas KB, Harned RK, Wu SR, Stein-Wexler R, Strain JD (2005) Giant cystic abdominal masses in children. Pediatr Radiol 35:1277–1288

Case 2: Gastric Duplication Cyst

Book

Jamieson D, Stringer D (2000) Small bowel. In: Decker BC (ed) Pediatric gastrointestinal imaging and intervention, 2nd edn. Decker Inc., Toronto, pp 311–445

Web Link

http://emedecine.medscape.com (article/933427-overview)

Articles

Azzie G, Beasley S (2003) Diagnosis and treatment of foregut duplications. Semin Pediatr Surg 12(1):46–54

Berrocal T, Hidalgo P, Gutiérrez J, Pablo L, Rodríguez-Lemos R (2004) Imagen radiológica de las duplicaciones del tubo digestivo. Radiologia 46(5):282–293

Carachi R, Azmy A (2002) Foregut duplications. Pediatr Surg Int 18(5–6):371–374

Cheng G, Soboleski D, Daneman A, Poenaru D, Hurlbur D (2005) Sonographic pitfalls in the diagnosis of enteric duplication cysts. AJR Am J Roentgenol 184(2):521–525

Granata C, Dell'Acqua A, Lituania M, Oddone M, Rossi U, Toma P (2003) Gastric duplication cyst appearance on prenatal US and MRI. Pediatr Radiol 33(2): 148–149

Hur J, Yoon CS, Kim MJ, Kim OH (2007) Imaging features of gastrointestinal tract duplications in infants and children: from esophagus to rectum. Pediatr Radiol 37:691–699

Lee NK, Kim S, Jeon TY, Kim HS, Kim DH, Seo H et al (2010) Complications of congenital and developmental abnormalities of the gastrointestinal tract in adolescents and adults: evaluation with multimodality imaging. Radiographics 30:1489–1507

Lim GY, Im SA, Chung JH (2008) Complication duplication cysts on the ileum presenting with a mesenteric inflammatory mass. Pediatr Radiol 38(4):467–470

Macpherson IR (1993) Gastrointestinal tract duplication: clinical, pathological, etiologic and radiologic considerations. Radiographics 13:1063–1080

Snivastava P, Gangopadhyay AN, Kumar V, Upadhyaya VD, Sarma SP, Jaiman R et al (2009) No communicating isolated enteric duplication cyst in childhood. J Pediatr Surg 44(7):9–10

Case 3: Meckel's Diverticulum

Book

Jamieson D, Stringer D (2000) Small bowel. In: Decker BC (ed) Pediatric gastrointestinal imaging and intervention, 2nd edn. Decker Inc., Toronto BC, pp 311–445

Web Link

http://emedecine.medscape.com/article/194776-overview

Articles

Daneman A, Myers M, Shuckett B, Alton D (1997) Sonographic appearances of inverted Meckel diverticulum with intussusception. Pediatr Radiol 27:295–298

Daneman A, Lobo E, Alton D, Shuckett B (1998) The value of sonography, CT and air enema for detection of complicated Meckel diverticulum in children with nonspecific clinical presentation. Pediatr Radiol 28:928–932

Elsayes K, Manias C, Harvin H, Francis I (2007) Imaging manifestations of Meckel's diverticulum. AJR Am J Roentgenol 189:81–88

Itagaki A, Uchida M, Ueki K, Kajii T (1991) Double targets sign in ultrasonic diagnosis of intussuscepted Meckel diverticulum. Pediatr Radiol 21:148–149

Levy AD, Hobbs CM (2004) From the archives of the AFIP. Meckel's diverticulum: radiologic features with pathologic correlation. Radiographics 24:565–587

Menezes M, Tareen F, Saeed A, Khan N, Puri P (2006) Symptomatic Meckel's diverticulum in children: a 16 years review. Pediatr Surg Int 24:575–577

Ojha S, Menon P, Rao KLN (2004) Meckel's diverticulum with segmental dilatation of the ileum: radiographic diagnosis in a neonate. Pediatr Radiol 34:649–651

Thurley P, Halliday KE, Somers JM, Al-Daraji W, Ilyas M, Broderick NJ (2009) Radiological features of Meckel's diverticulum and its complications. Clin Radiol 64:109–118

Tseng Y, Yang Y (2009) Clinical and diagnostic relevance of Meckel's diverticulum in children. Eur J Pediatr 168:1519–1523

Swaniker F, Soldes O, Hirschl RB (1999) The utility of technetium 99m pertechnetate scintigraphy in the evaluation of patients with Meckel's diverticulum. J Pediatr Surg 35(5):760–764

Bultron G, Latif U, Park A, Phatak U, Pashankar D, Husain SZ (2009) Acute pancreatitis in a child with celiac disease. J Pediatr Gastroenterol Nutr 49:137–138

Chavhan GB, Babyn PS, Manson D, Vidarsson L (2008) Pediatric MR cholangiopancreatography: principles, technique, and clinical applications. Radiographics 28:1951–1962

Darge K, Anupindi S (2009) Pancreatitis and the role of US, MRCP and ERCP. Pediatr Radiol 39:S153–S157

Delaney L, Applegate KE, Karmazyn B, Akisik MF, Jennings SG (2008) MR cholangiopancreatography in children: feasibility, safety, and initial experience. Pediatr Radiol 38:64–75

Flores J, Exiga E, Moran S, Martín J, Yamamoto A (2009) Acute pancreatitis in children with acute lymphoblastic leukemia treated with L-asparaginase. J Pediatr Hematol Oncol 31:790–793

Morinville VD, Barmada MM, Lowe ME (2010) Increasing incidence of acute pancreatitis at an American pediatric tertiary care center: is greater awareness among physicians responsible? Pancreas 39:5–8

Nievelstein RA, Robben SG, Blickman JG (2011) Hepatobiliary and pancreatic imaging in children techniques and an overview of non-neoplastic disease entities. Pediatr Radiol 41:55–75, Epub 2010 Oct 24

Nydegger A, Heine RG, Ranuh R, Gegati-Levy R, Crameri J, Oliver MR (2007) Changing incidence of acute pancreatitis: 10-year experience at the Royal Children's Hospital, Melbourne. J Gastroenterol Hepatol 22:1313–1316

Ozel A, Uysal E, Tufaner O, Erturk SM, Yalcin M, Basak M (2008) Duodenal duplication cyst: a rare cause of acute pancreatitis in children. J Clin Ultrasound 36:584–586

Case 4: Severe Acute Pancreatitis

Book

Babyn P, Siegel MJ (2008) Adrenal glands, pancreas, and other retroperitoneal structures. In: Siegel MJ, Babyn P, Lee EY (eds) Pediatric body CT, 2nd edn. Lippincott Williams & Wilkins, Philadelphia, pp 323–498

Web Link

http://emedicine.medscape.com/article/2014039-overview

Articles

Amodio J, Brodsky JE (2010) Pediatric Burkitt lymphoma presenting as acute pancreatitis: MRI characteristics. Pediatr Radiol 40:770–772

Case 5: Chronic Pancreatitis

Book

Morgan DE, Stanley RJ (2006) Pancreas. In: Lee JKT, Sagel SS, Stanley RJ, et al (eds) Computed body tomography with MRI correlation. Lippincott Williams & Wilkins, Philadelphia, pp. 1007–1100

Web Link

http://emedicine.medscape.com/article/2014039-overview

Articles

Akisik MF, Aisen AM, Sandrasegaran K, Jenning SG, Lin C, Sherman S et al (2008) Assessment of chronic pancreatitis: utility of diffusion-weighted MR imaging with secretin enhancement. Radiology 250:103–109

Chavhan GB, Babyn PS, Manson D, Vidarsson L (2008b) Pediatric MR cholangiopancreatography: principles, technique, and clinical applications. Radiographics 28:1951–1962

Darge K, Anupindi S (2009b) Pancreatitis and the role of US, MRCP and ERCP. Pediatr Radiol 39:S153–S157

Delaney L, Applegate KE, Karmazyn B, Akisik MF, Jennings SG (2008b) MR cholangiopancreatography in children: feasibility, safety, and initial experience. Pediatr Radiol 38:64–75

Refaat R, Harth M, Proschek P, Lindemayr S, Vogl TJ (2009) Autoimmune pancreatitis in an 11-year-old boy. Pediatr Radiol 39:389–392

Shah AP, Sahai S, Sugawa C, Macha S, Kamat D (2010) Recurrent pancreatitis in a child. Clin Pediatr 49:608–610

Shanbhogue A, Surabhi N, Doherty G, Shanbhogue D, Sethi S (2009) A clinical and radiologic review of uncommon types and causes of pancreatitis. Radiographics 29:1003–1026

Uchida H, Hirooka Y, Itoh A, Kawashima H, Hara K, Nonogaki K et al (2009) Feasibility of tissue elastography using transcutaneous ultrasonography for diagnosis of pancreatic diseases. Pancreas 38:17–22

Urushihara N, Fukumoto K, Fukuzawa H, Suzuki K, Matsuoka T, Kawashima S et al (2010) Recurrent pancreatitis caused by pancreatobiliary anomalies in children with annular pancreas. J Pediatr Surg 45:741–746

Zech CJ, Bruns C, Reiser MF, Herrmann KA (2008) Tumor-like lesion of the pancreas in chronic pancreatitis: imaging characteristics of computed tomography. Radiologe 48:777–784

balloon enteroscopy, magnetic resonance enterography, and abdominal US useful for evaluation of small-bowel disease in children with (suspected) Crohn's disease. Gastrointest Endosc 75:87–94

Dillman JR, Adler J, Zimmermann EM, Strouse PJ (2010) CT enterography of pediatric Crohn disease. Pediatr Radiol 40:97–105

Gallego JC, Echarri AI, Porta A, Ollero V (2011) Ileal Crohn's disease: MRI with endoscopic correlation. Eur J Radiol 80:e8–e12

Halligan S, Stoker J (2006) State of the art: imaging of fistula in ano. Radiology 239:18–33

Horsthuis K, Stoker J (2004) Pictorial essay: MRI of perianal Crohn's disease. AJR Am J Roentgenol 183:1309–1315

Levine A, Griffiths A, Markowitz J, Wilson DC, Turner D, Russell RK et al (2011) Pediatric modification of the Montreal classification for inflammatory bowel disease: the Paris classification. Inflamm Bowel Dis 17:1314–1321

Martínez MJ, Ripollés T, Paredes JM, Blanc E, Martí-Bonmatí L (2009) Assessment of the extensión and the inflammatory activity in Crohn's disease: comparison of ultrasound and MRI. Abdom Imaging 34:141–148

Rimola J, Rodríguez S, García-Bosch O, Ricart E, Pagès M, Pellisé M et al (2009) Role of 3.0-T MR colonography in the evaluation of inflammatory bowel disease. Radiographics 29:701–719

Tolan DJM, Greenhalgh R, Zealley IA, Halligan S, Taylor SA (2010) MR enterographic manifestations of small bowel Crohn disease. Radiographics 30:367–384

Case 6: Pediatric Crohn's Disease

Book

Rambla Vilar J, Sangüesa Nevot C (2011) Inflammatory bowel disease. In: Learning pediatric imaging. Springer, Berlin/Heidelberg, pp 108–110

Web Link

Endoscopia y Enfermedad Inflamatoria Intestinal. Atlas audiovisual, Resonancia. Unidad de EII-Digestivo C.H.A. Marcide. Area Sanitaria de Ferrol. http://www.endoinflamatoria.com/1_4.html

Articles

Bravo Bravo C, Martínez León MI (2011) Estudio con ecografía de la enfermedad inflamatoria intestinal en niños. Puesta al día en las técnicas. Pediatr Contin 9:55–59

De Rider L, Mensink PB, Lequin MH, Aktas H, de Krijger RR, van der Woude CJ, Escher JC (2012) Single-

Case 7: Hepatocellular Adenoma

Book

Federle MP (2004) Liver. Pocket radiologist abdomen: die 100 Top-diagnosen. Elsevier, München, pp 27–29

Web Link

http://emedicine.medscape.com/article/369104-overview. Accessed 6 Sept 2011

Articles

Dong Q, Xu W, Jiang B, Lu Y, Hao X, Zhang H et al (2007) Clinical applications of computerized tomography 3-D reconstruction imaging for diagnosis and surgery in children with large liver tumors or tumors at the hepatic hilum. Pediatr Surg Int 23:1045–1050

Jeremiah L, Deneve DO et al (2009) Liver cell adenoma: a multicenter analysis of risk factors for rupture and malignancy. Ann Surg Oncol 16:6408

Jha P, Chawla SC, Tavri S et al (2009) Pediatric liver tumors – a pictorial review. Eur Radiol 19:209–219

Litten JB, Tomlinson GE (2008) Liver tumors in children. Oncologist 13:812–820

Paulson EK, McClellan JS, Washington K et al (1994) Hepatic adenoma: MR characteristics and correlation with pathologic findings. AJR Am J Roentgenol 163:113–116

Resnick MB, Kozakewich HP, Perez-Atayde AR (1995) Hepatic adenoma in the pediatric age group: clinicopathological observations and assessment of cell proliferative activity. Am J Surg Pathol 19:1181–1190

Triantafyllopoulou M, Whitington PF, Melin-Aldana H, Benya EC, Brickman W (2007) Hepatic adenoma in an adolescent with elevated androgen levels. J Pediatr Gastroenterol Nutr 44:640–642

Touraine RL, Bertrand Y, Foray P et al (1993) Hepatic tumours during androgen therapy in Fanconi anaemia. Eur J Pediatr 152:691–693

von Riedenauer WB, Shanti CM, Abouljoud MS (2007) Resection of giant liver adenoma in a 17-year-old adolescent boy using venovenous bypass, total hepatic vascular isolation, and in situ cooling. J Pediatr Surg 42:E23–E27

Wheeler DA, Edmondson HA, Reynolds TB (1986) Spontaneous liver cell adenoma in children. Am J Clin Pathol 85:6–12

Case 8: Gastrointestinal Stromal Tumor (GIST) of Stomach in a Pediatric Patient

Book

Canon CL (2006) Gastrointestinal tract. In: Lee JKT, Stagel SS, Stanley RJ, Heiken JP (eds) Computed body tomography with MRI correlation, 4th edn. Lippincott Williams & Wilkins, Philadelphia, pp 771–828

Web Link

http://emedicine.medscape.com/article/278845-overview

Articles

Benesch M, Wardelmann E, Ferrari A, Brennan B, Verschuur A (2009) Gastrointestinal stromal tumors in children and adolescents: a comprehensive review of the current literature. Pediatr Blood Cancer 15(53):1171–1179

Egloff A, Lee E, Dillon J (2005) Gastrointestinal stromal tumor (GIST) of stomach in a pediatric patient. Pediatr Radiol 35:728–729

Horwitz B, Zamora G, Gallegos M (2011) Best cases from the AFIP: gastrointestinal stromal tumor of the small bowel. Radiographics 31:429–434

Hughes J, Cook J, Said A, Chong S, Town W, Reidy J (2004) Gastrointestinal stromal tumour of the duodenum in a 7-year-old boy. Pediatr Radiol 34:1024–1027

Kaemmer D, Otto J, Lassav L, Steinau G, Klink C, Junge K et al (2009) The GIST of literature on pediatric GIST:

review of clinical presentation. J Pediatr Hematol Oncol 31:108–112

Lau S, Tam KF, Kam CK, Lui CW, Siu C, Lam H et al (2004) Pictorial review. Imaging of gastrointestinal tumour (GIST). Clin Radiol 59:487–498

Levy AD, Remotti HE, Thompson WM, Sobin LH, Miettinen M (2003) Gastrointestinal stromal tumors: radiological features with pathologic correlation. Radiographics 23:283–294

Miettinen M, Lasota J (2001) Gastrointestinal stromal tumors: definition, clinical, histological, immunohistochemical and molecular genetic features and differential diagnosis. Virchows Arch 438:1–12

Muniyappa P, Kay M, Feinberg L, Mahajan L, Stallion A, Wyllie R (2007) The endoscopic appearance of gastrointestinal stromal tumor in a pediatric patient. J Pediatr Surg 42:1302–1305

Park J, Rubinas T, Fordham L, Phillips J (2006) Multifocal gastrointestinal stromal tumor (GIST) of the stomach in an 11-year-old girl. Pediatr Radiol 36:1212–1214

Case 9: Pancreatic Acinar Cell Carcinoma

Books

Morgan DE, Stanley RJ et al (2006) Pancreas. In: Lee JKT, Sagel SS, Stanley RJ (eds) Computed body tomography with MRI correlation. Lippincott Williams & Wilkins, Philadelphia, pp 1007–1100

Jaffe R (2002) The pancreas. In: Stocker J, Dehner L (eds) Pediatric pathology, 2nd edn. Lippincott Williams & Wilkins, Philadelphia, pp 797–834

Web Link

http://emedicine.medscape.com/article/36955-overview

Articles

Abraham SC, Wu TT, Hruban RH, Lee JH, Yeo CJ, Conlon K et al (2002) Genetic and immunohistochemical analysis of pancreatic acinar cell carcinoma: frequent allelic loss on chromosome 11p and alterations in the APC/beta-catenin pathway. Am J Pathol 160:953–962

Cantisani V, Mortele KJ, Levy A, Glickman JN, Ricci P, Passariello R et al (2003) MR imaging features of solid pseudopapillary tumor of the pancreas in adult and pediatric patients. AJR Am J Roentgenol 181:395–401

Chiou YY, Chiang JH, Hwang JI, Yen CH, Tsay SH, Chang CY (2004) Acinar cell carcinoma of the pancreas: clinical and computed tomography manifestations. J Comput Assist Tomogr 28:180–186

Chung EM, Travis MD, Conran RM (2006) Pancreatic tumors in children: radiologic-pathologic correlation. Radiographics 26:1211–1238

Johnson PR, Spitz L (2000) Cysts and tumors of the pancreas. Semin Pediatr Surg 9:209–215

McEvoy MP, Rich B, Klimstra D, Vakiani E, La Quaglia MP (2010) Acinar cell cystadenoma of the pancreas in a 9-year-old boy. J Pediatr Surg 45:7–9

Moholkar S, Sebire NJ, Roebuck DJ (2005) Solid-pseudopapillary neoplasm of the pancreas: radiological-pathological correlation. Pediatr Radiol 35:819–822

Park M, Koh KN, Kim BE, Im HJ, Kim DY, Seo JJ (2011) Pancreatic neoplasms in childhood and adolescence. J Pediatr Hematol Oncol 33:295–300

Xinghui Y, Xiqun W (2010) Imaging findings of pancreatoblastoma in 4 children including a case of ectopic pancreatoblastoma. Pediatr Radiol 40:1609–1614

Yu DC, Kozakewich HP, Perez-Atayde AR, Shamberger RC, Weldon CB (2009) Childhood pancreatic tumors: a single institution experience. J Pediatr Surg 44:2267–2272

Case 10: Omental Infarction in Children

Book

Siegel MJ (2008) Spleen, peritoneum and abdominal wall. In: Siegel MJ, Babyn P, Lee EY (eds) Pediatric body CT, 2nd edn. Lippincott Williams & Wilkins, Philadelphia, pp 217–250

Web Link

http://emedicine.medscape.com/article/191817-overview

Articles

Baldisserotto M, Maffazzoni DR, Dourado M (2005) Omental infarction in children: color Doppler sonography correlated with surgery and pathology findings. AJR Am J Roentgenol 184:156–162

Helmarath MA, Dorfman SR, Minifee PK, Bloss RS, Brandt ML, DeBakey ME (2001) Right lower quadrant pain in children caused by omental infarction. Am J Surg 182:729–732

Kamaya A, Federle M, Desser T (2011) Imaging manifestations of abdominal fat necrosis and its mimics. Radiographics 31:2021–2034

Pereira JM, Sirlin CB, Pinto PS, Jeffrey RB, Stella DL, Casola G (2004) Disproportionate fat stranding: a helpful CT sign in patients with acute abdominal pain. Radiographics 24(3):703–715

Pursyko AS, Remer E, Filho HL, Bittencourt LK, Lima R, Racy DJ (2011) Beyond appendicitis: common and uncommon gastrointestinal causes of right lower quadrant abdominal pain at multidetector CT. Radiographics 31:927–947

Puylaert JB (1992) Right-sided segmental infarction of the omentum: clinical, US, and CT findings. Radiology 185:169–172

Schlesinger A, Dorfman S, Braverman RM (1999) Sonographic appearance of omental infarction in children. Pediatr Radiol 29:598–601

Singh A, Gervais DA, Hahn PF, Sagar P, Mueller PR, Novelline RA (2005) Acute epiploic appendagitis and its mimics. Radiographics 25:1521–1534

Theriot JA, Sayat J, Franco S, Buchino J (2003) Childhood obesity: a risk factor for omental torsion. Pediatrics 112:460–463

Van Breda Vriesman AC, Loble PN, Coerkamp EG, Puylaert JB (1999) Infarction of omentum and epiploic appendage: diagnosis, epidemiology and natural history. Eur Radiol 9:1886–1892

Contents

M.I. Martínez-León et al., *Imaging for Pediatricians*, Imaging for Clinicians,
DOI 10.1007/978-3-642-28629-2_5, © Springer-Verlag Berlin Heidelberg 2012

Case 1: Bilateral Ureterocele

Luisa Ceres-Ruiz and María I. Martínez-León

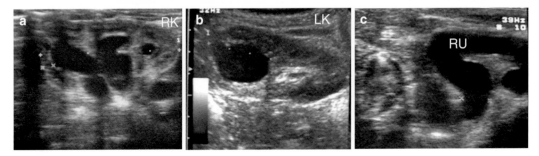

Fig. 5.1

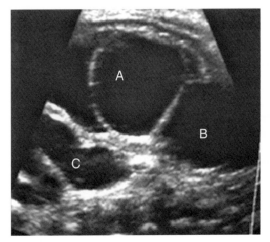

Fig. 5.2

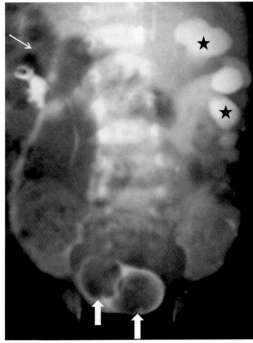

Fig. 5.3

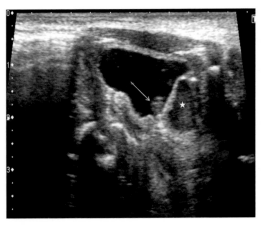

Fig. 5.4

A 1-month-old male of African origin with fever and evidence of pyuria.

The ureterocele (URC) is a congenital malformation consisting of a cystic dilatation of the terminal ureter, specifically the portion of intravesical ureteral submucosa. It arises from a weakness at the junction of the ureter with the bladder and also from a ureteral meatal stenosis. It occurs most often in women, with a ratio of 4:1, and it is associated to ureteral duplication (80%). Only 10% of cases are bilateral. It often accompanies other anomalies of the urinary and genital system whenever there is complete ureteral duplication, where URC is related to the hemi-kidney superior ureter following the Weigert-Meyer rule. There are two types of ureteroceles: the simple or "orthotopic" type, more common in adults, and the ectopic variety, in which the ectopic URC corresponds to a dual system located in a position distal to the trigone and can be projected inside the urethra (cecoureterocele). URCs show multiple anatomical variants and clinical presentations, most often associated with obstruction of the upper pole of duplicated collecting system. Ultrasounds show hydronephrosis and megaureter of the upper pole, which is often abnormal with little or no parenchyma. Bladder outlet obstruction may be present, causing bilateral hydronephrosis. There is high morbidity associated with URC. Prenatal diagnosis has allowed early indication of prophylactic antibiotics and has led to a decreased incidence of urinary tract infection from 70% to 80% historically to 3–15% at present. Early treatment also consists of intravesical endoscopic incision, significantly reducing morbidity.

(Fig. 5.1). Ultrasound (US). (a) Left kidney (LK): pelvicalyceal duplication with severely dilated upper pole; the lower pole is normal. (b) Right kidney (RK) with duplication and degree II/IV hydronephrosis in upper pole and less severe dilation in the lower pole with better preserved renal parenchyma and good corticomedullary differentiation. (c) Upper third right megaureter system (RU). (Fig. 5.2). US of the bladder, two large URCs are detected (A and B); B is trying to prolapse through the urethra. C: dilated right terminal ureter (Fig. 5.3). Intravenous urography: no contrast elimination at the level of right upper pole (*arrow*), with a marked separation of the inferior system to the midline. The left side shows good extraction and concentration of the contrast with hydronephrosis (*asterisk*) of the two collector hemi systems. In the bladder, two rounded filling defects are observed due to ureteroceles (*thick arrows*) (Fig. 5.4). After the incision of both ureteroceles, the left one (*arrow*) is retracted and the right one (*asterisk*) persists dilated with internal echoes due pyonephrosis. It is also prolapsed into the urethra.

Case 2: Posterior Urethral Valves

Carmina Duran Feliubadaló and Luis Riera Soler

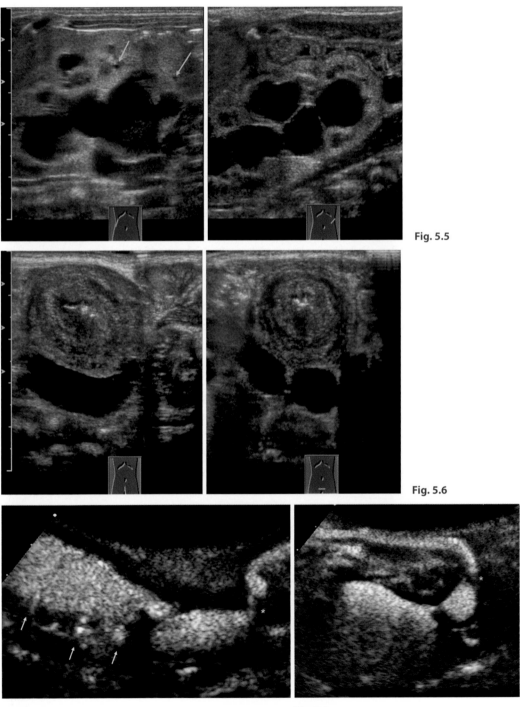

Fig. 5.5

Fig. 5.6

Fig. 5.7   Fig. 5.8

A newborn boy with a prenatal history of bilateral high-grade hydronephrosis and oligoamnios in the third trimester presented clinical and analytic signs of acute renal failure after induced delivery at 37 weeks' gestation.

Comments

With an incidence of 1 in every 5,000–8,000 newborn boys, posterior urethral valves (PUV) are the most common cause of pediatric obstructive uropathy, which leads to end-stage renal disease in males. The embryologic defect leading to the development of PUV is unknown. Many authors believe the anomaly is caused by abnormal integration of the Wolffian ducts into the urethra, while others consider it a result of persistence of the cloacal membrane.

The prenatal diagnosis of PUV remains a challenge, and the classic sonographic findings for PUV, which include a combination of megacystitis, thickened bladder wall, dilated posterior urethra (keyhole sign), and oligohydramnios, are rarely seen. Thus, most cases are detected after birth, with 50–70% diagnosed in the first year of life and only 25–50% diagnosed prenatally. Postnatal sonograms can show unilateral or bilateral hydronephrosis (obstruction or vesicoureteral reflux), morphological alterations in the bladder (megacystis, trabeculation…), and/or signs of renal dysplasia. Thus, PUV is the first cause to rule out in boys with these prenatal or postnatal findings.

The classical diagnostic approach to the diagnosis of PUV is voiding urethrocystography. Nowadays, another imaging technique, voiding urethrosonography, enables the diagnosis of PUV without using ionizing radiation.

Imaging Findings

(Fig. 5.5). B-mode sonography shows grade 3 bilateral hydronephrosis with dysplastic changes in the renal parenchyma, with increased parenchymal echogenicity and cortical microcysts (*arrows*).

(Fig. 5.6). Marked thickening of the bladder wall compatible with a trabeculated bladder.

(Fig. 5.7). Voiding urethrosonography using suprapubic transpelvic and interscrotal transperineal (Fig. 5.8) approaches shows the limited capacity of the bladder to distend, with very irregular walls and multiple diverticula (*arrows*). The bladder neck is hypertrophied, and the prostatic urethra is significantly dilated (10 mm) with stenosis (*) at the level of the external sphincter. The caliber of the anterior urethra is reduced, hindering the progress of the contrast material during voiding. These findings are consistent with PUV. The patient had no vesicoureteral reflux.

Case 3: Pyelonephritis in Newborns

Luisa Ceres-Ruiz

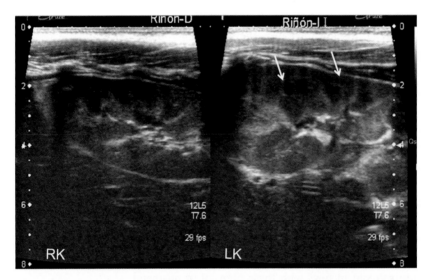

Fig. 5.9

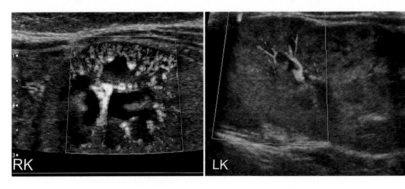

Fig. 5.10

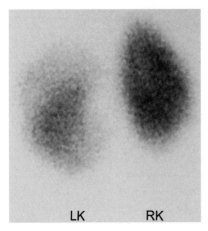

Fig. 5.11

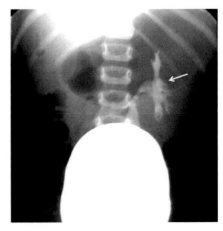

Fig. 5.12

A 15-day-old male with fever and vomiting; lab results showed a urinary infection.

In the pediatric population, urinary tract infections (UTIs) are second in frequency to that of respiratory tract infections. UTIs are often separated into the lower and the upper urinary tract. Infections of the upper tract are designated as pyelonephritis (PN). PN is an acute interstitial nephropathy which develops with an infection of the kidney parenchyma.

Age and sex are the most important factors. In newborns, the prevalence of UTI in preterm infants (2.5%) is greater than in term infants (0.8%). Sex has an impact on the prevalence of UTI: in the first 3 postnatal months, UTI is more common in boys and more in uncircumcised ones. Other risk factors include structural abnormalities of the kidneys and urinary tract. Up to 50% of infants may have an underlying structural or physiologic abnormality of the urinary tract. Vesicoureteral reflux is the most common and important risk factor. Several factors determine the intra-kidney inflammatory reaction: degree of the reflux, bacteria virulence, and host defenses. In the bloodstream infection, the damage starts at the surface of the kidney and then progresses into the medulla. The lesions are peripheral and multiple, and the usual bacterium is *Staphylococcus aureus*. In the retrograde infection, the most common bacterium is the *Escherichia coli*. It has an adhesive surface which allows it to go up the ureter and inside the parenchyma till the collecting ducts. In the parenchyma, the lesion has a triangular morphology, and in very severe infections, it can be spread all over the parenchyma.

An early and appropriate treatment is effective to prevent chronic renal lesions. Diagnosis based only on clinical findings and laboratory findings is hazardous. Ultrasound is the primary diagnostic tool. Identifying PN lesions requires experience, high quality equipment, and careful examination. It is the best method to detect congenital anomalies and also detect pyonephrosis and abscess.

Renal ultrasound shows an increase of the size of the left kidney with triangular hyper- or hypoechoic areas (*arrows*), loss of corticomedullary differentiation, hyperechoic renal sinus, and thickening of the pelvic urothelium (not shown) (Fig. 5.9). Power Doppler shows hypovascularized areas in the left kidney (Fig. 5.10), since the arteries are compressed by the adjacent edematous tissue. There is also a decrease in capitation in the DSMA (dimercaptosuccinic acid) in the initial phase of the PN (Fig. 5.11). But DMSA is postponed to assess permanent renal scars several months later. Voiding cystourethrogram (Fig. 5.12) shows left vesicoureteral reflux (*arrow*), the cause of PN.

Case 4: Acute Focal Nephronia

Luisa Ceres-Ruiz and
María I. Martínez-León

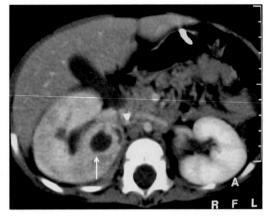

Fig. 5.14

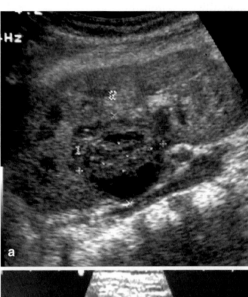

a

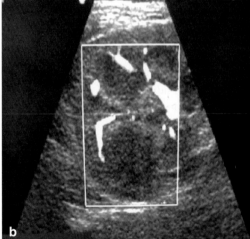

b

Fig. 5.13

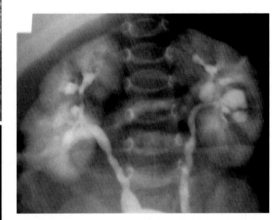

Fig. 5.15

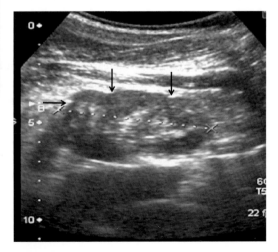

Fig. 5.16

Acute focal nephronia (AFN) is an acute bacterial infection localized in the kidney, also called acute focal bacterial nephritis or acute lobar nephronia. It has been defined as a renal mass caused by a localized infection without abscess. It is a rare entity; the clinic can be very insidious and requires a lengthy treatment. It is midway between uncomplicated acute pyelonephritis (APN) and a kidney abscess. AFN is an important differential diagnosis of lesions within the renal space. This entity should be distinguished from other noninfectious renal diseases, such as renal infarction, nephroblastomatosis, lymphoma, or Wilms tumor.

Histologically, in APN, there is diffuse edema and leukocyte infiltration. In AFN, these findings are similar, but more intense and localized. They can progress to tissue necrosis in the affected area and, eventually, produce a renal abscess. It is associated with a very high incidence of renal scarring, in comparison to APN, irrespective of the duration of antibiotic treatment. Scarring depends on the time of initiation of treatment, so early diagnosis is very important to minimize renal scars.

Escherichia coli is the most common pathogen associated with AFN. Adhesion of uropathogenic *E. coli* onto the epithelial cells has been recognized as the first event leading to various ascending UTIs, ranging from asymptomatic bacteriuria, cystitis, APN to the more severe AFN. Multiple virulence factors/capabilities may be associated with the pathogenesis of ALN and with host factors that can lead to serious infection of the parenchyma, such as immunosuppression, urinary tract abnormalities, etc. The most common abnormality is vesicoureteral reflux (VUR), especially when it has an intrarenal component.

Imaging Findings

The characteristic sonographic finding is that of a focal space-occupying lesion, hyperechoic, hypoechoic, or isoechoic, compared to renal parenchyma (depending on the evolutionary state, it is hyperechoic in early stages and hypoechoic in its evolution) (Fig. 5.13a), with disappearance of the corticomedullary differentiation in this area, poorly defined margins, with or without significant nephromegaly. Doppler ultrasound is very useful for detecting the presence of areas of hypoperfusion (Fig. 5.13b). CT is considered to have greater sensitivity and specificity for diagnosing. It shows ill-defined wedge-shaped areas, without enhancement after contrast administration (*arrow*) (Fig. 5.14). Its use is reserved for cases in which ultrasound is questionable and there is no adequate response to antibiotic treatment. Pediatric Voiding Cystourethrogram shows VUR grade III/V bilateral VUR with intrarenal component (Fig. 5.15), frequently associated with AFN. DMSA is necessary to follow up in 6 months to show the residual lesion; scars (*arrows*) can also be seen on ultrasound (Fig. 5.16) 2 years later.

Case 5: Testicular Rupture After Blunt Trauma

María I. Martínez-León and Antonio Jurado Ortiz

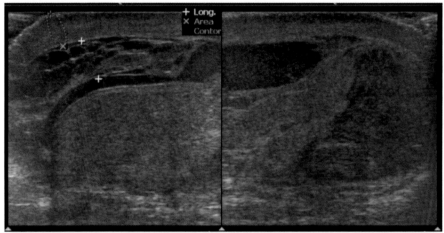

Fig. 5.17

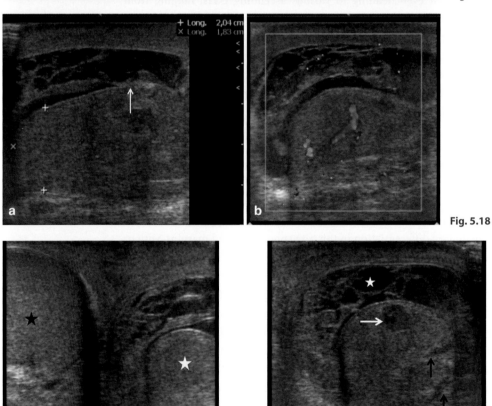

Fig. 5.18

Fig. 5.19   Fig. 5.20

A 16-year-old boy has suffered direct close scrotal trauma while practicing judo.

Testicular injury may result from direct impact against the testis, penetrating injury, or compression of the testis against the impacting object and the pubic arc. The early diagnosis of testicular rupture is important since only prompt surgery can salvage it.

Comments

Sonography (US) is the imaging procedure of choice in evaluating the acutely traumatized scrotum. There are some intra- and extratesticular US signs in this context:

1. Testicular rupture implies tearing of the fibrous tunica albuginea, a line with high echogenicity that is disrupted.
2. Secondary extrusion of testicular content into the scrotal sac.
3. The testicular rupture gives an alteration of the testicular contour or poorly defined testicular margins.
4. Focal alterations of intratesticular echogenicity correlating with areas of hemorrhage and/or infarction.
5. A discrete testicular fracture plane is identified in fewer than 20% of cases.
6. Alteration of the testicular perfusion showed with Doppler color sonography. In addition, Doppler US can display the undamaged residual parenchyma.
7. Hematocele, a complex fluid collection, originates from the bleeding of the leaves of the tunica vaginalis outside the tunica albuginea; the localization is extratesticular and intraescrotal.
8. Thickening of the scrotal wall.
9. Other infrequent presentations: intratesticular pseudoaneurysm, testicular torsion, testicular dislocation, post-traumatic epididymitis, and associated urethral lesion.

(Fig. 5.17). US compound imaging of a testicular longitudinal plane shows alterations of the echotexture of more than two fourths of the traumatic testicle, with extrusion of the testicular contents into the scrotal sac. Between cursors, complex hematocele with septa and clots. In green, thickening of the scrotal wall (Fig. 5.18). (a) Sonography, axial plane: the cursors display the superior part of the testicle, apparently untouched (between cursors). Disruption of the echogenic line that corresponds to tunica albuginea (*arrow*). (b) Color sonography of the same intact plane showing vascular patency (Fig. 5.19). Comparative axial plane of both testicles, *black asterisk*: right undamaged testicle and *white asterisk*: left traumatic testicle (Fig. 5.20). Transversal US plane of the blunt part of the testicle shows complex fluid collection within the leaves of the tunica vaginalis and outside the tunica albuginea (*asterisk*). Parenchymal heterogeneity with testicular fracture (*black arrows*) and intratesticular hematoma (*white arrow*).

Imaging Findings

Case 6: Nephrocalcinosis: Bartter's Syndrome

Luisa Ceres-Ruiz

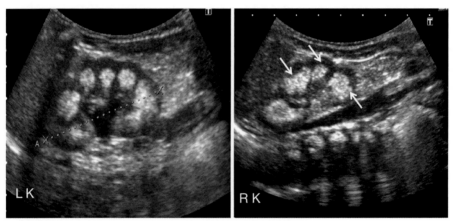

Fig. 5.21

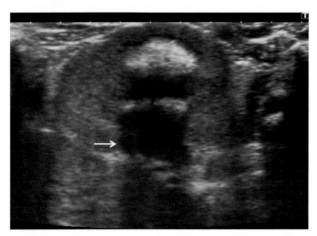

Fig. 5.22

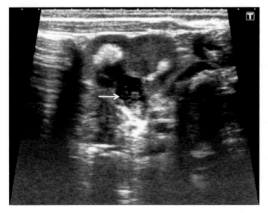

Fig. 5.23

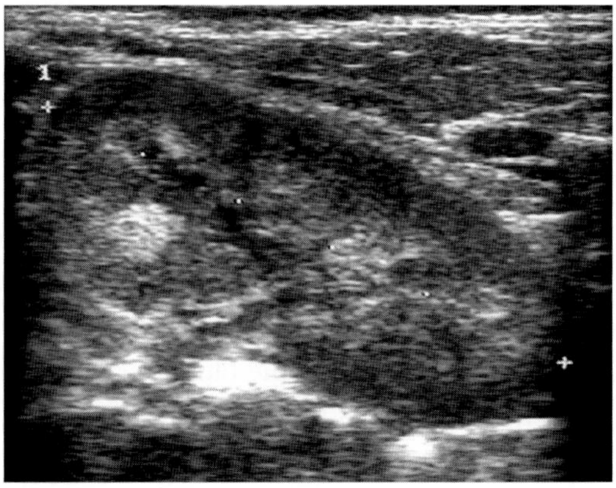

Fig. 5.24

A 3-year-old male suffering from growth retardation, polyuria, dehydration, vomiting, and suspicion of tubular acidosis. Later on, he was diagnosed with Bartter's syndrome.

Renal calcifications can be found through a pediatric ultrasound (US) study. They are nonspecific, and clinical and lab findings are needed to determine their etiology.

Comments

Nephrocalcinosis is calcium deposits in the renal parenchyma on focal or diffused distribution. The US does not allow to identify the etiology but can help to know whether it is located in the cortex or the medulla.

Medullar nephrocalcinosis in children, as in this case, is usually due to renal tubular acidosis (RTA) type I, sponge kidney (Cacchi Ricci), renal papillary necrosis, hyperparathyroidism, and, as the rarest cases, Bartter's syndrome.

Anderson-Carr-Randall's theory explains the mechanism by which calcium is deposited in the renal medulla. There is a high calcium concentration in the fluid surrounding the medullar tubules which drains in the lymphatic vessels. When its amount exceeds the lymphatic capacity, it is deposited in the papillae and in the margins of the medulla. In further stages, high-density symmetric calcifications in the medulla are found while the cortex is preserved.

Bartter's syndrome, a group of disorders that encompasses multiple genetic defects with similar clinical presentation, has been divided into six different genotypes, according to different genetic defects, and into three main clinical variants (or phenotypes).

Classic laboratory findings in all variants include hypochloremia, hypokalemia, and metabolic alkalosis with excessive excretion of chloride and potassium. It is characterized by stunted growth, hyperaldosteronism, normal blood pressure, a defect in the ability to concentrate, episodes of severe dehydration, hypercalciuria, and early-onset nephrocalcinosis.

Kidneys have a normal size in US, with hyperechogenic calcifications looking like dots with a symmetric distribution all over the medulla (*arrows*), encompassing all the pyramids while the cortex is preserved (Fig. 5.21).

Imaging Findings

Renal US done with a high-frequency transducer: an acoustic shadow (*arrow*) can be identified behind the calcium deposit of the highly echogenic pyramid (Fig. 5.22).

A bit of calcium inside the renal pelvis (*arrow*) (Fig. 5.23).

After 2 years of treatment, there is a significant decrease of the nephrocalcinosis with less echogenicity in the whole medulla (Fig. 5.24).

Case 7: Pediatric Urolithiasis

Carolina Fernández-Crehuet and María I. Martínez-León

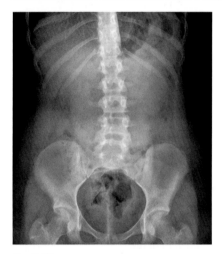

Fig. 5.25

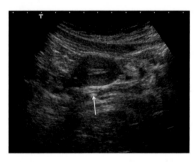

Fig. 5.27

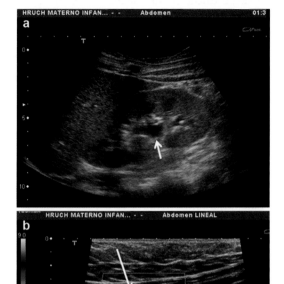

Fig. 5.26

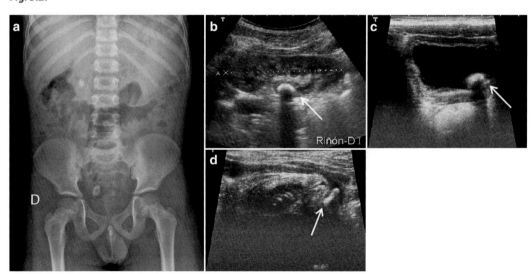

Fig. 5.28

Patient 1: A 13-year-old girl with a 4-day history of pain in the right iliac fossa. She was afebrile.

Patient 2: Oxalosis

Comments

Urinary lithiasis in pediatric age is uncommon. The development of urolithiasis is multifactorial, with wide variations depending on age, gender, diet, geographic location, inheritance, and anatomic/metabolic abnormalities. Incidence of urolithiasis and recurrences is higher in children with a positive family history.

Calculi formation is caused by a wide range of urologic, endocrine, and metabolic disorders. Congenital genitourinary malformations (pyeloureteral duplication is the most frequent) and endocrine-metabolic disorders (such as hypercalciuria and less common entities such as congenital oxalosis, hyperchloremic acidosis, distal renal tubular acidosis, etc.) must be excluded.

The most common calculi localization is in the renal pelvis. The majority of urinary stones in children contain not only calcium, but are mixed (phosphate, magnesium, oxalate, uric), with other elements such as cystine, xanthine, and glycine. Calcium oxalate is the most common component.

Urolithiasis should be suspected in children presenting with abdominal colic pain or macroscopic hematuria. Even if it is not common, it is an important entity to consider because it can lead to urinary tract infection or progressive renal damage.

Diagnosis is established with the clinical history and imaging studies. Ultrasonography is the ideal technique.

Treatment is focused on correcting the obstructive disease and the metabolic alterations; if medical treatment fails, less aggressive therapies such as lithotripsy may be associated; surgical management is reserved for exceptional cases.

Excessive urinary oxalate excretion, called hyperoxaluria, may arise from inherited or acquired diseases. The most severe forms are caused by increased endogenous production of oxalate related to one of several inborn errors of metabolism.

Imaging Findings

Patient 1 (Fig. 5.25) abdominal X-ray: Antalgic position of the spine to the right. There is no imaging of calcium along the right urinary system (Fig. 5.26). Ultrasound: (a) Grade I/IV hydronephrosis of the right kidney (*short arrow* in the minimally dilated pelvis). (b) Dilated right ureter in the location near the iliac vessels (*long arrow*) (Fig. 5.27). Ultrasound: dilated to its distal third, where there is a small stone (*arrow*).

Patient 2 (Fig. 5.28) oxalosis: Abdominal X-ray (a) shows three radiodense stones localized in the right renal pelvis, in the bladder, and in the proximal urethra. Corresponding ultrasound (b-d) shows the stones with the acoustic shadow in the right kidney, bladder, and urethra (*arrows* in b, c, d, respectively).

Case 8: Neurogenic Nonneurogenic Bladder

Luisa Ceres-Ruiz

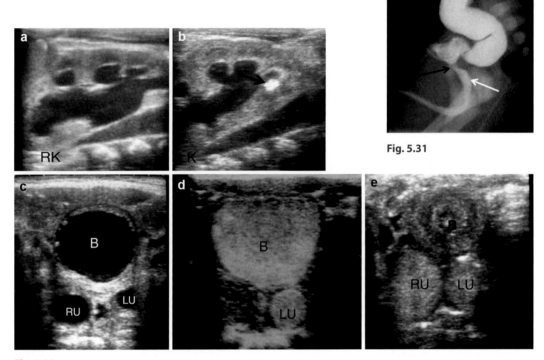

Fig. 5.31

Fig. 5.29

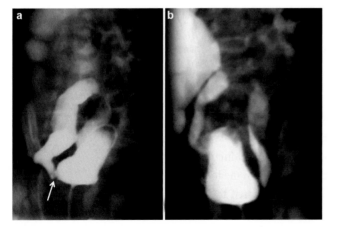

Fig. 5.30

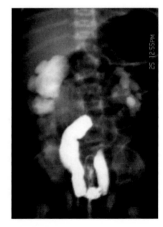

Fig. 5.32

A 6-month-old infant with urinary tract infection and previous history of mother's uncontrolled pregnancy.

Voiding dysfunction is a disorder of filling or emptying of the bladder whose origin can be neurogenic, myogenic, or functional. Neurogenic nonneurogenic bladder (NNNB) is defined as a voiding dysfunction without organic etiology, in which functional obstruction of the urinary tract is produced by alteration of bladder emptying and may initiate and perpetuate vesicoureteral reflux (VUR). There is increasing evidence to suggest that, in some infants, VUR is associated with congenital structural deficiency of the trigonal ureterovesical junction valve mechanism as well as aberrant lower urinary tract function.

VUR and NNBD are closely related, although a causal relationship has only been established for severe forms of detrusor-sphincter dyscoordination, causing abnormal urination or dysfunction characterized by low bladder capacity, high voiding pressure, and overactivity during filling.

Voiding dysfunction may require additional therapy. It has been associated with an increased incidence of urinary tract infection, kidney failure, and renal scarring associated with undiagnosed and untreated lower urinary tract dysfunction. The importance of recognizing the dysfunction must be emphasized, and radiologists should report signs of suspicion in voiding cystourethrogram (VCUG) and ultrasound and later perform a urodynamic study.

(Fig. 5.29). Ultrasound: (a, b) right and left kidneys (RK, LK) with hydronephrosis, lithogenic focus on the LK (*arrow*). (c) Bladder (B) with wall thickening and speculation; retrovesical ureters are dilated: right ureter (RU) and left ureter (LU). (d, e) Ultrasound contrast cystography, (d) bladder filling with reflux in the LU, (e) bladder contracted with marked thickening of the wall and massive reflux into both ureters, which show greater dilation than in the bladder filling phase.

(Fig. 5.30a, b). Cystography in the filling phase with bladder elongated and pear-shaped, bilateral VUR grades IV–V, and extravesicalization of the submucosal segment of the ureter (*arrow*).

(Fig. 5.31). Cystourethrogram in the voiding phase showing a contracted sphincter (*black arrow*) and moderately dilated posterior urethra (*white arrow*) while suffering from marked dilatation ureters; the bladder empties into the ureter, which constitutes a urinary anomaly known as detrusor-sphincter dyssynergia.

(Fig. 5.32). Post-voiding phase of the VCUG presenting a remarkable retention of urine (contrast) in the ureters due to voiding dysfunction.

Case 9: Nutcracker Syndrome

Marta García Ramírez and Luisa Ceres-Ruiz

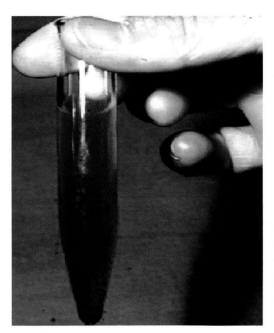

Fig. 5.33

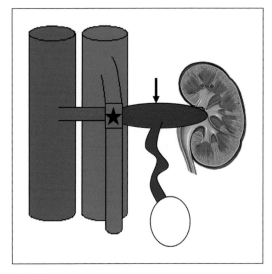

Fig. 5.34

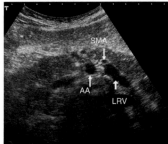

Fig. 5.35

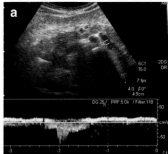

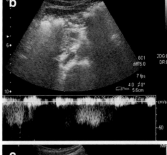

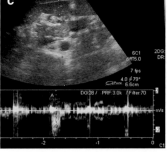

Fig. 5.36

Male, 5 years and 9 months old, hematuria of 3 months of evolution, bright red urine more intense at the beginning of urination and preceded by left flank pain, related to prior exercising and abundant fluid intake. The episodes were repeated at a frequency of 2–3 per week.

Nutcracker syndrome (NCS) is produced by compression of the left renal vein (LRV) between the aorta and the superior mesenteric artery (SMA). It usually occurs in young, previously healthy children. The compression leads to hypertension in the left renal vein, which can result in rupture of its thin wall in the fornix of the renal calyx, appearing clinically in the form of intermittent gross hematuria or microscopic hematuria.

Comments

This syndrome has a wide spectrum of clinical presentations and the diagnostic criteria are not well defined, often resulting in delayed or incorrect diagnosis. NCS is associated with hematuria that may even cause anemia and abdominal pain, classically on the left flank. Since the left gonad drains via the left renal vein, it can also lead to left testicular pain in men or to the left lower quadrant in women. Another manifestation that may be associated to NCS includes the formation of left varicocele.

Differential diagnosis must rule out stones, tumors of the urinary tract, and loin pain hematuria syndrome.

The diagnosis of NCS requires high clinical suspicion. Compression of the left renal vein between the SMA and the aorta is observed by all the radiological tools, but renal Doppler ultrasound is a test that avoids more invasive studies. The ability of color Doppler sonography to provide information about the reno-cava gradient is an important parameter to document the severity of the obstruction. Flow velocity should exceed 100 cm/s at the point of the obstruction, with a sensitivity of 78% and a specificity of 100%.

(Fig. 5.33). Hematuria every 2–3 days, sediment: gross hematuria with 20% of dysmorphia, no acanthocytes; leukocytes: 1–5 leuco/field, no bacteriuria (Fig. 5.34). Schema of the aorto/mesenteric clamp (A/M): dilation of the left renal vein (*arrow*) before crossing aortic/mesenteric localization (*asterisk*) (Fig. 5.35). Ultrasound: aorta (AA), superior mesenteric artery (SMA), left renal vein (LRV). A marked dilatation of the LRV is seen before the cross, showing similar caliber as the aorta (Fig. 5.36). (a) Doppler of the LRV (angle = 0°) before crossing A/M, showing a speed of 12 cm/s. (b) Doppler of the LRV after crossing A/M, without angle correction, presents a speed of 50 cm/s. (c) Doppler in the same place as (b) correcting the angle of insonation, reaching speeds up to 2 m/s. This gradient is sufficient for the diagnosis of nutcracker syndrome.

Imaging Findings

Case 10: Renal Cortical Necrosis

Luisa Ceres-Ruiz

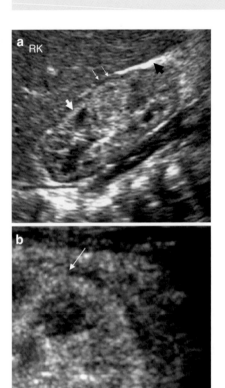

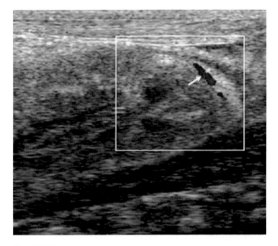

Fig. 5.38

Fig. 5.37

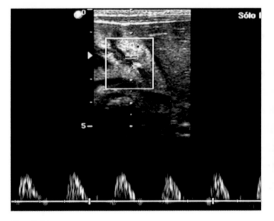

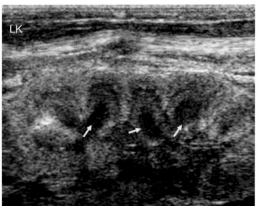

Fig. 5.39

Fig. 5.40

Preterm 3-day-old newborn (NB) with perinatal asphyxia, cerebral hemorrhage, and acute renal failure.

Acute renal failure (ARF) in the NB may be caused by a variety of congenital anomalies and can also be the result of acquired kidney injury, hypoxic-ischemic origin, or drug toxicity. ARF in neonates is suspected if the plasma creatinine level increases or fails to decrease during the first week of life. Plasma creatinine concentration should be above 15 mg/L for at least 24–48 h. Several studies have shown that ARF is common in the neonatal intensive care unit.

Blood flow is proportionally lower in infants than in older children in the neonatal period due to the increased peripheral resistance that exists in all organs, except the brain and the heart. This physiological decrease of flow is the basis of the risk factor for renal ischemia and hypoperfusion situations such as hypoxia, asphyxia, sepsis, surfactant deficiency, severe congenital heart disease, patent ductus arteriosus, and drugs that produce renal blood flow reduction (indomethacin, captopril, and totazoline hydrochloride). Impaired renal perfusion may lead to abnormalities of the pyramids, cortex, or renal vasculature, which include changes such as acute tubular necrosis, medullary or cortical necrosis, and renal vein thrombosis.

Renal cortical necrosis (RCN) is a rare cause of ARF secondary to ischemic necrosis of the cortex. RCN is usually extensive, although focal and localized forms can occur. Generally, the medulla, juxtamedullary cortex, and a thin rim of subcapsular cortex are spared. In these clinical situations, the power Doppler (PD) is used to evaluate conditions that alter renal blood flow distribution and understand the origin of the cortical and medullary ischemic necrosis.

(Fig. 5.37). (a) Ultrasound of a kidney with cortical necrosis: hypoechoic band surrounding the whole kidney. This vascular ring resulted from capsular vessels that try to compensate the ischemia (*thin arrows*). Hyperechoic and narrow band corresponding to the entire ischemic renal cortex and the columns of Bertin around the pyramids (*white thick arrow*). Hyperechoic band due to the edematous renal capsule for compensatory hyperemia of the renal cortex (*black arrow*). (b) Focus image (Fig. 5.38) power color Doppler capsular vessels (*arrow*) (Fig. 5.39). Color and pulsed Doppler of segmental renal arteries with low systolic spikes and absent diastolic flow due to poor renal perfusion (Fig. 5.40). Contralateral kidney: medullary ischemia. There is a hypoechoic band around the periphery of each pyramid and an anechoic central region extending down into the papilla (*arrows*), which has been identified as liquefaction necrosis.

Further Reading

Case 1: Bilateral Ureterocele

Book

Retik-Alan B (1990) Uréter Ectópico y Ureterocele. Campbell: Urología, 5ª edn. Tomo 11, Editorial Médica Panamericana, Buenos Aires, pp 2263–2278

Web Link

http://emedicine.medscape.com/article/1017202-overview

Articles

Bederti O, Scalercio F, Aprigliano D, Tsalikova E, Matrunola M, Principessa L (2000) Bilateral intravesical ureteroceles associated with hydroureteronephrosis and hyperechogenic spots in kidneys. Report of a neonatal case. Minerva Pediatr 52:69–73

Cooper CS, Passerini-Glazel G, Hutcheson JC, Iafrate M, Camuffo C, Milani C, Snyder HM (2000) Long-term follow-up of endoscopic incision of ureteroceles: intravesical versus extravesical. J Urol 164:1097–1100

Coplen DE (2001) Management of the neonatal ureterocele. Curr Urol Rep 2:102–105

Coplen DE, Duckett JW (1995) The modern approach to ureterocele. J Urol 153:166–171

Hochhauser L, Alton DJ (1986) Prolapse of an ectopic ureterocele into both urethra and ipsilateral orthotopic ureter. Pediatr Radiol 16:167–168

Merlini E, Lelli Chiesa P (2004) Obstructive ureterocele-an ongoing challenge. J Urol 22:107–114

Monfort G, Guys JM, Coquet M, Roth K, Louis C, Bocciardi A (1992) Surgical management of duplex ureteroceles. J Pediatr Surg 27:634–638

Nussbaum AR, Dorst JP, Jeffs RD, Gearhart JP, Sanders RC (1986) Ectopic ureter and ureterocele: their varied sonographic manifestations. Radiology 159:227–235

Roy GT, Desai S, Cohen RC (1997) Ureteroceles in children: an ongoing challenge. Pediatr Surg Int 12:448

Stunell H, Barrett S, Campbell N, Colhoun E, Torreggiani WC (2010) Prolapsed bilateral ureteroceles leading to intermittent outflow obstruction. JBR-BTR 93: 312–313

Case 2: Posterior Urethral Valves

Book

Dacher JN (2002) Abnormalities of the lower urinary tract and urachus. In: Fotter R (ed) Pediatric uroradiology, 2nd edn. Springer, Berlin/Heidelberg, pp 122–135

Web Link

Volberg F, Darge K, Paltiel H, McCarville B, Coley B, Fordham L, Bulas D (2012) Contrast-enhanced ultrasound task force. The society for pediatric radiology. Web site http://www.pedrad.org/displaycommon. cfm?an=1&subarticlenbr=707. Acceso el 3 de enero de 2012

Articles

Berrocal T, Gayá F, Arjonilla A (2005) Vesicoureteral reflux: can the urethra be adequately assessed by using contrast-enhanced voiding US of the bladder? Radiology 234:235–241

Darge K (2008) Voiding urosonography with US contrast agents for the diagnosis of vesicoureteric reflux in children. II. Comparison with radiological examinations. Pediatr Radiol 38:54–63, quiz 126–7

Darge K (2010) Voiding urosonography with US contrast agent for the diagnosis of vesicoureteric reflux in children: an update. Pediatr Radiol 40:956–962

Darge K (2011a) Contrast-enhanced US (CEUS) in children: ready for prime time in the United States. Pediatr Radiol 41:1486–1488

Darge K (2011b) Voiding urosonography: an additional important indication for use of US contrast agents. Radiology 259:614–615, author reply 615

Darge K, Grattan-Smith JD, Riccabona M (2010) Pediatric uroradiology: state of the art. Pediatr Radiol 41:82–91

Duran C, Valera A, Alguersuari A, Ballesteros E, Riera L, Martin C et al (2009) Voiding urosonography: the study of the urethra is no longer a limitation of the technique. Pediatr Radiol 39:124–131

Papadopoulou F, Anthopoulou A, Siomou E, Efremidis S, Tsamboulas C, Darge K (2009) Harmonic voiding urosonography with a second-generation contrast agent for the diagnosis of vesicoureteral reflux. Pediatr Radiol 39:239–244

Piscaglia F, Nolsøe C, Dietrich CF, Cosgrove DO, Gilja OH, Bachmann Nielsen M et al (2011) The EFSUMB guidelines and recommendations on the clinical practice of contrast enhanced ultrasound (CEUS): update 2011 on non-hepatic applications. Ultraschall in der Medizin 33:33–59

Ruano R (2011) Fetal surgery for severe lower urinary tract obstruction. Prenat Diagn 31:667–674

Case 3: Pyelonephritis in Newborns

Book

Risdon RA (1994) Pyelonephritis and reflux nephropathy. In: Tisher CC, Brenner BM (eds) Renal pathology with clinical and functional correlations, 2nd edn. Lippincott, Philadelphia, pp 852–854

Web Link

http://search.medscape.com/reference-search?newSearc
hHeader=1&queryText=pediatric+pyelonephritis

Articles

Berro Y, Baratte B, Seryer D, Boulu G, Slama M, Boudailliez B et al (2000) Comparison between scintigraphy, B-mode, and Doppler sonography in acute pyelonephritis in children. J Radiol 81:523–527

Dacher JN, Pfister Ch, Monroc M, Le Dosseur P (1996) Power Doppler sonographic pattern of acute pyelonephritis in children: comparison with CT. AJR Am J Roentgenol 166:1451–1455

Jakobson B, Berg U, Sevensson L (1994) Renal scarring after acute pyelonephritis. Arch Dis Child 70:111–115

Jakobsson B, Jacobson SH, Hjalmar K (1999) Vesico ureteric reflux and other risk factors for renal damage: identification of high and low risk children. Acta Paediatr Suppl 431:31–39

Jodal U, Winberg J (1987) Pyelonephritis: report of the 4th international symposium, Gotemborg, Sweden. Pediatr Nephrol 1:248–252

Lavocat MP, Granjon D, Allard D, Gay C, Frycon MT, Dubois F (1997) Imaging of pyelonephritis. Pediatr Radiol 27:159–165

Muro MD, Sangüesa C, Otero MC, Piqueras A, Lloret MT (2002) Pielonefritis aguda en la edad pediátrica: estudio comparativo entre la ecografía power-Doppler y el DMSA. Radiologia 44:237–242

Orellana P, Cavagnaro F et al (2002) Factores de riesgo de daño renal permanente en niños con infección del tracto urinario. Rev Méd Chile 130:1147–1153

Ozçelik G, Polat TB, Akta S, Cetinkaya F (2004) Resistive index in febrile urinary tract infections: predictive value of renal outcome. Pediatr Nephrol 19:148–152

Peters C, Rushton HG (2010) Vesicoureteral reflux associated renal damage: congenital reflux nephropathy and acquired renal scarring. J Urol 184:265–273

Case 4: Acute Focal Nephronia

Book

Kliegman R, Nelson WE (2011) Nelson textbook of pediatrics, 19th edn. Chapter 532. Saunders, Philadelphia

Web Link

http://rad.usuhs.edu/medpix/master.
php3?mode=single&recnum=2041

Articles

Cheng C, Tsau Y, Hsu S, Lee T (2004) Effective ultrasonographic predictor for the diagnosis of acute lobar nephronia. Pediatr Infect Dis J 23:11–14

Cheng CH, Su LH, Tsau YK, Lin TY (2011) Comparison of virulence variations on MDCK monolayers by *Escherichia coli* isolated from acute lobar nephronia and acute pyelonephritis. New Microbiol 34:65–72

Frieyro M, Martín M, Canals A, Nicova J, Camps J, Segarra F (2001) Nefronía lobar aguda. Aportación de tres nuevos casos. An Esp Pediatr 55:269–272

Granados A, Espino M, Gancedo A, Albulos J, Alvarez-Cortinas J, Molina C (2007) Nefronía focal aguda bacteriana: diagnóstico, tratamiento y evolución. An Pediatr 66:84–89

Hoddick W, Jeffrey RB, Goldberg HI, Federle MP, Laing FC (1983) CT and sonography of severe renal and perirenal infections. AJR Am J Roentgenol 140:517–520

Rosenfield AT, Quickman MG, Taylor KJ, Crade M, Hodson J (1979) Acute focal bacterial nephritis (acute lobar nephronia). Radiology 132:555–561

Seigel MJ, Glasier M (1981) Acute focal bacterial nephritis in children: significance of uretral reflux. AJR Am J Roentgenol 137:257–260

Seidel T, Kuwertz-Bröking E, Kaczmarek S et al (2007) Acute focal bacterial nephritis in 25 children. Pediatr Nephrol 22:1897–1901

Shimizu M, Katamaya K, Kato E, Miyayama S, Sugata T, Ohta K (2005) Evolution of acute focal bacterialnephritis into a renal abscess. Pediatr Nephrol 20:93–95

Uehling D, Hahnfel L, Scanlan K (2000) Urinary tract abnormalities in children with acute focal bacterial nephritis. BJU Int 85:885–888

Case 5: Testicular Rupture After Blunt Trauma

Book

Mirvis SE, Dunham CM (1992) Abdominal/pelvic trauma. In: Mirvis SE, Young JWR (eds) Imaging in trauma and critical care, 1st edn. Williams & Wilkins, Baltimore, pp 227–232

Web Link

Lonergan GJ (2007) Acute scrotum in children. http://www.radiologyassistant.nl/en/45c4a94292861

Articles

Bhatt S, Dogra VS (2008) Role of US in testicular and scrotal trauma. Radiographics 28:1617–1629

Buckley JC, McAninch JW (2006a) Diagnosis and management of testicular ruptures. Urol Clin North Am 33:111–116

Buckley JC, McAninch JW (2006b) Use of ultrasonography for the diagnosis of testicular injuries in blunt scrotal trauma. J Urol 175:175–178

Carkaci S, Ozkan E, Lane D, Yang WT (2010) Scrotal sonography revisited. J Clin Ultrasound 38:21–37

Deurdulian C, Mittelstaedt CA, Chong WK, Fielding JR (2007) US of acute scrotal trauma: optimal technique, imaging findings, and management. Radiographics 27:357–369

Guichard G, El Ammari J, Del Coro C, Cellarier D, Loock PY, Chabannes E et al (2008) Accuracy of ultrasonography in diagnosis of testicular rupture after blunt scrotal trauma. Urology 71:52–56

Lozano MC, Serrano C, Revilla Y, Miralles M, del Pozo G, López U (1998) Estudio ecográfico de la patología escrotal valorada como escroto agudo en una unidad de urgencia hospitalaria. Radiologia 40:33–42

Pace A, Powel C (2004) Testicular infarction and rupture after blunt trauma: use of diagnostic ultrasound. Scientific World Journal 4:437–441

Pavlica P, Barozzi L (2001) Imaging of the acute scrotum. Eur Radiol 11:220–228

Pepe P, Panella P, Pennisi M, Aragona F (2006) Does color Doppler sonography improve the clinical assessment of patients with acute scrotum? Eur J Radiol 60:120–124

Heffernan A, Steffensen TS, Gilbert-Barness E, Perlman S (2008) Bartter syndrome presenting as poor weight gain and abdominal mass in an infant. Fetal Pediatr Pathol 27:232–243

Katz M, Karlowicz M, Adelman RD, Werner A, Solhaug MJ (1994) Sonographic patterns, histological characteristics and clinical risk factors. J Ultrasound Med 13:777–783

Rodríguez Soriano J (1998) Bartter and related syndromes: the puzzle is almost solved. Pediatr Nephrol 12:315–327

Saarela T, Lanning P, Koivisto M (1999) Prematurity associated nephrocalcinosis and kidney function in early childhood. Pediatr Nephrol 13:886–890

Shalev H, Ohali M, Kachko L, Landau D (2003) The neonatal variant of Bartter syndrome and deafness: preservation of renal function. Pediatrics 112:628–633

Vieux R, Hamon I, Feldmann M, André JL, Hascoët JM (2009) Neonatal Bartter syndrome's special features in very premature newborns. Arch Pediatr 16:23–26

Case 6: Nephrocalcinosis: Bartter Syndrome

Book

Herrero JD, Ariceta G (2010) Síndromes de Bartter y Gitelman. In: Antón M, Rodríguez LM y Asociación Española de Nefrología Pediátrica (eds) Nefrología pediátrica, Manual práctico. Editorial Médica Panamericana, Madrid, pp 165–170

Web Link

www.revistanefrologia.com/modules. php?name=articulos...

Articles

Auron A, Alon US (2005) Resolution of medullary nephrocalcinosis in children with metabolic bone disorders. Pediatr Nephrol 20(8):1143–1145

Bartter FC, Pronove P, Gill JR, MacCardle RC (1962) Hyperplasia of the juxtaglomerular complex with hyperaldosteronism and hypokalemic alkalosis. A new syndrome. Am J Med 33:811–828

Dyer RB, Chen MYM, Zagoria RJ (1998) Abnormal calcifications in the urinary tract. Radiographics 18:1405–1424

Emma F, Pizzini C, Tessa A, Di Giandomenico S, Onetti-Muda A, Santorelli FM, Bertini E, Rizzoni G (2006) "Bartter-like" phenotype in Kearns-Sayre syndrome. Pediatr Nephrol 21:355–360

Case 7: Pediatric Urolithiasis

Book

Langman CB, Moore ES (1992) Pediatric urolithiasis. In: Edelmann CE, Spitzer A, Travis LB, Meadow SR (eds) Pediatric kidney disease, 2nd edn. Little Brown, Boston, pp 2005–2014

Web Link

Fathallah-Shaykh Sahar. Pediatric urolithiasis. Langman CB. http://emedicine.medscape.com/article/983884-overview

Articles

Bobrowski AE, Langman CB (2006) Hyperoxaluria and systemic oxalosis: current therapy and future directions. Expert Opin Pharmacother 7:1887–1896

Camacho Díaz JA, Casas Gómez J, Amat Barnés A, Giménez Llort A, García García L (1996) Litiasis renal en el niño. An Esp Pediatr 44:225–228

Erbagci A, Erbagci AB, Yilmaz M, Yagci F, Tarakcioglu M et al (2003) Pediatric urolithiasis, evaluation of risk factors in 95 children. Scand J Urol Nephrol 37:129–133

Fahlenkamp D, Noack B, Leberntrau S, Belz H (2008) Urolithiasis in children. Urolithiasis in children, rational diagnosis, therapy, and metaphylaxis. Urologe A 47:545–550

Gearhart JP, Herzberg GZ, Jeff RD (1991) Childhood urolithiasis: experiences and advances. Pediatrics 87:445–450

Hoppe B, Kemper MJ (2010) Diagnostic examination of the child with urolithiasis or nephrocalcinosis. Pediatr Nephrol 25:403–413

Lagomarsino D, Avila S, Baquedano P, Cavagnaro F, Céspedes P (2003) Litiasis urinaria en pediatría. Rev Chil Pediatr 74:381–388

Polinsky MS, Kaiser BA, Baluarte H (1987) Urolithiasis in childhood. Pediatr Clin North Am 34:683–710

Stapleton FB (1991) Pediatric urolithiasis: concepts and challenges. In: Straus J (ed) Pediatric nephrology. From old to new frontiers. University of Miami Press, Florida, pp 105–114

Watts RW (1990) What treatment do you advise for a small child with hyperoxaluria presenting with renal calculi? Pediatr Nephrol 4:99–100

Case 8: Neurogenic Nonneurogenic Bladder and Vesicoureteral Reflux

Book

Esposito C, Guys JM, Gough D, Savanelli A (eds) (2006) Pediatric neurogenic bladder dysfunction, diagnosis, treatment, long-term, follow-up. Springer, Berlin. ISBN 978-3-540-30866-9

Web Link

http://scielo.isciii.es/scielo.php?pid=S0210-48062004000200007

Articles

Acar B, Arikan FI, Germiyano lu C, Dallar Y (2009) Influence of high bladder pressure on vesicoureteral reflux and its resolution. Urol Int 82:77–80

Al Mosawi AJ (2007) Identification of nonneurogenic neurogenic bladder in infants. Urology 70:355–357

Hoang-Bohm J, Lusch A, Sha W, Alken P (2004) Biofeedback for urinary bladder dysfunctions in childhood. Indications, practice and the results of therapy. Urologe A 43:813–819

Hoebeke P, Everaert K, Van Laecke E, Vande Walle J, Van Gool J (1999) Assessment of lower urinary tract dysfunction in children with non-neuropathic bladder sphincter dysfunction. Eur Urol 35:57–69

Homsy YL (1994) Dysfunctional voiding syndromes and vesicoureteral reflux. Pediatr Nephrol 8:116–121

Johnson JF 3rd, Hedden RJ, Piccolello ML, Wacksman J (1992) Distention of the posterior urethra: association with nonneurogenic neurogenic bladder (Hinman syndrome). Radiology 185:113–117

Koff SA (1992) Relationship between dysfunctional voiding and reflux. J Urol 148:1703–1705

Martín-Crespo Izquierdo R, Luque Mialdea R (2003) Non-coordinated micturition syndrome mimicking posterior urethral valves in a male neonate. Cir Pediatr 16:134–138

Schewe J, Brands FH, Pannek J (2002) Voiding dysfunction in children: role of urodynamic studies. Urol Int 69:297–301

Vidal I, Héloury Y, Ravasse P, Lenormand L, Leclair MD (2009) Severe bladder dysfunction revealed prenatally or during infancy. J Pediatr Urol 5:3–7

Case 9: Nutcracker Syndrome

Book

García Blanco JM, del Rosa Hidalgo-Barquero (2006) Protocolo diagnóstico de la hematuria. In: García Nieto V, Santos Rodríguez F, Rodríguez-Iturbe B (eds) Nefrología pediátrica, 2nd edn. Grupo Aula médica, Madrid, pp 413–424

Web Link

http://www.aeped.es/sites/default/files/documentos/15_3.pdf

Articles

El Harrech Y, Jira H, Chafiki J, Ghadouane M, Ameur A, Abbar M (2009) Actitud expectante en el Síndrome del Cascanueces. Actas Urol Esp 33:93–96

Fitoz S, Ekim M, Ozcakac ZB, Elhan AH, Yalcinkaya F (2007) The role of upright position examination and superior mesenteric artery angle measurement in the diagnosis. J Ultrasound Med 26:573–580

Kurklinsky AK, Rooke TW (2010) Nutcracker phenomenon and nutcracker syndrome. Mayo Clin Proc 85:552–559

Mendizábal S, Román E, Serrano A, Berbel O, Simón J (2005) Síndrome de hipertensión vena renal izquierda. Nefrologia 25:141–146

Romera-Villegas A, Vila-Coll R, Cairols-Castellote M, Poveda-Monge R, Romera-Villegas A, Vila-Coll R, Cairols-Castellote M, Poveda-Monge R, Masuet-Aumatell C, Grinyo-Boira M (2009) The importance of a standing position in the diagnosis of nutcracker phenomenon by duplex sonography. Int Angiol 28:461–468

Shin JI, Park JM, Lee JS, Kim MJ (2007a) Morphologically improved nutcracker syndrome in an 11-year-old girl with hematuria. Pediatr Int 49:677–679

Shin JI, Park JM, Lee JS (2007b) Doppler ultrasonographic indices in diagnosing nutcracker syndrome in children. Pediatr Nephrol 22:409–413

Shin JI, Park JM, Lee JS, Kim MJ (2007c) Effect of renal Doppler ultrasound on the detection of nutcracker syndrome in children with hematuria. Eur J Pediatr 166:399–404

Takebayashi S, Ueki T, Ikeda N, Fujikawa A (1999) Diagnosis of the nutcracker syndrome with color Doppler sonography: correlation with flow patterns on retrograde left renal venography. AJR Am J Roentgenol 172:39–43

Vanegas Ruiz JJ, Baquero Rodríguez R, Arteaga Arteaga A, Vélez Moncada E et al (2009) Síndrome de Nutcracker como causa de hematuria en adolescentes: informe de dos casos y revisión de la literatura. NefroPlus 2:41–44

Case 10: Renal Cortical Necrosis

Book

Siegel MJ (ed) (1995) Pediatric sonography, 2nd edn. Raven, New York

Web Link

http://emedicine.medscape.com/article/983599-overview

Articles

Andreoli SP (2004) Acute renal failure in the newborn. Semin Perinatol 28:112–123

Brendridge AN, Chevalier RL, Kaiser DL (1986) Increased renal cortical echogenicity in pediatric renal disease: histopathologic correlations. J Clin Ultrasound 14: 595–600

Daneman A, Navarro OM, Somers GR, Mohanta A, Jarrín JR, Traubici J (2010) Renal pyramids: focused sonography of normal and pathologic. Radiographics 30:1287–1307

Gouyon JB, Guignard JP (2000) Management of acute renal failure in newborns. Pediatr Nephrol 14:1037–1044

Martinoli C, Derchi LE, Rizzatto G, Solbiati L (1998) Power Doppler sonography: general principles, clinical applications, and future prospects. Eur Radiol 8:1224–1235

Mercado-Deane MG, Beeson JE, John SD (2002) US of renal insufficiency in neonates. Radiographics 22:1429–1438

Riebel TW, Abraham K, Wartner R, Müller R (1993) Transient renal medullary hyperechogenicity in ultrasound studies of neonates: is it a normal phenomenon and what are the causes? J Clin Ultrasound 21:25–31

Slovis TL, Bernstein J, Gruskin A (1993) Hyperechoic kidneys in the newborn and young infant. Pediatr Nephrol 7:294–302

Smith LE, Adelman RD (1981) Early detection of renal cortical calcification in acute renal cortical necrosis in a child. Nephron 29:155–157

Wright NB, Blanch G, Walkinshaw S, Pilling DW (1996) Antenatal and neonatal renal vein thrombosis: new ultrasonic features with high frequency transducers. Pediatr Radiol 26:686–689

Contents

M.I. Martínez-León et al., *Imaging for Pediatricians*, Imaging for Clinicians,
DOI 10.1007/978-3-642-28629-2_6, © Springer-Verlag Berlin Heidelberg 2012

Case 1: Discoid Lateral Meniscus with Tear

Inés Solís Muñiz and Sergio Martínez Álvarez

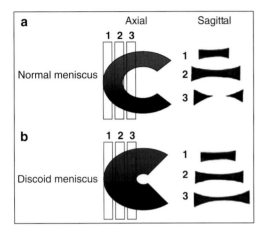

Fig. 6.1

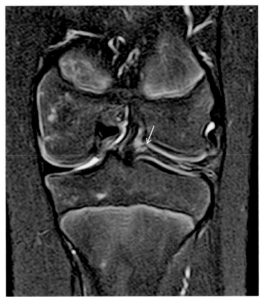

Fig. 6.3

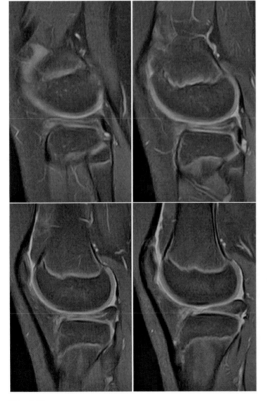

Fig. 6.2

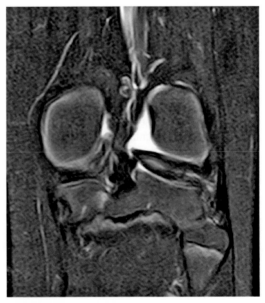

Fig. 6.4

A 11-year-old girl with knee pain and snapping on extension and internal rotation of the knee.

The lateral meniscus is a fibrocartilaginous structure which usually presents with a semilunar morphology in the axial plane. A discoid lateral meniscus (DLM) is a congenitally thick and wide meniscus with a reported prevalence of 1.5–4.5%. They are frequently bilateral (20%). The enlarged body of the meniscus extends medially toward the intercondylar notch and covers the articular surface of the tibial plateau, considering three types of DLM in arthroscopy: complete, incomplete (50–80% of coverage), and the Wrisberg variant (complete or incomplete with no capsular attachments).

The usual presentation is a young child (less than 10 years) with a catch or popping of the lateral side of the knee with motion. Sometimes patients describe true mechanical locking symptoms and painful or painless loss of motion. Clinical examination may show palpable, audible, and frequently visual hypermobile lateral meniscus instability. Effusion and loss of extension are common findings.

The MRI finding generally used as a criterion for discoid meniscus is the presence of three or more complete meniscal body segments (the "bow-tie" appearance) on continuous sagittal images, but the protocol used (usually 4–5 mm of thickness) and the smaller dimensions of menisci in children must be considered. It is reported that a DLM is present if its transverse width is greater than 13 mm, or 2 mm greater than the medial meniscus. DLM is also frequently asymmetric in height between the anterior and posterior horns.

Due to its abnormal morphology and mechanics, DLM is more frequently degenerated and torn than the normally C-shaped lateral meniscus. Most meniscal injuries in children under 10 years of age are related to DLM. Their tears are commonly horizontal and peripherally located.

Initial management is nonsurgical treatment that consists of activity modifications, anti-inflammatory medications, and swelling control (ice, rest, compression). If tear is present, and locking, loss of motion, or persistent pain and disability exist despite nonoperative management, surgery is indicated. The surgical management is arthroscopic meniscoplasty.

A normal C-shaped meniscus shows less than three body segments on continuous sagittal images (Fig. 6.1a). Three or more "bow ties" are seen on sequential sagittal slices in discoid meniscus (Fig. 6.1b). Sequential sagittal proton density-weighted fat-saturated images show the presence of meniscal body segments in four continuous slices. A horizontal tear extending through body and both horns of the meniscus is also seen (Fig. 6.2). Coronal PD-weighted image with fat saturation of the left knee demonstrates the body of the lateral meniscus extending into the intercondylar notch (*arrow*), consistent with complete discoid meniscus (Fig. 6.3). Coronal image through the posterior horn demonstrates its increased height and linear high signal intensity of the horizontal tear (Fig. 6.4).

Case 2: Glenohumeral Dysplasia Following Neonatal Brachial Plexus Palsy

Ignacio Barber Martínez de la Torre and Francisco Soldado Carrera

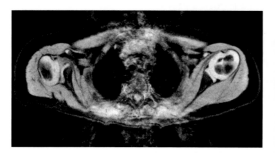

Fig. 6.5

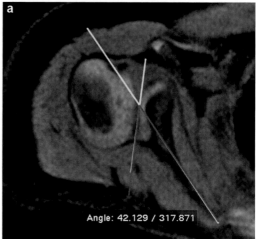

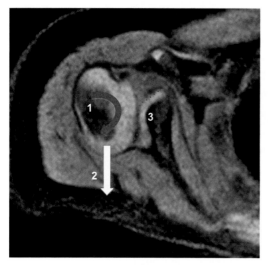

Fig. 6.6

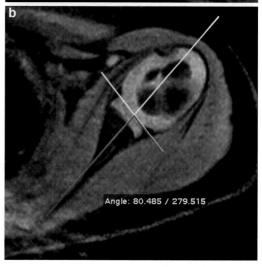

Fig. 6.7

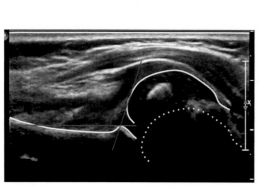

Fig. 6.8

A 14-month-old girl with residual right brachial plexus birth palsy (BPBP) presented with an internal rotation posture of the shoulder. On physical exam, an apparently shorter arm with asymmetric skin folds and minus 60° passive external rotation was present.

Ten to 30% of BPBP evolve into an incomplete recovery that can result in subscapularis muscle contracture. The internal rotation contracture of the shoulder leads to a progressive glenohumeral deformity characterized by posterior displacement of the humeral head on a progressive dysplastic glenoid. On clinical evaluation, a shoulder joint deformity should be suspected if passive external rotation with the arm adducted and the scapula stabilized is less than neutral.

Current recommended imaging studies for the evaluation of shoulders include ultrasonography and MR. US is a useful tool for the evaluation of glenohumeral joint posterior subluxation and has been proposed as a screening tool in infants. MR offers more anatomic detail and allows both joint and muscle assessment. In 1998, Waters et al. established a standardization of GHD findings in VII radiographic types. The measurements were based on axial CT and MR images of both shoulders and included the glenoscapular angle (glenoid version) and the percentage of the humeral head anterior to the scapular line (drawn from the medial aspect of the scapula to the humeral head through the middle of the glenoid fossa). Current recommended treatment is a surgical anterior capsule and upper subscapularis tendon release to relocate the humeral head in the original glenoid facet. The reduced position in abduction and external rotation is kept for some weeks with the use of a shoulder splint. Joint deformity remodels overtime and the child can recover overhead active motion.

(Figs. 6.5 and 6.6). Axial MR imaging of both shoulders and detailed image of the right shoulder obtained with a 3D GE T2-weighted sequence that shows right global muscle volume loss, more severely affecting the subscapularis; internal rotation (1) and posterior subluxation (2) of the right humeral head and secondary glenoid dysplasia with a posterior false glenoid (3) (waters type IV dysplasia). (Fig. 6.7a,b). Measurement of the version angle demonstrates retroversion of the right glenoid of −58° (42–90°). A normal −10° retroversion of the left glenoid is shown (80–90°). (Fig. 6.8). Transversal posterior US image of the right shoulder obtained below the scapular spine shows an echogenic line representing the scapula, ending in the posterior margin of the glenoid. The partially ossified humeral head shows posterior subluxation. An alpha angle is obtained: 62° (normal <30°). The discontinuous line shows the normal position of the humeral head.

Case 3: Transient Lateral Patellar Dislocation

Inés Solís Muñiz and Sergio Martínez Álvarez

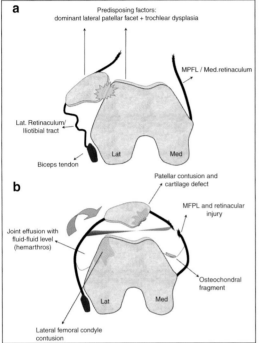

Fig. 6.9

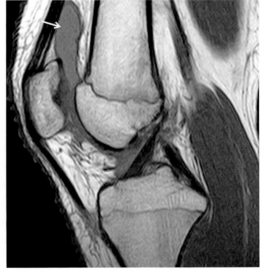

Fig. 6.11

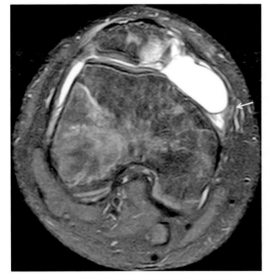

Fig. 6.10

Fig. 6.12

A 15-year-old boy with knee pain and swelling after traumatic event.

Patellar instability in children and adolescents usually involves an episode of complete dislocation of the patella from the trochlear groove. There are two types of patella dislocation: acute traumatic patella dislocation and atraumatic dislocation-subluxation secondary to ligamentous laxity. Traumatic dislocation of the patella occurs almost exclusively in the lateral direction. Lateral patellar dislocation (LPD) typically occurs in young patients between 10 and 17 years of age. The mechanism of injury usually results from a twisting motion: a flexed position and internal rotation on a fixed foot with a valgus component. It might be unsuspected and most dislocations (50–75%) spontaneously relocate, making clinical assessment and differentiation from other more common traumatic injuries often difficult.

There are characteristic MRI findings for this entity, which include contusion of the inferomedial patellar border and the anterolateral margin of the lateral femoral condyle, injury to medial stabilizers (MPFL and medial retinaculum), joint effusion (frequently hemarthros), and possible osteochondral fragments. Injury of the medial patellofemoral ligament (MPFL) occurs in 94–100% of LPD, with tears more frequently located at the femoral attachment. It is the main passive restraint against LPD and can be difficult to discern from the medial retinaculum in MRI.

Traumatic events rarely cause patellar dislocations in patients without predisposing anatomic factors for patellar instability, such as trochlear dysplasia, dominant lateral patellar facet, high position of the patella, and lateralization of the tibial tuberosity. Trochlear dysplasia is found in up to 85% of patients with LPD.

Initial management of LPD after reduction is with a knee immobilizer, analgesia and crutch walking for 4 weeks. Once symptoms have resolved, the focus of conservative treatment turns to providing dynamic stability through strengthening (quadriceps and hamstrings). Operative treatment is indicated for first-time patellar dislocation that fails to reduce, osteochondral damage (larger than 1 cm in diameter), removal of a loose body, or dislocations that fail bracing and physical therapy. Surgical management consists in the repair of osteochondral lesions and reconstruction of MCFL.

Schematic diagram of LPD mechanism of injury, initially (Fig. 6.9a) and subsequently (Fig. 6.9b). Axial proton density-weighted image with fat saturation of the right knee shows osteochondral defect of the inferomedial patellar margin and bone edema resulting from contusion against the lateral condyle. Detachment of the femoral MPFL insertion (*arrow*), with irregularity of the ligament and surrounding edema, as well as joint effusion, are noted (Fig. 6.10). Coronal PD-weighted with fat saturation MRI depicts the free osteochondral fragment (*arrow*) located next to the edematous lateral femoral condyle due to contusion against the medial patella. Joint effusion and edema of the inferior portion of the vastus medialis obliquus muscle are also seen (Fig. 6.11). Sagittal T1-weighted image shows high intensity of the joint effusion (*arrow*) consistent with hemarthros (Fig. 6.12).

Case 4: Osteochondritis Dissecans of the Knee

Miguel A. López Pino and Ana Ramírez Barragán

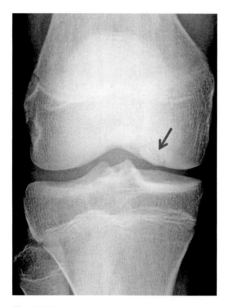

Fig. 6.13

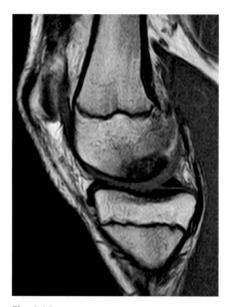

Fig. 6.14

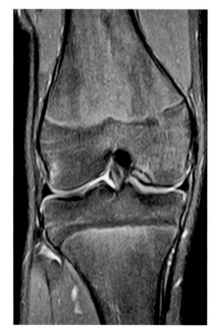

Fig. 6.15

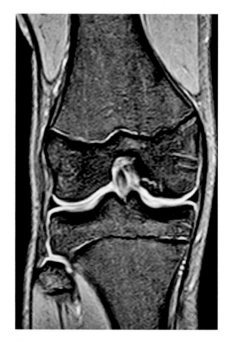

Fig. 6.16

A 13-year-old boy with poorly localized knee pain, stiffness with activity, and occasional swelling.

Osteochondritis dissecans (OCD) is an acquired, potentially reversible disorder of the subchondral bone that can secondarily affect the overlying articular cartilage and may, in some cases, lead to cartilage separation and fragmentation.

Juvenile OCD describes an OCD lesion found in skeletally immature children with a maximum incidence occurring between the ages of 10 and 20. It is found more frequently in children who are athletically active and is twice as common in males as in females. It usually affects the lateral aspect of the medial femoral condyle (MFC) but can also affect the weight-bearing surface of the lateral femoral condyle. Possible causative factors include repetitive microtrauma, ischemia, and genetic and endocrine factors. The most common complaint is aching and activity-related knee pain.

Successful imaging characterizes the lesion, determines prognosis of nonoperative management, and predicts the ultimate status of the lesion. Initial plain films should include anteroposterior and lateral views of the knee. The classic OCD lesion of the MFC is best seen on the tunnel view. In conventional radiological studies, the necrotic fragment appears like a radiolucent half-moon detached from the rest of the epiphyseal bone. OCD can be diagnosed using plain radiographs alone, but they are poor at establishing the stability of the lesion. Magnetic resonance imaging (MRI) can detect the presence of OCD in the early stages of the disease process when radiographs only show subtle changes. MRI also provides useful information about the size, location, and presence of loose bodies, the underlying cartilage, and stability of OCD. Stability is the single most important prognostic factor for determining the likelihood of an OCD lesion. Chondral fragments are best seen on fat-saturated fast spin-echo images. MR arthrography improves visualization of fluid across articular cartilage surfaces, thus helping determine whether the lesion is stable or unstable.

Treatment is dependent upon age at presentation, fragment size, fragment location, and stability. Stable lesions in skeletally immature patients are generally amenable to conservative management.

Knee AP film (Fig. 6.13) radiographs demonstrating an OCD on the MFC (*arrow*). Sagittal T1 MRI (Fig. 6.14) demonstrating an OCD lesion in the posterolateral aspect of the MFC. Coronal fat-suppressed T2- (Fig. 6.15) and T2-GE-weighted (Fig. 6.16) MRI show no disruption of low-signal-intensity subchondral bone plate at edges of OCD. The lesion is clearly demarcated from underlying subchondral bone and an intact articular mantle.

Case 5: Hemophilic Arthropathy and Magnetic Resonance Imaging

María I. Martínez-León
and Angeles Palomo Bravo

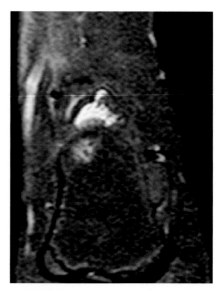

Fig. 6.18

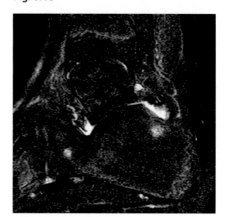

Fig. 6.19

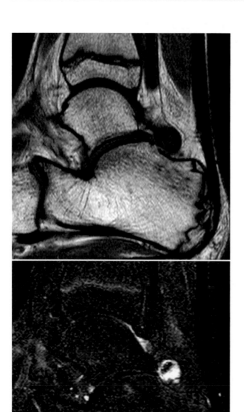

Fig. 6.17

Compatible MRI scale	Denver MRI scale	European MRI scale
Effusion/ hemarthrosis		
Small	1	
Moderate	2	
Large	3	
Synovial hypertrophy		
Small	4	1
Moderate	5	2
Large	6	3
Hemosiderin		1
Small	4	
Moderate	5	
Large	6	
Changes of subchondral bone or joint margins		
Any surface erosion	7	1
Any surface erosion in at least 2 bones		1
Half or more of the articular surface eoded in al least 1 bone	8	1
Half or more of the articular surface eoded in at least 2 bone		1
At least 1 subchondral cyst	7	1
More than 1 subchondral cyst	8	1
Subchondral cysts in at least 1 bones		1
Multiple subchondral cysts in each of at least 1 bones		1
Cartilage loss		
Any loss of joint cartilage height	9	1
Any loss of joint cartilage height in at least2 bones		1
Any loss of joint cartilage height involving more than 1/3 of the joint surface in at least 1 bone		1
Any loss of joint cartilage height involving more than 1/3 of the joint surface in at least 2 bones		1
Full-thickness loss of joint cartilage involves at least some area in at least 1 bone	10	1
Full-thickness loss of joint cartilage involves at least some area in at least 2 bones		1
Full-thickness loss of joint cartilage involves at least 1/3 of the joint surface in at least 1 bone		1
Full-thickness loss of joint cartilage involves at least 1/3 of the joint surface in at least 2 bonse		1

Fig. 6.20

A 13-year-old boy with moderate hemophilia A (1.2% FVIII baseline), with secondary prophylaxis (recombinant factor VIII).

Arthropathy is one of the most disabling consequences of hemophilia. The management of this condition has been improved by the introduction of prophylactic treatment. In order to monitor the benefits of this treatment, the severity of the joint disease needs to be accurately assessed. Diagnostic imaging is used to objectively evaluate HA, and there are several established scoring systems for grading hemophilic arthropaty (HA) based on conventional radiography and MRI.

Even though the diagnosis of hemophilia is essentially clinical and laboratory based, imaging has become an important tool for diagnostic confirmation, evaluation of complications, and/or complementation and therapeutic follow-up in HA. In addition to the conventional Magnetic Resonance Imaging (MRI) modalities, new imaging techniques (diffusion-weighted imaging, blood oxygen level dependent, T1 and T2 mapping MRI, and ultrasmall superparamagnetic iron-oxide contrast-enhanced, among others) hold promise for the assessment of HA.

The "progressive" Denver MRI scale, classifies arthropathy in different stages in relation to the most severe finding, with a maximum value of 10. The "additive" European MRI scale classifies the HA in relation to the addition of the lesions, with a maximum value of 20. Both scales make up the actual Compatible MRI scale.

MRI can be a very valuable tool that will help improve management of patients with hemophilia and optimize the outcome of treatment. The goal is to clearly differentiate the osteoarticular status of hemophilic patients cross-sectionally in either early or late stages. Some lesions are potentially reversible (temporal lesions), such as effusion, hemarthrosis, synovial hypertrophy, and hemosiderin, and others are potentially irreversible (permanent lesions), such as cartilage and osseous lesions. This information has to be well defined in the radiological report.

The common target joints in HA are ankles, knees, and elbows.

Sagittal T1- and STIR-weighted MR localized images of the ankle show low-signal-intensity material in the posterior recess of the joint, due to effusion with small hypertrophic synovium with hemosiderin deposition (Fig. 6.17). Coronal STIR-weighted MRI shows a bright medullar lesion of the margins in the superior-lateral and posterior aspect of the calcaneus (Fig. 6.18). Sagittal STIR-weighted MRI shows the same intramedullar lesion with minimum superficial erosion (Fig. 6.19). The ankle lesions described in Compatible MRI scale (Fig. 6.20) correspond to 7 points in Denver MRI score and 3 points in European MRI score.

Case 6: Osteomyelitis

Sara Inmaculada Sirvent Cerdá
and Javier Alonso Hernández

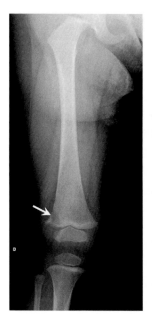

Fig. 6.21

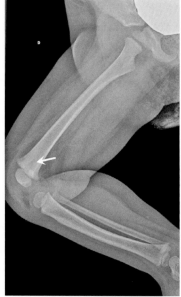

Fig. 6.22

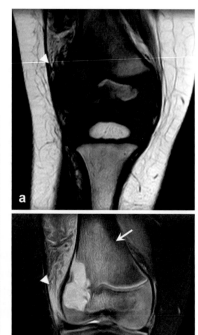

Fig. 6.23

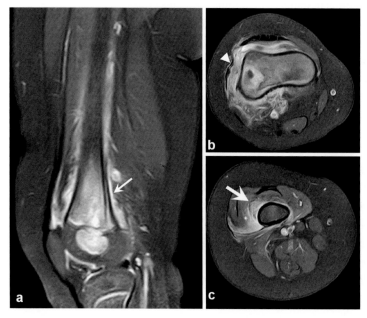

Fig. 6.24

A 9-month-old infant with pain and swelling in the right knee. No fever.

Osteomyelitis is an infection of cortical bone and/or bone marrow. It can have an acute, subacute or chronic course. The vast majority of cases are caused by *Staphylococcus aureus*, followed by *Streptococcus species*.

The most frequent route of infection is hematogenous, but direct inoculation or spread from contiguous structures is occasionally seen. Hematogenous osteomyelitis usually affects the metaphysis of long bones or the metaphyseal equivalents. During the first 18 months of life, infection can easily reach the epiphysis and joint cavity. After that age, transphyseal vessels are severed so joint involvement is uncommon.

Acute infection consists in extensive inflammatory response associated with cortical destruction, periosteal elevation, and spread of infection to soft tissues. Subacute infection remains localized in the bone with no or few soft tissue involvement. Chronic infection is limited to bone structures.

Clinical presentation consists of pain, swelling, tenderness, erythema, and fever with or without abnormal biochemical markers. But pediatric osteomyelitis can be clinically silent during the initial course of the disease, especially in neonates and infants.

The most common bones involved are the distal femur and the proximal tibia.

Diagnostic imaging may be performed to confirm clinical suspicion and to define the extent of infection. The first imaging technique is usually plain film. It has low sensitivity, but it is useful to exclude other pathologies. Ultrasound demonstrates soft tissue swelling and periosteal elevation. Scintigraphy using 99m Tc-methylene diphosphonate has high sensitivity (80%) and low specificity (50%), but it has the advantage of imaging the whole body. Magnetic resonance (MR) is considered the best technique to diagnose and follow up bone infections in children. It has whole-body imaging capability as well and does not use ionizing radiation.

The majority of pediatric cases respond to antibiotic therapy. Prompt diagnosis and treatment are essential to avoid late sequelae.

Anteroposterior (Fig. 6.21) and lateral (Fig. 6.22) radiographs of the right knee show a relatively well-defined lytic lesion in the medial aspect of the distal metaphysis of the femur (*arrows*). Coronal T1-WI (Fig. 6.23a) and DP-WI with fat saturation (Fig. 6.23b) MR demonstrate diffuse bone marrow edema (*arrow*) surrounding a focal lesion and extensive soft tissue swelling (*arrowhead*). Sagittal (Fig. 6.24a) and axial (Fig. 6.24b, c) fat-suppressed postgadolinium T1-WI demonstrate a fluid halo around the cortex limited by the periosteum (*thin arrow*), infiltration of the medial retinaculum (*arrowhead*), and marked inflammation of the deep quadriceps (*thick arrow*).

Case 7: Intramuscular Venous Malformation

Miguel A. López Pino
and Daniel Azorín Cuadrillero

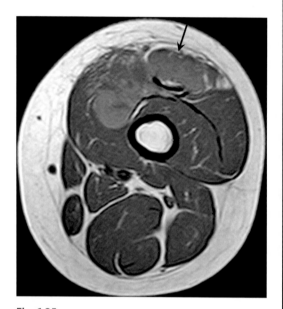

Fig. 6.25

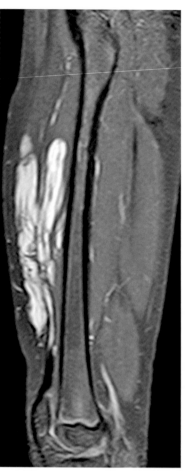

Fig. 6.27

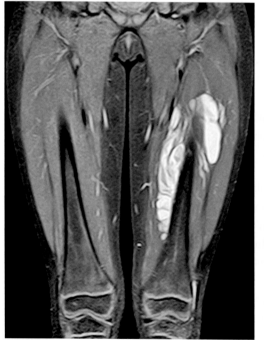

Fig. 6.26

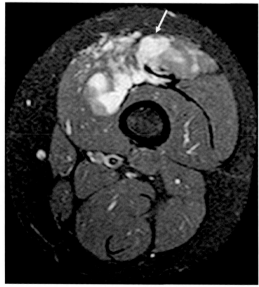

Fig. 6.28

An 11-year-old girl with intermittent episodes of pain and swelling in the left thigh.

Vascular anomalies comprise a wide spectrum of lesions involving all parts of the body. A good knowledge of the classification and clinical characteristics of vascular anomalies is necessary. However, confusion with respect to terminology and imaging guidelines continues to result in improper diagnosis and treatment.

Vascular anomalies are classified as hemangiomas and vascular malformations. Venous malformations (VM) are the most common vascular malformations. A VM is defined as a simple malformation with slow flow and an abnormal venous network. VM are usually seen at birth and increase in size as the child grows.

VM are characterized by a soft, compressible, nonpulsatile tissue mass. The overlying skin usually has a bluish tint. The main locations are the head and neck (40% of cases), extremities (40%), and trunk (20%). They often enlarge during puberty (due to hormonal influence) and do not regress. Symptoms are related to size and location. Most venous malformations are solitary.

The differential diagnosis must include hemangiomas and other slow-flow vascular malformations (lymphatic or venolymphatic malformations). Hemangiomas have rapid postnatal growth followed by spontaneous involution. Slow-flow vascular malformations grow concomitantly with the child. Doppler US and magnetic resonance imaging (MRI) allow classification of vascular anomalies and are useful in clinically uncertain cases to establish the correct diagnosis.

VM are managed conservatively. The indications for treatment are pain, articular involvement, and disfigurement. Interventional radiology plays a major role in the treatment of VM with the increasing efficacy of sclerotherapy.

In most cases, Doppler US demonstrates a large heterogeneous hypervascular solid soft tissue mass with monophasic, low-velocity flow.

MRI demonstrates a nonencapsulated lesion with mixed architecture. VM are usually hypointense on T1-W MRI (*arrow*) (Fig. 6.25) and markedly hyperintense on T2-W. Coronal (Fig. 6.26) and sagittal (Fig. 6.27) STIR MRI clearly show a high-signal-intensity mass within the quadriceps and the extension of the malformation into adjacent structures. Phleboliths show signal voids with all image sequences. Abnormal veins can be observed in the area of the malformation. Fat-suppressed fast spin-echo T1-weighted imaging (Fig. 6.28) should be performed after contrast material injection to evaluate perfusion of the malformation. Partial heterogeneous enhancement (*arrow*) suggests partial thrombosis of the VM.

Case 8: Infantile Fibrosarcoma (IFS)

Sara Inmaculada Sirvent Cerdá
and Alvaro Lassaletta Atienza

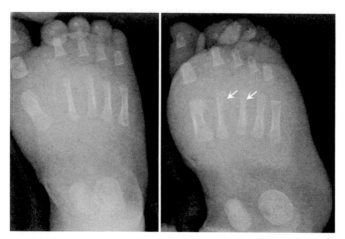

Fig. 6.29

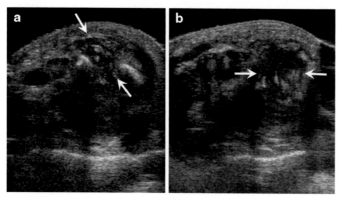

Fig. 6.30

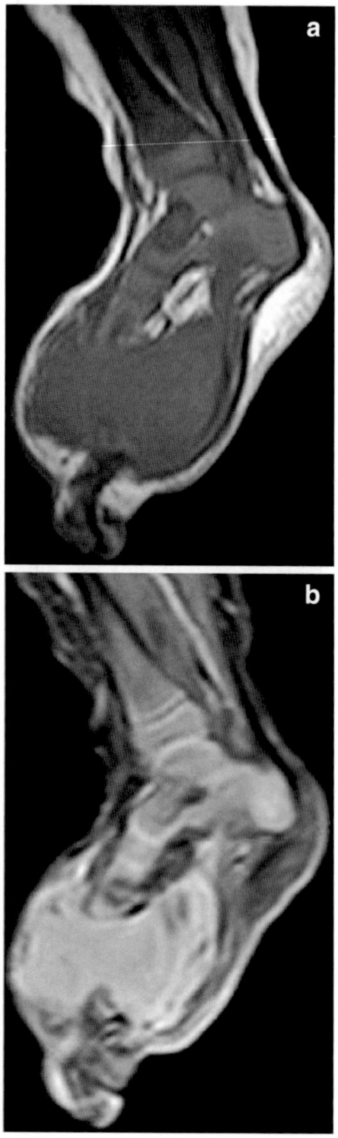

Fig. 6.32

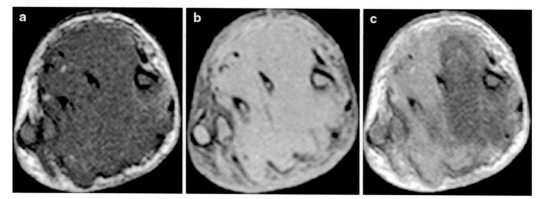

Fig. 6.31

A 1-month-old male infant presented with a rapid swelling of his foot to the emergency department. Physical examination revealed a firm warm mass in his left forefoot.

Fibrosarcomas are malignant tumors that predominantly arise in soft tissues. They are characterized by a cellular proliferation reproducing fibroblasts and are classified, when they occur in children, in the heterogeneous group of nonrhabdomyosarcoma malignant mesenchymal tumors. IFS occurs in the first 5 years of life, predominantly during the first year (approximately 5–10% of all sarcomas in infants younger than the age of 1 year), and in one-third of the cases is present at birth. Overall, IFS has a good prognosis; more than 80% of patients are usually cured. Metastatic spread is very rare, comprising 8% of reported pediatric cases, but local recurrence is a common problem, with a rate of 32%. There is no gender predilection. This tumor usually presents as a painless and rapidly enlarging mass with overlying reddish and/or ulcerated skin. The most frequent primary sites are the limbs, more common in the lower limb, and the trunk.

Ultrasound (US) shows a large heterogeneous hypervascular solid soft tissue mass with some cystic areas. Magnetic resonance imaging (MRI) demonstrates a nonencapsulated lesion with mixed architecture, heterogeneous intensity, and heterogeneous enhancement. The lesion is usually iso- to hypointense in T1WI and hyperintense on T2WI. IFS sometimes affects underlying bone with cortical thickening or osseous erosion; it also can infiltrate vasculonervous structures. These nonspecific imaging features can lead to misdiagnosis, and a biopsy must be done for diagnosis.

The differential diagnosis must include hemangioma and slow-flow vascular malformations (venolymphatic malformations). Hemangiomas have rapid postnatal growth followed by spontaneous involution. Slow-flow vascular malformations grow concomitantly with the child. US and MRI facilitate the differential diagnosis.

Although complete resection is rarely feasible at diagnosis, conservative surgery remains the mainstay treatment for infantile fibrosarcoma. Chemotherapy with an alkylating agent-free and anthracycline-free regimen is usually effective and should be chosen as first-line treatment for inoperable tumors.

Anteroposterior and oblique plain films of the right foot (Fig. 6.29a, b) show diaphyseal thinning of the second and third metatarsals with cortical erosion (*arrows*). TTransversal US in two differents planes ((Fig. 6.30a, b) depicts an ill-margined soft tissue mass in the first and second intermetatarsal spaces (*arrows*). Axial MRI demonstrates a huge tumor encasing and thinning the first three metatarsals; it is hypointense in T1-WI (Fig. 6.31a), hyperintense in DP-WI (Fig. 6.31b), and heterogeneous enhancement with a cystic/necrotic area (Fig. 6.31c). MRI demonstrates dorsoplantar extension of the soft tissue mass (Fig. 6.32a, b).

Case 9: Chondroblastoma

Pedro Torres Rubio and Daniel Azorín Cuadrillero

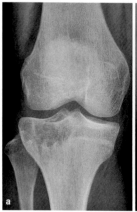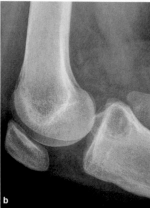

Fig. 6.33

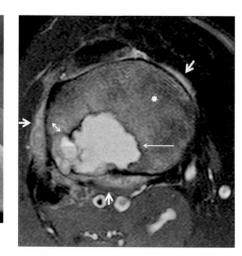

Fig. 6.35

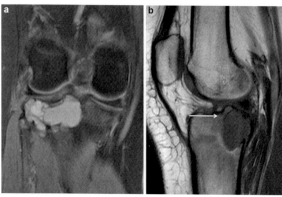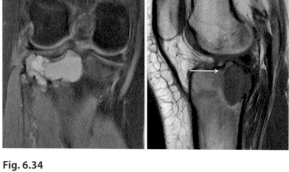

Fig. 6.34

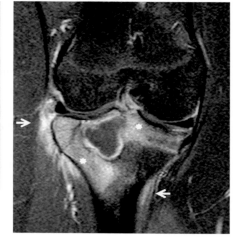

Fig. 6.36

A 14-year-old girl with knee pain.

Chondroblastoma is a benign, cartilage-producing neoplasm usually arising in the epiphysis and apophysis of skeletally immature patients. It is the third most common benign cartilaginous tumor, after enchondroma and osteochondroma. The most frequent locations are femur, tibia, and humerus. Clinical presentation usually includes local pain, swelling, and limited range of motion of the adjacent joint. These lesions are also common incidental findings.

Comments

In radiography, chondroblastoma is a well-defined osteolytic, geographic, subcortical lesion, mostly confined to the epiphysis with variable secondary metaphyseal extension. Diaphyseal and intracortical involvement is extremely rare. CT is useful to highlight the thin sclerotic rim, matrix mineralization, and chondroid calcifications. Other features are cortical bulging or erosion and, in some cases, transcortical extension. In MRI, the hallmark features are homogeneous hypointensity in T1-WI and heterogeneous, predominantly low signal, in T2-WI. T2 hypointense foci might correspond to immature chondroid matrix, hypercellularity of chondroblasts, calcifications, and hemosiderin deposition. T2 hyperintensity represents islands of hyaline cartilage or secondary aneurismal bone cyst (ABC in 15–30% of cases in some reviews). The enhancement within the tumor is not as marked as that of the surrounding reactive bone. Postcontrast enhancement might have a lobular, marginal, or septal pattern, the latter if there is a secondary ABC. Potentially misleading features are related to inflammatory changes in surrounding tissue: extensive perilesional edema and metaphyseal thick solid or laminated periosteal reaction (even in exclusive epiphyseal involvement). Soft tissue edema and joint effusion can also be present.

The differential diagnosis includes osteomyelitis, avascular necrosis, eosinophilic granuloma, giant cell tumor, and clear cell chondrosarcoma. The overlap of imaging features does not allow a reliable differentiation between chondroblastoma and clear cell chondrosarcoma, but chondrosarcoma is extremely rare in pediatric populations. The treatment consists of extensive curettage and replacement with bone graft.

(Fig. 6.33a, b). AP (a) and LAT (b) radiographs of the knee demonstrate a well-defined, geographic, and osteolytic lesion in the posterolateral aspect of tibial epiphysis. No periosteal reaction or soft tissue mass is depicted. (Fig. 6.34a). Coronal T2-WI with fat saturation shows a hyperintense lobulated lesion. (Fig. 6.34b). Sagittal PD demonstrates a homogeneous hypointense lesion with a peripheral dark rim (*long arrow*). (Fig. 6.35). Axial T2-WI with fat saturation illustrates the lobular margins of the lesion with extensive perilesional edema (star) and soft tissue involvement (*thick arrow*). There is also a secondary aneurysmal bone cyst with fluid-fluid level (*double arrowhead*). The peripheral hypointense rim is well depicted (*long arrow*). (Fig. 6.36). Coronal T1-WI with fat saturation postgadolinium shows a marked peripheral enhancement of the lesion. Extensive perilesional edema (*star*) and soft tissue involvement (*thick arrow*) with marked enhancement.

Imaging Findings

Case 10: Extraskeletal Chondroma

Miguel A. López Pino and Daniel Azorín Cuadrillero

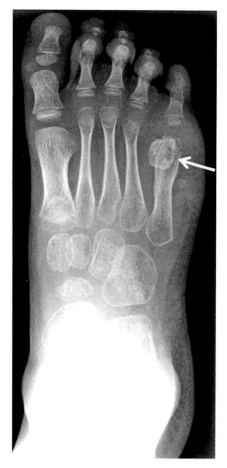

Fig. 6.37

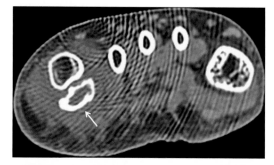

Fig. 6.38

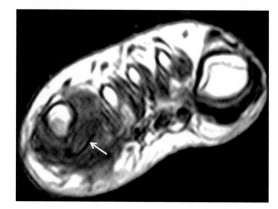

Fig. 6.39

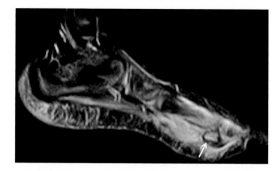

Fig. 6.40

A 6-year-old boy presented with a painful mass at the lateral aspect of the foot. Physical examination showed a firm, tender, and non-mobile mass. There was no history of trauma. The local temperature was normal, and the overlying skin was supple, with no dilated veins.

Comments

Soft tissue chondroma or extraskeletal chondroma is a relatively rare benign soft tissue tumor that usually occurs adjacent to periarticular tissues or tendosynovium, but unattached to bone.

Patients usually present with a slowly growing soft tissue mass. In approximately 20% of the patients, the lesion is painful and tender. The tumor mainly affects 30–60-year-old adults, but patients range in age from less than 1 year to more than 85 years of age.

Lesions are typically well demarcated and rarely exceed 2 cm in greatest dimension. The majority of extraskeletal chondromas are solitary. The most frequent sites are the hands and feet.

Chondromas are primarily cartilaginous lesions. They contain focal or diffuse calcification, and some of them show ossification.

The imaging features depend on the amount of calcification and the response of the surrounding tissues. Calcification is seen in 33–70% of lesions. Mineralization may be central or peripheral. Adjacent bone may show evidence of secondary remodeling. Plain films and CT scans nicely demonstrate the osseous nature of the mass. MRI shows a lobulated soft tissue mass of predominantly high signal intensity on T2-weighted images and signal void in calcified areas.

The differential diagnosis of soft tissue tumors with calcification includes several entities such as myositis ossificans, soft tissue chondrosarcoma, and synovial sarcoma. Typical chondroid calcifications can limit the differential diagnosis to cartilaginous tumors.

Marginal surgical excision is the treatment of choice. Recurrence is not uncommon (up to 18%). Recurrent tumors are best treated with reexcision.

Imaging Findings

Foot AP plain film (Fig. 6.37) demonstrates a soft tissue mass with calcification adjacent to the base of the fifth metatarsal (*arrow*).

Coronal CT scan (Fig. 6.38) shows the osseous mass with peripheral calcification (*arrow*).

Coronal T1-weighted MRI (Fig. 6.39) shows a well-defined, heterogeneous mass isointense to muscle (*arrow*). The mass displays high signal intensity on fat-suppressed T2-weighted MRI (*arrow*) (Fig. 6.40). The areas of decreased signal intensity on both pulse sequences correspond to calcifications.

Further Reading

Case 1: Discoid Lateral Meniscus with Tear

Book

Stoller DW et al (2004a) Discoid meniscus. Diagnostic imaging orthopaedics, 1st edn. Amirsys Inc, Salt Lake City, pp 5.2–5.5

Web Link

Emedicine. Discoid Meniscus. http://emedicine.medscape.com/article/1249111-overview#a0101

Articles

Anderson MW (2002) MR imaging of the meniscus. Radiol Clin North Am 40:1081–1094

Araki Y, Ashikaga R, Fujii K et al (1998) MR imaging of meniscal tears with discoid lateral meniscus. Eur J Radiol 27(2):153–160

Fox MG (2007) MR imaging of the meniscus. Radiol Clin North Am 45:1033–1053

Good CR, Green DW, Griffith MH et al (2007) Arthroscopic treatment of symptomatic discoid meniscus in children: classification, technique, and results. Arthroscopy 23:157–163

Rao SP, Rao SK, Paul R (2001) Clinical, radiologic, and arthroscopic assessment of discoid lateral meniscus. Arthroscopy 17:275–277

Rohren EM, Kosarek FJ, Helms CA (2001) Discoid lateral meniscus and the frequency of meniscal tears. Skeletal Radiol 30:316–320

Ryu KN, Kim IS, Kim EJ et al (1998) MR imaging of tears of discoid lateral menisci. Am J Roentgenol 171:963–967

Samoto N, Kozuma M, Tokuhisa T, Kobayasi K (2002) Diagnosis of discoid lateral meniscus of the knee on MR imaging. Magn Reson Imaging 20:59–64

Sanchez R, Strouse PJ (2009) The knee: MR imaging of uniquely pediatric disorders. Rad Clin North Am 47:1009–1028

Strouse PJ (2010) MRI of the knee: key points in the pediatric population. Pediatr Radiol 40:447–452

Case 2: Glenohumeral Dysplasia Following Neonatal Brachial Plexus Palsy

Book

Rockwood CA (2004) The shoulder, 3rd edn. Saunders, Philadelphia

Web Link

http://www.orthosupersite.com/view.aspx?rid=64872

Articles

Hogendoorn S, van Overvest KL, Watt I, Duijsens AH, Nelissen RG (2010) Structural changes in muscle and glenohumeral joint deformity in neonatal brachial plexus palsy. J Bone Joint Surg Am 92:935–942

Kozin SH (2004) Correlation between external rotation of the glenohumeral joint and deformity after brachial plexus birth palsy. J Pediatr Orthop 24:189–193

Kozin SH, Chafetz RS, Shaffer A, Soldado F, Filipone L (2010) Magnetic resonance imaging and clinical findings before and after tendon transfers about the shoulder in children with residual brachial plexus birth palsy: a 3-year follow-up study. J Pediatr Orthop 30:154–160

Pearl ML (2009) Shoulder problems in children with brachial plexus birth palsy: evaluation and management. J Am Acad Orthop Surg 17:242–254

Pearl ML, Edgerton BW (1998) Glenoid deformity secondary to brachial plexus birth palsy. J Bone Joint Surg Am 80:659–667

Pöyhiä TH, Nietosvaara YA, Remes VM, Kirjavainen MO, Peltonen JI, Lamminen AE (2005) MRI of rotator cuff muscle atrophy in relation to glenohumeral joint incongruence in brachial plexus birth injury. Pediatr Radiol 35:402–409

Pöyhiä TH, Lamminen AE, Peltonen JI, Kirjavainen MO, Willamo PJ, Nietosvaara Y (2010) Brachial plexus birth injury: US screening for glenohumeral joint instability. Radiology 254:253–260

Soldado F, Kozin SH (2005) The relationship between the coracoid and glenoid after brachial plexus birth palsy. J Pediatr Orthop 25:666–670

Van Gelein Vitringa VM, van Kooten EO, Mullender MG, van Doorn-Loogman MH, van der Sluijs JA (2009) An MRI study on the relations between muscle atrophy, shoulder function and glenohumeral deformity in shoulders of children with obstetric brachial plexus injury. J Brachial Plex Peripher Nerve Inj 4:5

Waters PM, Smith GR, Jaramillo D (1998) Glenohumeral deformity secondary to brachial plexus birth palsy. J Bone Joint Surg Am 80:668–677

Case 3: Transient Lateral Patellar Dislocation

Book

Kan JH, Kleinman PK (2007) Case 1. Acute lateral patellar dislocation. Pediatric and adolescent musculoskeletal MRI – a case based approach, 1st edn. Springer Science + Business Media LLC, New York, pp 1–6

Web Link

Emedicine. Patellar Injury and Dislocation. http://emedicine.medscape.com/article/90068-overview

Articles

Arnbjornsoson A, Egund N, Ryding O et al (1992) The natural history of recurrent dislocation of the patella: long-term results of conservative and operative treatment. J Bone Joint Surg 74B:140–142

Balcarek P et al (2011) Patellar dislocations in children, adolescents and adults: a comparative MRI study of medial patellofemoral ligament injury patterns and trochlear groove anatomy. Eur J Radiol 79:415–420. doi:10.1016/j.ejrad.2010.06.042

Buncher M, Baudendistel B, Sabo D et al (2005) Acute traumatic primary patellar dislocation: long-term results comparing conservative and surgical treatment. Clin J Sport Med 15:62–66

Davis KW (2010) Imaging pediatric sports injuries: lower extremity. Radiol Clin North Am 48: 1213–1235

Diederichs G, Issever AS, Scheffler S (2010) MR imaging of patellar instability: injury patterns and assessment of risk factors. Radiographics 30:961–981

Elias DA, White LM, Fithian DC (2002) Acute lateral patellar dislocation at MR imaging: injury patterns of medial patellar soft tissue restraints and osteochondral injuries of the inferomedial patella. Radiology 225:736–743

Kirsch MD, Fitzgerald SW, Friedman H, Rogers L (1993) Transient lateral patellar dislocation: diagnosis with MR imaging. Am J Radiol 161:109–113

Nomura E, Horiuchi Y, Inoue M (2002) Correlation of MR imaging findings and open exploration of medial patella femoral ligament injuries in acute patellar dislocations. Knee 9:139–143

Sanchez R, Strouse PJ (2009) The knee: MR imaging of uniquely pediatric disorders. Rad Clin North Am 47:1009–1028

Sanders TG, Paruchuri NB, Zlatkin MB (2006) MRI of osteochondral defects of the lateral femoral condyle: incidence and pattern of injury after transient lateral dislocation of the patella. Am J Roentgenol 187(5):1332–1337

Case 4: Osteochondritis Dissecans of the Knee

Book

Lane Donnelly (2005) Osteochondritis dissecans. Diagnostic imaging: pediatrics. 1st ed. Elsevier-Masson, Estados Unidos, p 6/166–6/169

Web Link

http://www.mayoclinic.com/health/osteochondritis-dissecans/DS00741

Articles

Bohndorf K (1998) Osteochondritis (osteochondrosis) dissecans: a review and new MRI classification. Eur Radiol 8:103–112

Cain EL, Clancy WG (2001) Treatment algorithm for osteochondral injuries of the knee. Clin Sports Med 20:321–342

Chambers HG, Shea KG, Carey JL (2011) AAOS Clinical Practice Guideline: diagnosis and treatment of osteochondritis dissecans. J Am Acad Orthop Surg 19:307–309

Flynn JM, Kocher MS, Ganley TJ (2004) Osteochondritis dissecans of the knee. J Pediatr Orthop 24:434–443

Gold GE, McCauley TR, Gray ML, Disler DG (2003) Special focus session: what's new in cartilage? RadioGraphics 23:1227–1242

Kijowski R, Blankerbaker DG, Shinki K et al (2008) Juvenile versus adult osteochondritis dissecans of the knee: appropriate MR imaging criteria for instability. Radiology 248:571–578

Kocher MS, Tucker R, Ganley TJ, Flynn JM (2006) Management of osteochondritis dissecans of the knee: current concepts review. Am J Sports Med 34:1181–1191

O'Connor MA, Palaniappan M, Khan N, Bruce CE (2002) Osteochondritis dissecans of the knee in children: a comparison of MRI and arthroscopic findings. J Bone Joint Surg Br 84:258–262

Pill SG, Ganley TJ, Milam RA, Lou JE, Meyer JS, Flynn JM (2003) Role of magnetic resonance imaging and clinical criteria in predicting successful nonoperative treatment of osteochondritis dissecans in children. J Pediatr Orthop 23:102–108

Robertson W, Kelly BT, Green DW (2003) Osteochondritis dissecans of the knee in children. Curr Opin Pediatr 15:38–44

Case 5: Hemophilic Arthropaty and Magnetic Resonance Imaging

Book

Roberts HR (2007) Haemophilia and haemostasis: a case-based approach to management, 1st edn. Blackwell, Malden

Web Link

Haemophilia. The official journal of the world federation of haemophilia. http://www.wiley.com/bw/journal.asp?ref=1351-8216

Articles

Dardzinski BJ, Schmithorst VJ, Klosterman L, Graham TB (2002) Mapping T2 relaxation time in the pediatric knee: feasibility with a clinical 1.5-T MR imaging system. Radiology 225:233–239

Doria AS (2010) State-of-the-art imaging techniques for the evaluation of haemophilic arthropathy: present and future. Haemophilia 16(Suppl 5):107–114

Doria AS, Babyn PS, Lundin B, Kilcoyne RF, Miller S, Rivard GE et al (2006) Reliability and construct validity of the compatible MRI scoring system for evaluation of haemophilic knees and ankles of haemophilic children. Expert MRI working group of the international prophylaxis study group. Haemophilia 12:503–513

Gold GE, McCauley TR, Gray ML, Disler DG (2003) Special focus session: what's new in cartilage? RadioGraphics 23:1227–1242

Jelbert A, Vaidya S, Fotiadis N (2009) Imaging and staging of haemophilic arthropathy. Clin Radiol 64:1119–1128

Kerr R (2003) Imaging of musculoskeletal complications of hemophilia. Semin Musculoskelet Radiol 7:127–136

Lundin B, Babyn P, Doria AS, Kilcoyne R, Ljung R, Millar S et al (2005) Compatible scales for progressive and additive MRI assessments of haemophilic arthropathy. Haemophilia 11:109–115

Martínez León MI (2009) El diagnóstico de la artropatía inicial en niños hemofílicos. Diagnóstico por imagen: RM. VI Jornadas de Hemostasia. Haematologica (Spanish Ed) 94(suppl 2):21–23

Querol Fuentes F, Aparisi Rodríguez F (2007) Unificación de criterios de valoración de la resonancia magnética en hemofilia. Haematologica (Spanish Ed) 92:31–41

Soler R, López Fernández F, Rodríguez E, Marino M (2002) Hemophilic arthropathy. A scoring system for magnetic resonance imaging. Eur Radiol 12:836–843

Case 6: Osteomyelitis

Book

Stoller DW et al (2004b) Osteomyelitis, elbow. Diagnostic imaging orthopaedics, 1st edn. Amirsys Inc, Salt Lake City, pp 2.98–2.101

Web link

http://www.posna.org/education/StudyGuide/gn_infection.asp

Articles

Averill LW, Hernandez A, Gonzalez L, Peña AH, Jaramillo D (2009) Diagnosis of osteomyelitis in children: utility of fat-suppressed contrast-enhanced MRI. Am J Roetgenol 192:1232–1238

Browne LP, Mason EO, Kaplan SL, Cassady CI, Krishnamurthy R, Guillerman RP (2008) Optimal imaging strategy for community-acquired *Staphylococcus aureus* musculoskeletal infections in children. Pediatr Radiol 38:841–847

Harik NS, Smeltzer MS (2010) Management of acute hematogenous osteomyelitis in children. Expert Rev Anti Infect Ther 8:175–181

Jaramillo D (2011) Infection: musculoskeletal. Pediatr Radiol 41:S127–S134

Jennin F, Bousson V, Parlier C, Jomaah N, Khanine V, Laredo JD (2011) Bony sequestrum: a radiologic review. Skeletal Radiol 40:963–975

Johson DP, Hernanz-Schulman M, Martus JE, Lovejoy SA, Yu C, Kan JH (2011) Significance of epiphyseal cartilage enhancement defects in pediatric osteomyelitis identified by MRI with surgical correlation. Pediatr Radiol 41:355–361

Kao FC, Lee ZL, Kao HC, Hung SS, Huang YC (2003) Acute primary hematogenous osteomyelitis of the epiphysis: report of two cases. Chang Gung Med J 26:851–856

McGuinness B, Wilson N, Doyle AJ (2007) The "penumbra sign" on T1-weighted MRI for differentiating musculoskeletal infection from tumour. Skeletal Radiol 36:417–421

Offiah AC (2006) Acute osteomyelitis, septic arthritis and discitis: differences between neonates and older children. Eur J Radiol 60:221–232

Pruthi S, Thapa MM (2009) Infectious and inflammatory disorders. Radiol Clin North Am 47:911–926

Case 7: Intramuscular Venous Malformation

Book

Weiss SW, Goldblum JR (2008a) Benign tumors and tumor-like lesions of blood vessels. In: Weiss SW, Goldblum JR (eds) Enzinger & Weiss's soft tissue tumors. Mosby Elsevier, St. Louis, pp 633–679

Weblink

http://www.novanews.org/

Articles

Dubois J, Alison M (2010) Vascular anomalies: what a radiologist needs to know. Pediatr Radiol 40:895–905

Fayad L, Hazirolan T, Bluemke D, Mitchell S (2006) Vascular malformations in the extremities: emphasis on MR imaging features that guide treatment options. Skeletal Radiol 35:127–137

Fishman SJ, Mulliken JB (1993) Hemangiomas and vascular malformations of infancy and childhood. Pediatr Clin North Am 40:1177–1200

Hein KD, Mulliken JB, Kozakewich HPW, Upton J, Burrows PE (2002) Venous malformations of skeletal muscle. Plast Reconstr Surg 110:1625–1635

Hyodoh H, Hori M, Akiba H, Tamakawa M, Hyodoh K, Hareyama M (2005) Peripheral vascular malformations: imaging, treatment approaches, and therapeutic issues. Radiographics 25:159–171

Paltiel HJ, Burrows PE, Kozakewich HP, Zurakowski D, Mulliken JB (2000) Soft-tissue vascular anomalies: utility of US for diagnosis. Radiology 214:747–754

Rivas S, López-Gutiérrez JC, Díaz M, Andrés AM, Ros Z (2006) Malformaciones venosas. Importancia de su diagnóstico y su tratamiento en la infancia. Cir Pediatr 19:77–80

Steven M, Kumaran N, Carachi R, Desai A, Bennet G (2007) Haemangiomas and vascular malformations of the limb in children. Pediatr Surg Int 23:565–569

Theruvil B, Kapoor V, Thalava R, Nag HL, Kotwal PP (2004) Vascular malformations in muscles around the knee presenting as knee pain. Knee 11:155–158

Trop I, Dubois J, Guibaud L et al (1999) Soft-tissue venous malformations in pediatric and young adult patients: diagnosis with Doppler US. Radiology 212:841–845

so-called fibrohistiocytic, muscular, lymphomatous, neurogenic, hair matrix, and uncertain origin. Radiographics 29, e-36. http://radiographics.rsna.org/content/29/4/e36.full

Navarro OM, Laffman EE, Ngan B (2009) Pediatric soft-tissue tumors and pseudotumors: MR imaging features with pathognomonic correlation. Part1. Imaging approach, pseudotumors, vascular lesions, and adipocytic tumors. Radiographics 29:887–906

Orbach D, Rey A, Cecchetto G, Oberlin O, Casanova M, Thebaud E et al (2010) Infantile fibrosarcoma: management based on the European experience. J Clin Oncol 28:318–323

Sultan I, Casanova M, Al-Jumaily U, Meazza C, Rodriguez-Galindo C, Ferrari A (2010) Soft tissue sarcomas in the first year of life. Eur J Cancer 46:2449–2456

Wu JS, Hochman MG (2009) Soft-tissue tumors and tumorlike lesions: a systematic imaging approach. Radiology 253:297–316

Case 8: Infantile Fibrosarcoma (IFS)

Book

Okcu M, Pappo A, Hicks J, Million L, Anddrassy R, Spunt S (2011) The nonrhabdomyosarcoma soft tissue sarcomas. In: Pizzo P, Poplack D (eds) Principles and practice of pediatric oncology, 6th edn. Lippincott Williams and Wilkins, Philadelphia, pp 954–986

Web Link

http://www.cancer.gov/cancertopics/pdq/treatment/child-soft-tissue-sarcoma/HealthProfessional

Articles

Alymlahi E, Dafiri R (2004) Congenital-infantile fibrosarcoma: imaging features and differential diagnoses. Eur J Radiol 51:37–42

Canale A, Vanel DS, Couanet D, Patte C, Caramella C, Dromain C (2009) Infantile fibrosarcoma: magnetic resonance imaging findings in six cases. Eur J Radiol 72:30–37

Demir HA, Akyüz C, Varan A, Ergen FB, Büyükpamukçu M (2010) Right foot congenital infantile fibrosarcoma treated only with chemotherapy. Pediatr Blood Cancer 54:618–620

Fink AM, Stringer DA, Cairns RA, Nadel HR, Magee JF (1995) Pediatric case of the day. Congenital fibrosarcoma (CFS). Radiographics 15:243–246

Kurkubasche AG, Halvorson EG, Forman EN, Terek RM, Ferguson WS (2000) The role of preoperative chemotherapy in the treatment of infantile fibrosarcoma. J Pediatr Surg 35:880–883

Laffan EE, Ngan B, Navarro OM (2009) Pediatric soft-tissue tumors and pseudotumors: MR imaging features with pathognomonic correlation. Part 2. Tumors of fibroblastic/myofibroblastic,

Case 9: Chondroblastoma

Book

Greenspan A, Jundt G, Remagen W (2007) Cartilage (chondrogenic) lesions. In: Differential diagnosis in orthopedic oncology, 2nd edn. Lippincott Williams & Wilkins, Philadelphia, pp 199–207

Web Link

Emedicine. Chondroblastoma Imaging. http://emedicine.medscape.com/article/388632-overview

Articles

Azorín D, González-Mediero I, Colmenero I, De Prada I, López-Barea F (2006) Diaphyseal chondroblastoma in a long bone: first report. Skeletal Radiol 35:49–52

Blancas C, Llauger J, Palmer J, Valverde S (2008) Manifestaciones radiológicas del condroblastoma. Radiologia 50:416–423

Jee WH, Park YK, McCauley TR et al (1999) Chondroblastoma: MR characteristics with pathologic correlation. J Comput Assist Tomogr 23:721–726

Kaim AH, Hügli R, Bonél HM, Jundt G (2002) Chondroblastoma and clear cell chondrosarcoma: radiological and MRI characteristics with histopathological correlation. Skeletal Radiol 31:88–95

Kilpatrick SE, Parisien M, Bridge JA (2002) Chondroblastoma. In: Fletcher CDM, Unni KK, Mertens F (eds) World Health Organization classification of tumours. Pathology and genetics of tumours of soft tissue and bone. IARC Press, Lyon, pp 241–242

Maheshwari AV, Jelinek JS, Song AJ, Nelson KJ, Murphey MD, Henshaw RM (2011) Metaphyseal and diaphyseal chondroblastomas. Skeletal Radiol 40:1563–1573

Rybak LD, Rosenthal DI, Wittig JC (2009) Chondroblastoma: radiofrequency ablation–alternative to surgical resection in selected cases. Radiology 251:599–604

Suneja R, Grimer RJ, Belthur M, Jeys L, Carter SR, Tillman RM et al (2005) Chondroblastoma of bone long – term results and functional outcome after intralesional curettage. J Bone Joint Surg Br 87:974–978

Weatherall PT, Maale GE, Mendelsohn DB, Sherry CS, Erdman WE, Pascoe HR (1994) Chondroblastoma: classic and confusing appearance at MR imaging. Radiology 190:467–474

Wootton-Gorges SL (2009) MR imaging of primary bone tumors and tumor-like conditions in children. Radiol Clin North Am 47:957–975

Case 10: Extraskeletal Chondroma

Book

Weiss SW, Goldblum JR (2008b) Cartilagineous soft tissue tumors. In: Weiss LM, Goldblum JR (eds) Enzinger and Weiss's soft tissue tumours, 5th edn. Mosby, St Louis, pp 1017–1023

Web Link

http://www.iarc.fr/en/publications/pdfs-online/pat-gen/index.php

Articles

Bansal M, Goldman AB, DiCarlo EF, McCormack R (1993) Soft tissue chondromas: diagnosis and differential diagnosis. Skeletal Radiol 22:309–315

Chung EB, Enzinger FM (1978) Chondroma of soft parts. Cancer 41:1414–1424

Dahlin DC, Salvador AH (1974) Cartilaginous tumors of the soft tissues of the hands and feet. Mayo Clin Proc 49:721–726

Demir MK, Unlu E, Usta U (2008) A curious mass of the anterior compartment in the knee. Br J Radiol 82:435–437

González-Lois C, García-de-la-Torre P, SantosBriz-Terrón A, Vilá J, Manrique-Chico J, Martínez-Tello J (2001) Intracapsular and para-articular chondroma adjacent to large joints: report of three cases and review of the literature. Skeletal Radiol 30:672–676

Kransdorf MJ, Meis JM (1993) From the archives of the AFIP. Extraskeletal osseous and cartilaginous tumors of the extremities. Radiographics 13:853–884

Kudawara I, Ueda T, Araki N (2001) Extraskeletal chondroma around the knee. Clin Radiol 56:779–782

Liu ZJ, Zhao Q, Zhang LJ (2010) Extraskeletal osteochondroma near the hip: a pediatric case. J Pediatr Orthop B 19:524–528

Papagelopoulos PJ, Savvidou OD, Mavrogenis AF, Chloros GD, Papaparaskeva KT, Soucacos PN (2007) Extraskeletal chondroma of the foot. Joint Bone Spine 74:285–288

Sheff JS, Wang S (2005) Extraskeletal osteochondroma of the foot. J Foot Ankle Surg 44:57–59

Contents

M.I. Martínez-León et al., *Imaging for Pediatricians*, Imaging for Clinicians,
DOI 10.1007/978-3-642-28629-2_7, © Springer-Verlag Berlin Heidelberg 2012

Case 1: Percutaneous Ultrasound-Guided Liver Biopsy

Carmen Gallego Herrero and Enrique Medina Benítez

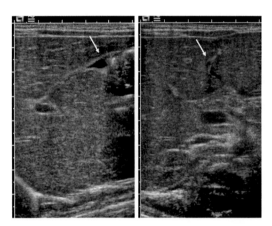

Fig. 7.1

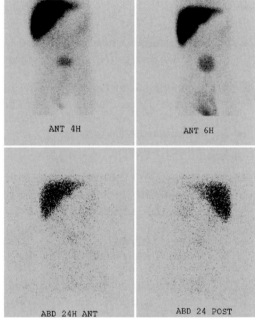

Fig. 7.2

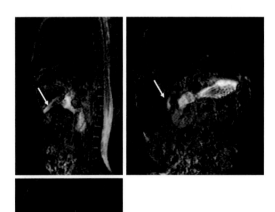

Fig. 7.4

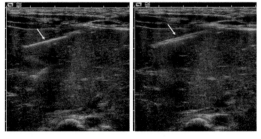

Fig. 7.3

A 1-month 3-week-old infant with a history of neonatal jaundice, cholestasis, and acholia is admitted to our hospital to rule out biliary atresia and further treatment. Physical examination demonstrates mild mucocutaneous jaundice and hepatomegaly.

Comments

Neonatal jaundice is a frequent problem for pediatricians and neonatologists. Most children have unconjugated hyperbilirubinemia of benign and physiologic nature. By contrast, conjugated bilirubinemia greater than 1.5–2 mg/dl or more than 20% of total bilirubinemia is pathologic and termed neonatal cholestasis. Cholestasis refers to impairment of bile flow anywhere along its pathway, from secretion by the hepatocyte to its delivery to the duodenal lumen. Most common etiologies of neonatal cholestasis include sepsis, total parenteral nutrition, and/or drug induced in the premature infant, extrahepatic biliary atresia, idiopathic neonatal hepatitis, α-1-antitrypsin deficiency, and intrahepatic cholestasis syndromes (progressive familial intrahepatic cholestasis and others). Biliary atresia consists in obliteration or discontinuity of the biliary system that leads to obstruction to bile flow. It is the most common neonatal cholestatic disorder, with a disease prevalence of 1/800 Asian to 1/18,000 European live births, and the leading cause of liver transplant in children. Moderate elevations of total bilirubin are typical, with direct (conjugated) bilirubin representing around 50–60% of total. GGT and transaminases are elevated. Acholia after birth or some weeks later is typical. Congenital forms of BA may associate situs inversus or heterotaxia syndromes.

Imaging Findings

Ultrasound may demonstrate an absent or hypoplastic gallbladder remnant (*arrow*) (Fig. 7.1), but both sensitivity and specificity are less than 80%. Although hepatic nuclear scintiscan (Fig. 7.2) with TC-labeled DISIDA demonstrates absence of intestinal excretion of the radiolabel, it may have a false-positive and false-negative rate of around 10%. MR (Fig. 7.3) can also help in diagnosis, although false positives have been reported in some series due to the small spatial resolution of the technique, the small size of the bile ducts (*gallbladder, arrows*) and motion artifacts. Percutaneous liver biopsy is regarded as the most useful single procedure in the evaluation of neonatal cholestasis with low morbidity rates, especially in the absence of coagulopathy. Ultrasound-guided liver biopsy is nowadays preferred to the blind technique. A safe area of the liver is selected by ultrasound scanning, and the biopsy (*arrows*) is performed under ultrasound guidance (Fig. 7.4). Intraoperative cholangiography demonstrates the patency of the biliary system. It is performed when the results of the biopsy are equivocal or suggest an obstruction or when the scintiscan fails to demonstrate patency of the bile ducts.

Case 2: Sonographically Guided Transrectal Drainage

Carmen Gallego Herrero and María López Díaz

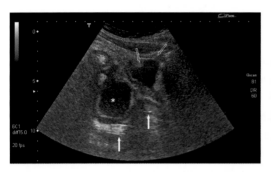

Fig. 7.5

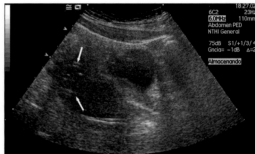

Fig. 7.7

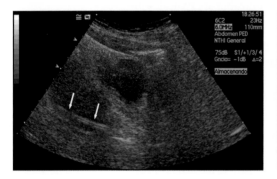

Fig. 7.6

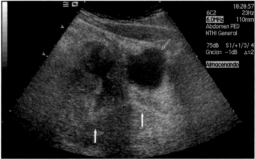

Fig. 7.8

An 11-year-old boy is admitted to the emergency department with fever and malaise 15 days after laparoscopic surgery for gangrenous appendicitis. Abdominal ultrasound demonstrates an abscess at Douglas' pouch. A sonographically guided transrectal drainage of the abscess is performed under general anesthesia.

Douglas' pouch abscesses are infrequent in children and most of them secondary to perforated appendicitis.

Treatment of peritoneal abscesses consists in a combination of antibiotics and drainage. Only small abscesses (<1–3 cm) would benefit from antibiotherapy alone. Drainage is indicated when signs of infection, pain, constipation, or bowel obstruction are present, whether the fluid collection is infected or not. A few contraindications are found for radiologically guided drainage: coagulation anomalies can be corrected before the procedure; unsafe access route to fluid collection is the only contraindication of the technique. Transrectal drainage is a well-known technique among surgeons, who used to perform it blindly: a drain is advanced from the anus through the rectum into the abscess. However, many surgeons do not feel confident with a blind technique and would rather drain those abscesses by opening the peritoneum a second time.

Abdominal US-guided transrectal drainage increases the safety of the technique. With a single-step trocar, the whole process can be controlled with transabdominal ultrasound, obviating the use of radiation; it also avoids complications such us peritoneal fecal spillage with needle withdrawal and dilatation, which would potentially happen with a Seldinger technique.

Transrectal drains are well tolerated by children when awake. The catheter is secured to the patient's thigh and may be locked to prevent dislodgement. Retrieval is done according to the surgeon's criteria. Spontaneous dislodgement during a bowel movement may occur, especially if the catheter is left unlocked. For that reason, draining as much pus as possible during the procedure is advisable.

(Fig. 7.5). A unilocular abscess (*asterisk*) is seen in the rectovesical space. *White arrows*: rectum; *white opened arrows*: bladder. The drainage catheter and trocar (*arrows*) is advanced through the rectum into the lower part of the abscess (Fig. 7.6). The trocar and stylet are removed and the catheter coils (*arrows*) in the upper part of the abscess (Fig. 7.7). A complete resolution of the abscess is demonstrated after drainage of a total of 50 cc of purulent material (Fig. 7.8). *Opened white arrows*: bladder; *solid white arrows*: rectum.

Case 3: Percutaneous Cecostomy

Mark J. Hogan

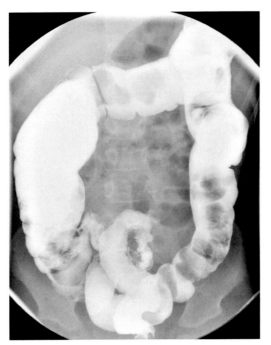

Fig. 7.9

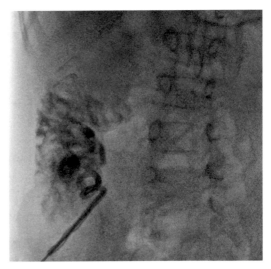

Fig. 7.11

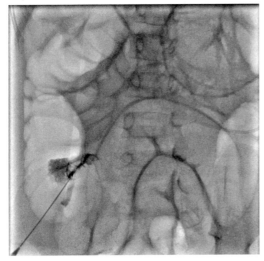

Fig. 7.10

Fig. 7.12

A 6-year-old male with myelomeningocele presenting with constipation. He currently takes polyethylene glycol 3350 orally and receives rectal enemas every evening, but it is difficult on the family and it may take several hours before a bowel movement.

Encopresis can be a difficult condition to treat. Etiologies include spinal cord abnormalities (myelomeningocele, caudal regression, tethered cord, and posttraumatic injury), anatomic colonic pathology, physiologic abnormalities, and behavioral issues. Colonic issues are seen in patients with prior surgery for imperforate anus or Hirschsprung's disease. Pseudoobstruction and other motility problems can also be causative. Symptoms may be from the difficulty in defecation such as abdominal distension or bleeding from rectal fissures, or the patient may have fecal soiling from liquid stool bypassing the retained feces. Multiple treatments are often attempted including dietary modification, laxatives, enemas, and digital disimpaction; however, these are not universally successful. The MACE (Malone antegrade continence enema) procedure was invented to provide for better elimination by irrigating the entire colon in an antegrade approach from the cecum. Since the colon usually takes a day to refill with stool, the risk of fecal soiling is greatly reduced. Percutaneous cecostomy was then developed to provide the same access to the cecum, but avoiding laparotomy. It has similar excellent results as the MACE procedure, but less invasive. Prior to performance of the procedure, a barium enema is obtained to confirm the cecal position. Outpatient consultation is then performed to explain the procedure and the risks and benefits. The patient is on a clear liquid diet for 2 days prior to the procedure. The colon is cleaned out with a laxative. The patient is placed on antibiotics immediately before the procedure, and these are continued for 48 h. Anesthesia or sedation is required.

A barium enema prior to the procedure confirms the position of the cecum (Fig. 7.9). During the procedure, an enema tip is placed in the colon for insufflation. Glucagon is provided for bowel paralysis. Local anesthesia is administered. The colon is then inflated, and a needle is advanced into the colon (Fig. 7.10). The position is confirmed by injecting contrast. After deployment of two suture anchors, the tract is dilated over a wire and a pigtail catheter placed into the colon (Fig. 7.11). The patient remains in the hospital until taking adequate enteral nutrition and completing the antibiotic course. Sutures are cut at 1 week, and at 6 weeks the pigtail catheter is exchanged for a button device (Fig. 7.12).

Case 4: Ultrasound-Guided Corticosteroid Injection Therapy for Juvenile Idiopathic Arthritis

Mabel García-Hidalgo
and Begoña Losada

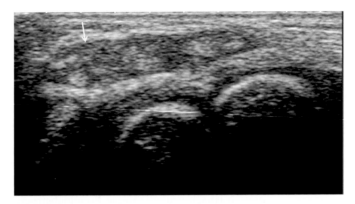

Fig. 7.13

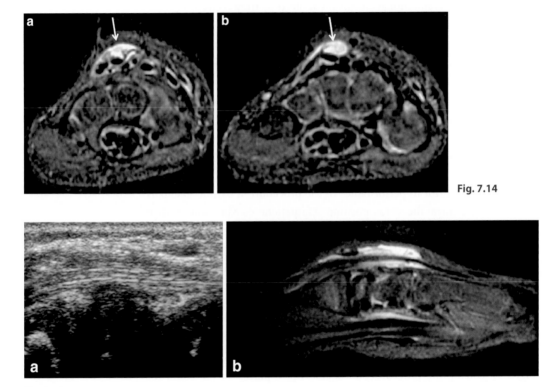

Fig. 7.14

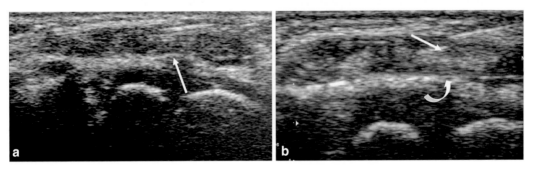

Fig. 7.15

Fig. 7.16

A 3-year-old girl with juvenile idiopathic arthritis (JIA) presented with left elbow, bilateral knee, and bilateral wrist involvement. Initial treatment was oral ibuprofen followed by arthrocentesis and intra-articular steroid injections into both knees. Clinical improvement was seen in all areas except the left wrist. Dorsal left wrist pain and swelling, refractory to methotrexate therapy, prompted ultrasound (US) and magnetic resonance (MR) imaging that showed inflammation in the common extensor tendon sheaths of the fingers. Ultrasound-guided corticosteroid injection of the tendon sheath was performed with immediate and prolonged symptom relief.

Comments

JIA is the most common pediatric rheumatologic condition. Symptoms vary depending on the type of JIA but principally include debilitating joint pain, stiffness, and occasionally deformity that limits physical and social activity.

Diagnostic US is useful to demonstrate pannus, joint effusions, articular erosions, extra-articular soft tissue swelling, and tendon sheath inflammation. It helps to localize the source of the inflammation, especially in children. US is also useful therapeutically to guide articular, tendon sheath, and occasionally bursal corticosteroid injections. The procedure is done under sedation, injecting triamcinolone acetonide without local anesthetic. US guidance helps ensure that the steroids are injected into the source of the inflammation.

Although tendon sheaths can be treated without image guidance, direct puncture of the tendon with intratendinous infiltration of corticosteroid may cause tendon injury that can be permanent. Direct US visualization of the needle tip in the tendon sheath during the injection helps to avoid this complication.

US-guided corticosteroid injection is beneficial as a targeted adjunctive therapy for patients with arthritic symptoms refractory to systemic therapy. It greatly reduces local joint inflammation and can help to limit toxicities of systemic medical therapy.

Imaging Findings

Transverse US of the left wrist demonstrates significant inflammation in the common extensor tendon sheath of the fingers (*arrow*) (Fig. 7.13). Corresponding axial STIR MR images display similar findings (*arrows*) (Fig. 7.14a, b). Longitudinal US of the wrist (Fig. 7.15a) and sagittal STIR MR image (Fig. 7.15b) show fluid and pannus surrounding the extensor tendons. US images show 25-G needle (*straight arrow*) in the tendon sheath (Fig. 7.16a) avoiding the body of the tendon and injection of echogenic corticosteroid (*curved arrows*) (Fig. 7.16b). Triamcinolone drops are very echogenic and easily seen by US.

Case 5: Osteoid Osteoma

James W. Murakami

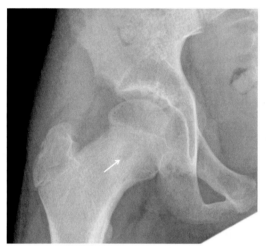

Fig. 7.17

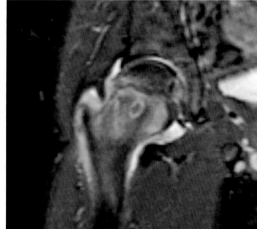

Fig. 7.18

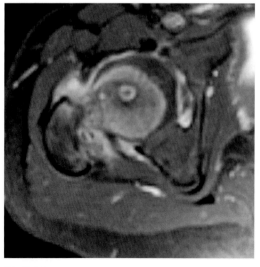

Fig. 7.19

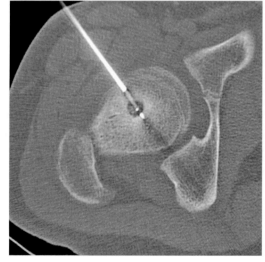

Fig. 7.20

A 14-year-old boy presents with a 6-month history of progressive right hip pain.

An osteoid osteoma (OO) is a small painful bone tumor most often found in children and young adults. These lesions characteristically cause bone pain, which is worse at night and is relieved, at least initially, by nonsteroidal anti-inflammatory agents.

On plain film and CT, an OO commonly appears as a small lucent nidus occasionally with internal calcifications and surrounding sclerosis and periostitis. Profound increased uptake of radiotracer is usually observed with radionuclide skeletal scintigraphy. On MR, there is usually a large area of bone edema and enhancement around the nidus. The nidus can be hard to see on MR if there is central mineralization. Imaging differential diagnosis includes osteomyelitis with a small abscess and a stress fracture.

An OO can be managed medically with anti-inflammatory drugs, but it is usually managed surgically due to the relatively long time before symptom regression. Historically, treatment was surgical resection. Current operative management is more commonly carried out by interventional radiologists employing image-guided radiofrequency (RF) ablation. First described in 1989, this technique uses CT guidance to place a 14-G guiding needle into the nidus. After obtaining a bone biopsy, an RF electrode with a relatively short burning tip, such as a 10 mm tip, is inserted across the center of the nidus and heated to 90°C for approximately 6 min. Complete clinical success with RF ablation is around 90% with a single treatment.

Comments

Right hip radiograph shows 8-mm lucent nidus with central mineralization in the femoral metaphysis with surrounding sclerosis (*arrow*) (Fig. 7.17). Edema is seen throughout the femoral neck and a hip effusion is evident on coronal STIR MR image (Fig. 7.18). Axial contrast-enhanced T1-weighted MR image shows extensive enhancement of the femoral neck and synovium (Fig. 7.19). CT image during RF ablation demonstrates RF electrode placed through the guiding needle and across the nidus (Fig. 7.20).

Imaging Findings

Case 6: Percutaneous Sclerosis of Lymphangioma

Carmen Gallego Herrero and Dolores Delgado

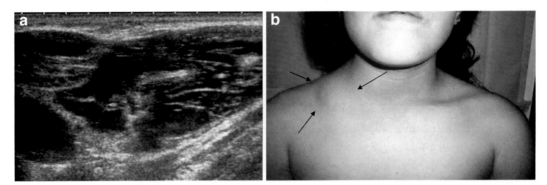

Fig. 7.21

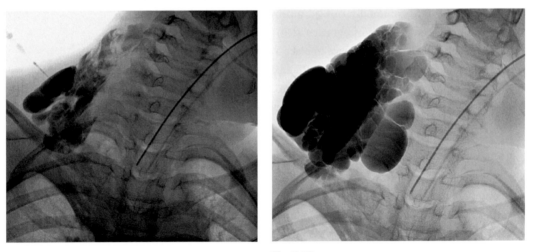

Fig. 7.22   Fig. 7.23

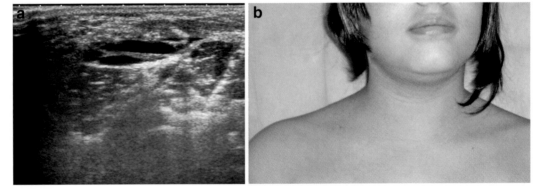

Fig. 7.24

A 6-year-old girl with a sudden onset of a lump in the neck, related to complicated cystic lymphangioma, is admitted to our hospital to perform a percutaneous sclerosis of the malformation.

Lymphangiomas are localized congenital malformations of the lymphatic channels, consisting of fluid-filled lymphatic spaces. They can be divided into macrocystic and microcystic, depending on the predominant cyst size (> or < than 1 cm). Although present at birth, they may manifest later in infancy. Around 70–80% are located in the head/neck and axillary regions. They present as ill-defined asymptomatic subcutaneous lesions that grow overtime. Pain and tenderness is usually secondary to complications such as bleeding or infection. Other complications depend on the size and location of the lymphangioma: airway obstruction, dysphagia, poor dental hygiene, skeletal hypertrophy, cutaneous oozing, vaginal discharge, or subcutaneous hypertrophy. Radiological studies help confirm the diagnosis. Ultrasound demonstrates the predominant cystic size and the absence of flow in the cysts. Vascular flow is only seen within the septa of the malformation. MRI delineates the extent of the disease and may distinguish between venous and lymphatic components in cases of complex combined low flow malformations such as in Klippel-Trenaunay syndrome. Treatment of these lesions can be frustrating and complex. A multidisciplinary approach is advisable. Surgery, sclerosis, laser ablation, and radiofrequency ablation are commonly used either alone or combined, depending on size and location of the lymphangioma. Sclerosing agents are varied and include alcohol, bleomycin, doxycycline, detergents such as sodium tetradecyl sulfate, sodium morrhuate, ethoxisclerol, and ok432. The use of image-guided access to those lesions helps to prevent many local complications of the sclerosants like inadvertent endovascular injection or extravasation and pain, skin necrosis or retraction, neuropathy, and myoglobulinuria.

Comments

(Fig. 7.21). Ultrasound shows multiple cysts greater than 1 cm located in the right supraclavicular fossa related to macrocystic lymphangioma (a). A lump (*arrows*) is observed above the right clavicle but the overlying skin is not involved (b). (Fig. 7.22). After US-guided access to the malformation, a cystography is performed. Diluted contrast is introduced in the lymphangioma to determine the communication between the cysts, and the extent and volume of the malformation. (Fig. 7.23). The maximal capacity of the malformation helps to determine the amount of the sclerosant employed for sclerotherapy. (Fig. 7.24). Follow-up ultrasound (a) after sclerosis demonstrates a minimal residual cystic cavity that does not cause a bump in the neck (b).

Imaging Findings

Case 7: Venous Malformation

Gustavo Albi Rodríguez

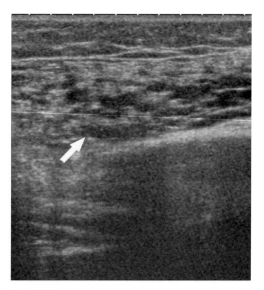

Fig. 7.26

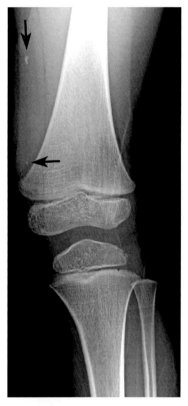

Fig. 7.25

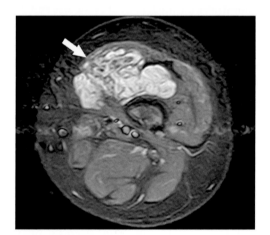

Fig. 7.27

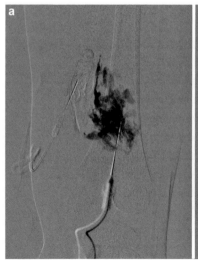
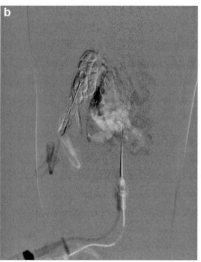

Fig. 7.28

An asymptomatic soft tissue mass is noticed at the right knee in a 6-year-old boy.

Venous malformations (VMs) have an estimated incidence of 1–2 cases per 10,000 births and a prevalence of 1%. In 1982, Mulliken classified vascular anomalies into two groups, hemangiomas and vascular malformations. In 1993, Jackson proposed a classification based on the flow pattern. VMs are considered low-flow malformations. VMs are made up of abnormal clusters of veins, of varying diameters and thick walls. They are usually less defined than hemangiomas. Although present at birth, they grow in proportion with the child and most are diagnosed in adolescence or early adulthood. Superficial VMs are soft tissue bluish compressible masses that increase with Valsalva maneuvers. They typically do not show local increase in temperature, pulsatility, or thrill like arteriovenous malformations (AVMs).

Comments

Imaging is used for confirmation, assessment of deeply seated lesions, or when clinical findings are confusing. The presence of phleboliths in plain X ray films (*arrows*) is considered pathognomonic for VMs (Fig. 7.25), although they may not be present. Ultrasound is the initial technique for vascular anomaly assessment (*arrows*) because of its wide availability and lack of ionizing radiation. Color Doppler US helps to distinguish between arteriovenous malformations, hemangiomas, and VMS. With color Doppler US, venous flow is detected in 84% of VMs; the rest may be either thrombosed or may have undetectable flow. US is also used for biopsy and percutaneous guided sclerotherapy. MRI is the technique of choice to characterize and determine their extent (*arrow*) (Fig. 7.26). VMs are usually iso- or hypointense on T1, though some hyperintense signal can be present if there is fatty tissue between the abnormal veins. Heterogeneity can also be due to hemorrhage or thrombosis. VMs behave as hyperintense on T2WI (Fig. 7.27). Signal voids at all sequences are related to phleboliths. Uptake of gadolinium can be homogeneous or heterogeneous. Direct percutaneous phlebography, despite being the gold standard imaging technique, is currently used only for therapy (Fig. 7.28a). It determines the extent and volume of the lesion and detects venous drainage into the systemic circulation. Percutaneous sclerosis (Fig. 7.28b) is the treatment of choice for MVs: the aim is the permanent disappearance of the vessel with obliteration of the lumen and fibrosis. There are multiple substances available for sclerosis (alcohol, aethoxysclerol, sodium tetradecyl sulfate, etc.). Results of sclerotherapy are good in the short term, with variable success rates in the long term. Complications of sclerotherapy are infrequent and include pain, soft tissue swelling, cutaneous changes, and proximal embolization of the sclerosing agent. Management of these drugs should be performed by experienced radiologists.

Imaging Findings

Case 8: Brain Arteriovenous Malformation

Pedro Navia and Ana Plá

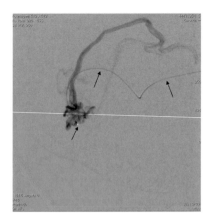

Fig. 7.30

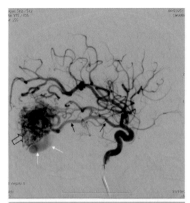

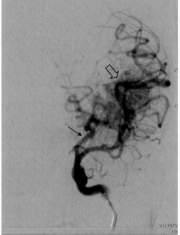

Fig. 7.29

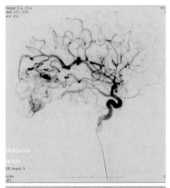

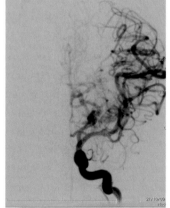

Fig. 7.31

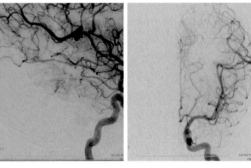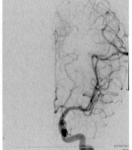

Fig. 7.32

A 4-year-old asymptomatic infant. A brain arteriovenous malformation (AVM) was incidentally found on a CT scan performed for a head lump. The study was completed with a brain MRI and a cerebral angiography.

Brain AVMs are very rare lesions and occur in less than 1% of the general population but are of special concern because of the damage they cause when they bleed. The risk of bleeding is 4% per year, and the risk of bleeding over one's lifetime may be high especially if the AVM is discovered in a child or a young person. Approximately 50% of the bleeds are significant, with permanent disability in half of these cases and death in the other half, so treatment is offered to prevent bleeding from the AVM.

The risks of the natural history of the untreated lesion must be weighted against the risks of treatment, evaluating its location, size, venous drainage, and the extent of anticipated possible deficit associated with the treatment.

There are three modalities of treatment available: endovascular techniques, radiosurgery, and standard neurosurgery. Treatment of brain AVM has been greatly enhanced by adopting a team approach with combined modality treatment, offering the lowest risk and providing the highest chance of obliterating the lesion.

Endovascular treatment involves advancing, under general anesthesia, a microcatheter into the arterial feeders of the AVM and injecting liquid adhesive material into the nidus and the feet of the veins of the AVM to block off the abnormal vessels. Chances of cure with embolization alone are between 20% and 40%.

If blood flow persists through a portion of the AVM after the endovascular treatment, the patient remains at risk of hemorrhage. A subsequent operation is made significantly easier than if the embolization had not been performed.

(Fig. 7.29). The figure is the diagnostic cerebral angiography that shows a 4 cm left occipital AVM (*open arrow*), with main feeders from left posterior cerebral artery (*black arrows*) and venous drainage to the transverse venous sinus (*white arrows*).

(Fig. 7.30). Endovascular treatment consisted of selective microcatheterization of three feeders of the AVM and embolization with liquid embolics (cyanoacrylate glue and ethylene-vinyl-alcohol). The figure shows a contrast injection with a 1.3-Fr. microcatheter in the nidus of the AVM (*arrows*).

(Fig. 7.31). It shows the control angiography after the endovascular treatment, achieving obliteration of 85% of the AVM.

(Fig. 7.32). Cerebral angiography done after subsequent complete surgical resection of the lesion with no arterial to venous shunting.

There were no complications in either intervention and the patient was asymptomatic at discharge.

Case 9: Percutaneous Varicocele Embolization

Carmen Gallego Herrero and Ricardo San Román Manso

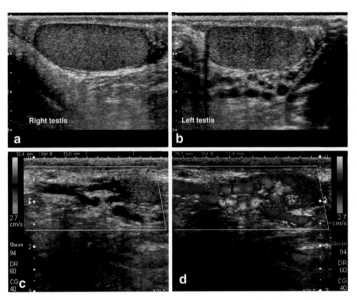

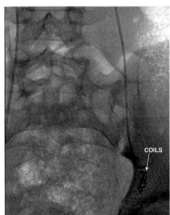

Fig. 7.35

Fig. 7.33

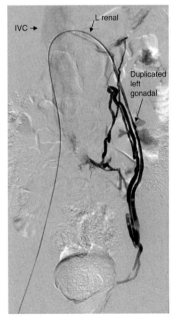

Fig. 7.34

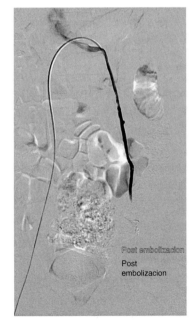

Fig. 7.36

An 11-year-old boy with past clinical episodes of left scrotal pain, varicocele grade 2, and asymmetry in size of testes (the left smaller) is admitted to our hospital for a percutaneous left gonadal vein embolization.

Comments

Varicocele is an abnormal dilatation of the pampiniform plexus that occurs in around 6% of boys at age 10 and 13% of adolescents. Left varicocele is by far more common (70–90%) than right varicocele. It is presumed to be secondary to retrograde blood flow, favored by the anatomic disposition of the left gonadal vein at square angles with the left renal vein. Varicocele seems to cause a time-dependent decline on semen quality and in fact around 35% of men with primary infertility and 80% with secondary infertility have varicocele. At clinical examination, varicocele can be graded into three groups. In grade 1, varicocele only presents with Valsalva; in grade 2 it presents without Valsalva, and in grade 3 it is visible through the skin. The major indication for treatment in children is testicular growth arrest. Other indications include high-grade varicocele with abnormal results at semen analysis, symptomatic (pain, heaviness, swelling), and bilateral varicoceles. There are two treatment options: surgical internal spermatic vein ligation and percutaneous left gonadal vein embolization. The aim of treatment is to obstruct the refluxing venous drainage to the testis while maintaining arterial inflow and lymphatic drainage.

Imaging Findings

Ultrasound demonstrates the asymmetry in size (Fig. 7.33a, b) and the presence of tortuous anechogenic dilated tubular structures along the spermatic cord (Fig. 7.33c). Doppler and pulsed-wave ultrasound demonstrate the venous flow pattern and the presence of reflux during Valsalva maneuver (Fig. 7.33d).

Percutaneous embolization of the internal spermatic vein is a safe, cost-effective technique with long-term success rates that is gaining acceptance among pediatric surgeons as the primary therapeutic option for varicocele. A catheter is advanced from the femoral vein into the left renal vein and left gonadal vein and a venogram is performed to demonstrate the varicocele (Fig. 7.34). Once a catheter is advanced to the distal spermatic vein (above the inguinal ligament), embolization is performed with either coils (Fig. 7.35), sclerosants, or both. Postembolization venograms demonstrate the absence of venous reflux into the distal spermatic vein (Fig. 7.36). Complication rates of the procedure are few and mild and include thrombophlebitis of the pampiniform plexus when sclerosants are used, coil migration, and groin hematoma. Varicocele embolization is a safe minimally invasive outpatient procedure that permits the patient to resume normal activity in 1–2 days and exercise in 2 weeks.

Case 10: Renovascular Hypertension

Carmen Gallego Herrero and Ricardo San Román Manso

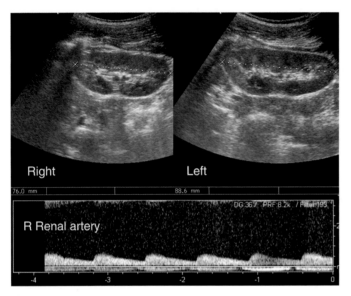

Fig. 7.37

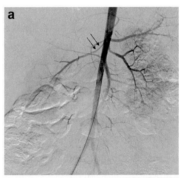

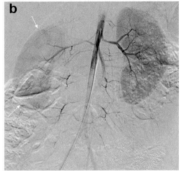

Fig. 7.38

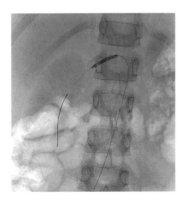

Fig. 7.39

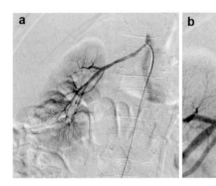

Fig. 7.40

An 8-year-old boy with renovascular hypertension for at least the past 4 years. Four years ago, he was admitted to our hospital with abdominal pain, headache, syncope, and BP 200/140. Actually, his blood pressure is normal under triple-drug therapy.

Most childhood hypertension is secondary to underlying disease, particularly in preadolescent patients. Renal parenchymal (around 60%) and renovascular disease (around 10%) are the most common causes of hypertension in children under 12 years of age. In renovascular disease, hypertension results from a lesion that impairs optimal flow to one or both kidneys. The most common cause of this impairment of flow is uni- or bilateral fibromuscular disease affecting both main renal arteries and intrarenal branches. The diagnostic workup in a child who has hypertension should include an ultrasound to rule out parenchymal disease and a Doppler ultrasound to rule out main renal or segmental stenosis. Scintigraphy with DMSA labeled with technetium-99 and MR renal angiography or contrast-enhanced CT and selective renal vein renin sampling determine the location and extent of the stenosis prior to surgery or angioplasty. Treatment options include medical management, surgery (aortorenal bypass, renal reimplantation, nephrectomy), or percutaneous angioplasty or embolization. Medical management has been the standard therapy, but despite combined drug therapy, sometimes it is impossible to control blood pressure. Indications for renal angioplasty are to decrease the burden of drug therapy, to delay or avoid complex surgical revascularization, and to offer a chance of kidney salvation in extensive arterial disease. Outcomes of renal angioplasty vary, but around 60% of patients experience an improvement in blood pressure control. Complications of angioplasty include thrombosis and distal embolization, intimal dissection, groin hematoma, and arterial rupture and pseudoaneurysm formation.

Doppler ultrasound (Fig. 7.37) shows a small right kidney, and a parvus tardus spectral pattern on the right renal artery. An aortogram (Fig. 7.38) is performed under general anesthesia. It demonstrates a long stenosis at the proximal third of the right renal artery (*black arrows*) (Fig. 7.38a), and a small right kidney with delayed parenchymal enhancement (*white arrows*) (Fig. 7.38b). A mild stenosis of the left renal artery is also seen (not amenable to dilation with the same procedure). A guidewire is introduced into the distal right renal artery and a 3-mm balloon is advanced over the wire and inflated at the stenotic site (Fig. 7.39). Postangioplasty selective arteriography of the right kidney shows a reasonably good morphological result (Fig. 7.40a). Mild contour irregularity (Fig. 7.40b) of the vessel secondary to recent dilation is a common postprocedural finding.

Further Reading

Case 1: Percutaneous Ultrasound-Guided Liver Biopsy

Book

Maller ES, Altschuler S (1996) Biliary atresia and cholestasis. In: Spitzer AE (ed) Intensive care of the fetus and neonate, 1st edn. Mosby-Year Book, St Louis, pp 875–887

Web Link

http://www.merckmanuals.com/professional/pediatrics/gastrointestinal_disorders_in_neonates_and_infants/neonatal_cholestasis.html

Articles

Amaral JG, Schwartz J, Chait P, Temple M, John P, Smith C et al (2006) Sonographically guided percutaneous liver biopsy in infants: a retrospective review. AJR Am J Roentgenol 187(6):W644–W649

Azzam RK, Alonso EM, Emerick KM, Whitington PF (2005) Safety of percutaneous liver biopsy in infants less than three months old. J Pediatr Gastroenterol Nutr 41:639–643

Copel L, Sosna J, Kruskal JB, Kane RA (2003) Ultrasound-guided percutaneous liver biopsy: indications, risks, and technique. Surg Technol Int 11:154–160

Hays DM, Woolley MM, Snyder WH, Reed GB, Gwinn JL, Landing BH (1967) Diagnosis of biliary atresia: relative accuracy of percutaneous liver biopsy, open liver biopsy, and operative cholangiography. J Pediatr 71:598–607

Jensen MK, Biank VF, Moe DC, Simpson PM, Li SH, Telega GW (2012) HIDA, percutaneous transhepatic cholecysto-cholangiography and liver biopsy in infants with persistent jaundice: can a combination of PTCC and liver biopsy reduce unnecessary laparotomy? Pediatr Radiol 42:32–39

Metreweli C, So NMC, Chu WCW, Lam WWM (2004) Magnetic resonance cholangiography in children. Br J Radiol 77:1059–1064

Neimark E, Leleiko NS (2011) Early detection of biliary atresia raises questions about etiology and screening. Pediatrics 128(6):e1598–e1599

Pietrobattista A, Fruwirth R, Natali G, Monti L, Devito R, Nobili V (2009) Is juvenile liver biopsy unsafe? Putting an end to a common misapprehension. Pediatr Radiol 39:959–961

Sokol RJ, Mack C, Narkewicz MR, Karrer FM (2003) Pathogenesis and outcome of biliary atresia: current concepts. J Pediatr Gastroenterol Nutr 37:4–21

Sporea I, Popescu A, Sirli R (2008) Why, who and how should perform liver biopsy in chronic liver diseases. World J Gastroenterol 14:3396–3402

Case 2: Sonographically Guided Transrectal Drainage

Book

Scott GC, Letourneau JG, Berman JM, Beidle TR (1997) Drainage of abdominal abscesses. In: Castañeda Zúñiga W (ed) Interventional radiology, vol 2, 3rd edn. Williams & Wilkins, Baltimore, pp 1745–1785

Web Link

Percutaneous abscess drainage. http://emedicine.medscape.com/article/1821039-overview

Articles

Alexander AA, Eschelman DJ, Nazarian LN, Bonn J (1994) Transrectal sonographically guided drainage of deep pelvic abscesses. AJR Am J Roentgenol 162:1227–1230

Chung T, Hoffer FA, Lund DP (1996) Transrectal drainage of deep pelvic abscesses in children using a combined transrectal sonographic and fluoroscopic guidance. Pediatr Radiol 26:874–878

Gervis DA, Hahn PF, O'Neill MJ, Mueller PR (2000) CT-guided transgluteal drainage of deep pelvic abscesses in children: selective use as an alternative to transrectal drainage. AJR Am J Roentgenol 175:1393–1396

Gervais DA, Brown SD, Connolly SA, Brec SL, Harisinghani MG, Mueller PR (2004) Percutaneous imaging guided abdominal and pelvic abscess drainage in children. Radiographics 24:737–754

Jamieson DH, Chait P, Filler R (1997) Interventional drainage of appendiceal abscesses in children. AJR Am J Roentgenol 169:1619–1622

Koral K, Derinjuyu B, Gargan L, Lagomarsino RM, Murphy JT (2010) Transrectal ultrasound and fluoroscopy-guided drainage of deep pelvic collections in children. J Pediatr Surg 45:513–518

Nadler EP, Reblock KK, Vaughan KG, Meza MP, Ford HR, Gaines BA (2004) Predictors of outcome for children with perforated appendicitis initially treated with non-operative management. Surg Infect (Larchmt) 5:349–356

Pereira JK, Chait PG, Miller SF (1996) Deep pelvic abscesses in children: transrectal drainage under radiologic guidance. Radiology 198:393–396

Potet J, Franchi-Abella S, Al Issa M, Fayard C, Pariente D (2010) Drainage pour la voie transrectale sous contrôle échographique sus-pubienne des abscès du Douglas chez-l'enfant: technique et résultats. J Radiol 91:221–225

Rao S, Hogan MJ (2009) Trocar transrectal abscess drainage in children: a modified technique. Pediatr Radiol 39:982–984

Case 3: Percutaneous Cecostomy

Book

Loening-Baucke V, Wyllie R, Hyams JS, (eds) (2011) Constipation and fecal incontinence. In: Pediatric gastrointestinal and liver disease, 4th edn. Elsevier, Philadelphia, pp 127–136

Web Site

http://www.nationwidechildrens.org/percutaneous-cecostomy

Articles

Becmeur F, Demarche M, Lacreuse I, Molinaro F, Kauffmann I, Moog R, Donnars F, Rebeuh J (2008) Cecostomy button for antegrade enemas: survey of 29 patients. J Pediatr Surg 43:1853–1857

Chait PG, Shlomovitz E, Connolly BL, Temple MJ, Restrepo R, Amaral JG et al (2003) Percutaneous cecostomy: updates in technique and patient care. Radiology 222:246–250

Donkol RA, Al-Nammi A (2010) Percutaneous cecostomy in the management of organic fecal incontinence in children. World J Radiol 2:463–467

Lorenzo AJ, Chait PG, Wallis MC, Raikhlin A, Farhat WA (2007) Minimally invasive approach for treatment of urinary and fecal incontinence in selected patients with spina bifida. Urology 70:568–571

Lykke J, Hansen MB, Meisner S (2006) Fecal incontinence treated with percutaneous endoscopic cecostomy. Endoscopy 38:950

Lynch CR, Jones RG, Hilden K, Wills JC, Fang JC (2006) Percutaneous endoscopic cecostomy in adults: a case series. Gastrointest Endosc 64:279–282

Mousa HM, van den Berg MM, Caniano DA, Hogan M, Di Lorenzo C, Hayes J (2006) Cecostomy in children with defecation disorders. Dig Dis Sci 51:154–160

Sierre S, Lipsich J, Questa H, Bailez M, Solana J (2007) Percutaneous cecostomy for management of fecal incontinence in pediatric patients. J Vasc Interv Radiol 18:982–985

Tomikashi K, Nomura Y, Miyawaki K, Shimada A, Kanemitsu D, Takashima H et al (2008) A case of hepatic encephalopathy successfully treated by antegrade glycerin enema through percutaneous endoscopic cecostomy. Nihon Shokakibyo Gakkai Zasshi 105:60–67

Yamout SZ, Glick PL, Lee YH, Yacobucci DV, Lau ST, Escobar MA, Caty MG (2009) Initial experience with laparoscopic Chait Trapdoor cecostomy catheter placement for the management of fecal incontinence in children: outcomes and lessons learned. Pediatr Surg Int 25:1081–1085

Case 4: Ultrasound-Guided Corticosteroid Injection Therapy for Juvenile Idiopathic Arthritis

Book

Peterson JJ, Fenton DS, Czervionke LF (2008) Image-guided musculoskeletal intervention. Saunders Elsevier, Philadelphia

Web Link

http://emedicine.medscape.com/article/392850-overview

Articles

Balint PV, Kane D, Hunter J, McInnes IB, Field M, Sturrock RD (2002) Ultrasound guided versus conventional joint and soft tissue fluid aspiration in rheumatology practice: a pilot study. J Rheumatol 29:2209–2213

Cahill AM, Cho SS, Baskin KM, Beukelman T, Cron RW, Kaye RD et al (2007) Benefit of fluoroscopically guided intraarticular, long-acting corticosteroid injection for subtalar arthritis in juvenile idiopathic arthritis. Pediatr Radiol 37:544–548

Furtado RN, Oliveira LM, Natour J (2005) Polyarticular corticosteroid injection versus systemic administration in treatment of rheumatoid arthritis patients: a randomized controlled study. J Rheumatol 32:1691–1698

Louis LJ (2008) Musculoskeletal ultrasound intervention: principles and advances. Radiol Clin North Am 46:515–533, vi

Marti P, Molinari L, Bolt IB, Serger R, Saurenmann RK (2008) Factors influencing the efficacy of intra-articular steroid injections in patients with juvenile idiopathic arthritis. Eur J Pediatr 167:425–430

Padeh S, Passwell JH (1998) Intraarticular corticosteroid injection in the management of children with chronic arthritis. Arthritis Rheum 41:1210–1214

Ravelli A, Martini A (2007) Juvenile idiopathic arthritis. Lancet 369:767–778

Raza K, Lee CY, Pilling D, Heaton S, Situnayake RD, Carruthers DM et al (2003) Ultrasound guidance allows accurate needle placement and aspiration from small joints in patients with early inflammatory arthritis. Rheumatology 42:976–979

Reach JS, Easley ME, Chuckpaiwong B et al (2009) Accuracy of ultrasound guided injections in the foot and ankle. Foot Ankle Int 30:239–242

Sibbit WL Jr, Peisajovich A, Michael AA et al (2009) Does sonographic needle guidance affect the clinical outcome of intraarticular injections? J Rheumatol 36:1892–1902

Case 5: Osteoid Osteoma

Book

Torriani M, Rosenthal DI (2007) Percutaneous radiofrequency ablation of osteoid osteoma. In: Schweitzer MA, Laredo JD (eds) New techniques in interventional musculoskeletal radiology. Informa Healthcare, New York, pp 293–303

Web Links

http://www.radiology.ucsf.edu/patient-care/services/osteoid-osteoma

Article

Akhlaghpoor S, Aziz Ahari A, Arjmand Shabestari A, Alinaghizadeh MR (2010) Radiofrequency ablation of osteoid osteoma in atypical locations: a case series. Clin Orthop Relat Res 468:1963–1970

Becce F, Theumann N, Rochette A, Larousserie F, Campagna R, Cherix S et al (2010) Osteoid osteoma and osteoid osteoma-mimicking lesions: biopsy findings, distinctive MDCT features and treatment by radiofrequency ablation. Eur Radiol 20:2439–2446

Bosschaert PP, Deprez FC (2010) Acetabular osteoid osteoma treated by percutaneous radiofrequency ablation: delayed articular cartilage damage. JBR-BTR 93:204–206

Donkol RH, Al-Nammi A, Moghazi K (2008) Efficacy of percutaneous radiofrequency ablation of osteoid osteoma in children. Pediatr Radiol 38:180–185

Jankharia B, Burute N (2009) Percutaneous radiofrequency ablation for osteoid osteoma: how we do it. Indian J Radiol Imaging 19:36–42

Martel Villagran J, Bueno Horcajadas A, Ortiz Cruz EJ (2009) Percutaneous radiofrequency ablation of benign bone tumors: osteoid osteoma, osteoblastoma, and chondroblastoma. Radiologia 51:549–558

Motamedi D, Learch TF, Ishimitsu DN, Motamedi K, Katz MD, Brien EW et al (2009) Thermal ablation of osteoid osteoma: overview and step-by-step guide. Radiographics 29:2127–2141

Mylona S, Patsoura S, Galani P, Karapostolakis G, Pomoni A et al (2010) Osteoid osteomas in common and in technically challenging locations treated with computed tomography-guided percutaneous radiofrequency ablation. Skeletal Radiol 39:443–449

Rybak LD, Gangi A, Buy X, La Rocca Vieira R, Witting J (2010) Thermal ablation of spinal osteoid osteomas close to neural elements: technical considerations. AJR Am J Roentgenol 195:W293–W298

Virayavanich W, Singh R, O'Donnell RJ, Horvai AE, Goldsby RE, Link TM (2010) Osteoid osteoma of the femur in a 7-month-old infant treated with radiofrequency ablation. Skeletal Radiol 39:1145–1149

Case 6: Percutaneous Sclerosis of Lymphangioma

Book

Lee BB, Laredo J, Seo JM, Neville RF (2009a) Treatment of lymphangiomas. In: Mattassi R, Loose DA, Vaghi Massimo (eds) Hemangiomas and vascular malformations: an atlas of diagnosis and treatment. Springer, New York, pp 231–250

Web Link

Lymphatic vascular malformations. http://emedicine.medscape.com/article/1296163-overview

Articles

Alomari AI, Karian VE, Lord DJ, Padua HM, Burrows PE (2006) Percutaneous sclerotherapy for lymphatic malformations: a retrospective analysis of patient-evaluated improvement. J Vasc Interv Radiol 17:1639–1648

Burrows PE, Mitri RK, Alomari AI, Padua HM, Lord DM, Sylvia MB, Fishman SJ et al (2008) Percutaneous sclerotherapy of lymphatic malformations with doxycycline. Lymphat Res Biol 6:209–216

Dubois J, Alison M (2010) Vascular anomalies: what a radiologist needs to know. Pediatr Radiol 40:895–905

Garzon MC, Huang JT, Enjolras O, Frieden IJ (2007a) Vascular malformations. Part I. J Am Acad Dermatol 56:353–370

Garzon MC, Huang JT, Enjolras O, Frieden IJ (2007b) Vascular malformations. Part II. J Am Acad Dermatol 56:541–564

Lee BB (2005) New approaches for the treatment of congenital vascular malformations (CVMs): a single center experience. Eur J Vasc Endovasc Surg 30:184–197

Mulliken JB, Glowacki J (1982) Hemangiomas and vascular malformations in infants and children: a classification based on endothelial characteristics. Plast Reconstr Surg 69:412–420

Puig S, Casati B, Staudenherz A, Paya K (2005) Vascular low flow malformations in children: current concepts for classification, diagnosis and therapy. Eur J Radiol 53:35–45

Shiels WE II, Kenney BE, Caniano DA, Besner GE (2008) Definitive percutaneous treatment of lymphatic malformations of the trunk and extremities. J Pediatr Surg 43:136–140

Shiels WE II, Kang R, Murakami JW, Hogan MJ, Wiet GJ (2009) Percutaneous treatment of lymphatic malformations. Otolaryngol Head Neck Surg 141:219–224

Case 7: Venous Malformation

Book

Lee BB, Laredo J, Seo JM, Neville RF (2009b) Treatment of lymphangiomas. In: Mattassi R, Loose DA, Vaghi Massimo (eds) Hemangiomas and vascular malformations: an atlas of diagnosis and treatment. Springer, New York, pp 231–250

Web Link

http://emedicine.medscape.com/article/1296303-overview

Articles

Blaise S, Charavin-Cocuzza M, Riom H et al (2011) Treatment of low-flow vascular malformations by ultrasound-guided sclerotherapy with polidocanol foam: 24 cases and literature review. Eur J Vasc Endovasc Surg 41:412–417

Boll DT, Merkle EM, Lewin JS (2004) Low-flow vascular malformations: MR-guided percutaneous sclerotherapy in qualitative and quantitative assessment of therapy and outcome. Radiology 233:376–384

Burrows PE, Mason KP (2004) Percutaneous treatment of low flow vascular malformations. J Vasc Interv Radiol 15:431–445

Cabrera J, Cabrera J, Garcia-Olmedo MA, Redondo P (2003) Treatment of venous malformations with sclerosant in microfoam form. Arch Dermatol 139:1409–1416

Donnelly LF, Adams DM, Bisset GS (2000) Vascular malformations and hemangiomas: a practical approach in a multidisciplinary clinic. AJR Am J Roentgenol 174:597–608

Ernemann U, Kramer U, Miller S et al (2010) Current concepts in the classification, diagnosis and treatment of vascular anomalies. Eur J Radiol 75:2–11

Hammer F, Boon L, Mathurin P, Vanwijck R (2001) Ethanol sclerotherapy of venous malformations: evaluation of systemic ethanol contamination. J Vasc Interv Radiol 12:595–600

Hyodoh H, Hori M, Akiba H, Tamakawa M, Hyodoh K, Hareyama M (2005) Peripheral vascular malformations: imaging, treatment approaches, and therapeutic issues. Radiographics 25(Suppl 1):S159–S171

Legiehn GM, Heran MKS (2008) Venous malformations: classification, development, diagnosis, and interventional radiologic management. Radiol Clin North Am 46:545–597

Li L, Zeng XQ, Li YH (2010) Digital subtraction angiography-guided foam sclerotherapy of peripheral venous malformations. AJR Am J Roentgenol 194:W439–W444

Articles

Berenstein A, Ortiz R, Niimi Y, Elijovich L, Fifi J, Madrid M et al (2010) Endovascular management of arteriovenous malformations and other intracranial arteriovenous shunts in neonates, infants, and children. Childs Nerv Syst 26:1345–1358

Brown RD, Flemming KD, Meyer FB, Cloft HJ, Pollock BE, Link MJ (2005) Natural history, evaluation, and management of intracranial vascular malformations. Mayo Clin Proc 80:269–281

Huisman TAGM, Singhi S, Pinto PS (2010) Non-invasive imaging of intracranial pediatric vascular lesions. Childs Nerv Syst 26:1275–1295

Karel G, Brugge T (1999) Neurointerventional procedures in the pediatric age group. Childs Nerv Syst 15:751–754

Kondziolka D, Kano H, Yang H, Flickinger JC, LLunsford L (2010) Radiosurgical management of pediatric arteriovenous malformations. Childs Nerv Syst 26:1359–1366

Krings T, Geibprasert S, Terbrugge K (2010) Classification and endovascular management of pediatric cerebral vascular malformations. Neurosurg Clin N Am 21:463–482

Ozanne A, Alvarez H, Krings T, Lasjaunias P (2007) Pediatric neurovascular malformations: vein of Galen arteriovenous malformations (VGAM), pial arteriovenous malformations (pial AVM), dural sinus malformations (DSM). J Neuroradiol 34:145–166

Smith ER, Butler WE, Ogilvy CS (2002) Surgical approaches to vascular anomalies of the child's brain. Neurology 15:165–171

Starke RM, Komotar RJ, Otten ML, Hahn DK, Fischer LE, Hwang BY et al (2009) Adjuvant embolization with N-butyl cyanoacrylate in the treatment of cerebral arteriovenous malformations: outcomes, complications, and predictors of neurologic deficits. Stroke 40:2783–2790

Thiex R, Williams A, Smith E, Scott RM, Orbach DB (2010) The use of Onyx for embolization of central nervous system arteriovenous lesions in pediatric patients. AJNR Am J Neuroradiol 31:112–120

Case 8: Brain Arteriovenous Malformation

Book

Lasjaunias P, TerBrugge KG, Berenstein A (2006) Surgical neuroangiography, vol 3, 2nd edn, Clinical and interventional aspects in children. Springer, Berlin

Web Link

Guía de Malformaciones Vasculares Cerebrales del Grupo Español de Neurorradiología Intervencionista (GENI). http://www.neurointervencionismo.com

Case 9: Percutaneous Varicocele Embolizaton

Book

Qian Z, Comhaire F, Kunnen M, Hunter DW, Amplatz K, Castañeda-Zuñiga WR, Castañeda Zúñiga W (ed) (1997) Varicocele embolization. In: Interventional radiology, vol 2, 3rd edn. Williams & Wilkins, Baltimore, pp 1414–39

Web Link

http://en.wikipedia.org/wiki/Varicocele

Articles

Ayechu-Díaz A, Oscoz-Lizarbe M, Pérez-Martínez A, Pisón-Chacón J, Esparza J, Bento L (2009) Treatment of adolescent varicocele: is percutaneous embolization better? Cir Pediatr 2:134–138

Beecroft JRD (2007) Percutaneous varicocele embolization. Can Urol Assoc J 1:278–280

Calama Santiago JA, Penedo Cobos JM, Molina López MY, González Ruiz C, García Mollá R, Sierra Díaz F (2008) Paediatric varicocele embolization dosimetric study. Actas Urol Esp 32:833–842

Canning DA (2003) Percutaneous embolization of varicocele in children: a Canadian experience. J Urol 170:328

Garel L, Dubois J, Rypens F, Ouimet A, Yazbeck S (2004) Anatomic variations of the spermatic vein and endovascular treatment of left varicoceles: a pediatric series. Can Assoc Radiol J 55:39–44

Glassberg KI, Badalato GM, Poon SA, Mercado MA, Raimondi PM, Gasalberti A (2011) Evaluation and management of the persistent/recurrent varicocele. Urology 77:1194–1198

Lord DJ, Burrows PE (2003) Pediatric varicocele embolization. Tech Vasc Interv Radiol 6:169–175

Piñera JG, Fernández-Córdoba MS, Anselmi EH, Mollá EJ, Jiménez MJ, Cabañero AG, Baró A (2009) Results of the percutaneous retrograde embolization as the first choice in the treatment of varicocele. Cir Pediatr 22:128–133

Reinberg O, Meyrat BJ (2007) Children and adolescent varicocele. Rev Med Suisse 5(3):2779–2780

Villar Esnal R, Sánchez Guerrero A, Pamplona Casamayor M, Fernández Sáez R, Parga López G, García-Hidalgo Castilla E (2004) Varicocele's radiological endovascular occlusion. Arch Esp Urol 57:941–950

Case 10: Renovascular Hypertension

Book

Tegtmeyer CJ, Selby JB, Jr, Ferral H, Castañeda Zúñiga W (ed) (1997) Percutaneous transluminal angioplasty of the renal arteries. In: Interventional radiology, vol 1, 3rd edn. Williams & Wilkins, Baltimore, pp 483–502

Web Link

Pediatric hypertension. http://emedicine.medscape.com/article/889877-overview

Articles

Inn T, Shimazaki S, Kaneko K, Yabuta K, Yamaguchi H, Kaneko K (1994) Multiple spasms of renal arteries following percutaneous transluminal renal angioplasty in children. Pediatr Nephrol 8:129–132

Lacombe M (2011) Surgical treatment of renovascular hypertension in children. Eur J Vasc Endovasc Surg 41:770–777

Lindblad B (2011) Renovascular hypertension in children: time to further centralise handling? Eur J Vasc Endovasc Surg 41:778–779

Mali WP, Puijlaert CB, Kouwenberg HJ, Klinge J, Donckerwolcke RA, Geijskes BG et al (1987) Percutaneous transluminal renal angioplasty in children and adolescents. Radiology 165:391–394

Martin EC, Diamond NG, Casarella WJ (1980) Percutaneous transluminal angioplasty in non-atherosclerotic disease. Radiology 135:27–33

Shroff R, Roebuck DJ, Gordon I, Davies R, Stephens S, Marks S, Chan M et al (2006) Angioplasty for renovascular hypertension in children: 20-year experience. Pediatrics 118:268–275

Srinivasan A, Krishnamurthy G, Fontalvo-Herazo L, Nijs E, Keller MS, Kaplan B et al (2010) Angioplasty for renal artery in pediatric patients: an 11-year retrospective experience. J Vasc Interv Radiol 21:1672–1680

Stanley JC, Zelenock GB, Messina LM, Wakefield TW (1995) Pediatric renovascular hypertension: a thirty-year experience of operative treatment. J Vasc Surg 21:212–227

Towbin RB, Pelchovitz DJ, Cahill AM, Baskin KM, Meyers KE, Kaplan BS et al (2007) Cutting balloon angioplasty in children with resistant renal artery stenosis. J Vasc Interv Radiol 18:663–669

Tullus K (2011) Renal artery stenosis: is angiography still the gold standard in 2011? Pediatr Nephrol 26:833–837

Contents

M.I. Martínez-León et al., *Imaging for Pediatricians*, Imaging for Clinicians,
DOI 10.1007/978-3-642-28629-2_8, © Springer-Verlag Berlin Heidelberg 2012

Case 1: Acute Cerebellitis

Alba Martínez Broquetas and María I. Martínez-León

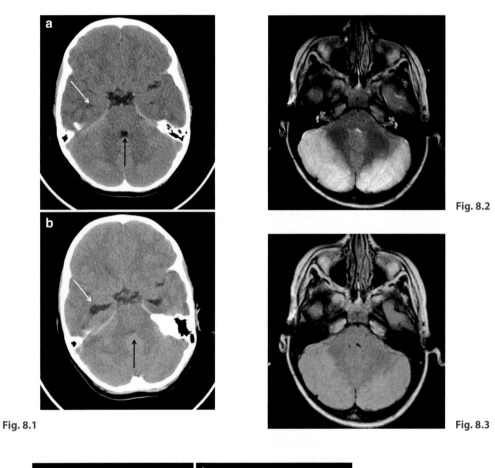

Fig. 8.1

Fig. 8.2

Fig. 8.3

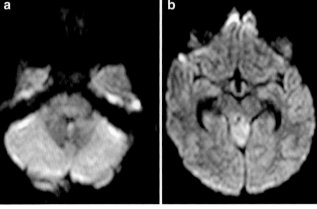

Fig. 8.4

A 10-year-old patient with a headache for a week, without any other signs or symptoms.

Acute cerebellitis is one of the main causes of acute cerebellar dysfunction in childhood. The etiology is usually infectious, postinfectious, or after vaccination. The most frequent infectious organisms are the varicella-zoster virus, mumps, mycoplasma, and Epstein-Barr virus.

Although many patients may by asymptomatic, they frequently present a triad of severe headache, preventing sleep, vomiting, and changing consciousness. Occasionally, this is associated with increased intracranial pressure due to cerebellar swelling and secondary obstructive hydrocephalus.

The diagnosis of acute cerebellitis can sometimes be difficult because the patient may present only mild cerebellar signs and the examination of cerebrospinal fluid may be normal.

The main differential diagnosis includes acute intoxication, demyelinating processes, lead poisoning, Lhermitte-Duclos disease, and vasculitis.

Although usually benign and self-limiting, acute cerebellitis may develop a fulminant course, resulting in cerebellar atrophy or sudden death.

Neuroimaging, especially MRI, demonstrates the early signs and is an important tool in the diagnosis of acute cerebellitis, particularly in cases with nonspecific or vague symptoms and normal cerebrospinal fluid.

Steroids, or acyclovir in some cases, are the first line of treatment when symptoms are moderate to severe, although most patients will recover without any specific treatment. In severe cases, an emergency decompression with external ventricular drainage may be necessary.

First brain CT without contrast shows normal size of temporal horns (*white arrow*) and IV ventricle (*black arrow*) (Fig. 8.1a). One week later, a new brain CT without contrast shows IV ventricle narrowing and enlargement of the temporal horns of the lateral ventricles, indicating mild hydrocephalus (Fig. 8.1b). Axial T2-weighted (Fig. 8.2) and FLAIR (Fig. 8.3) MR images show hyperintensity in both sequences due to bilateral hemispheric cerebellar swelling. Axial diffusion-weighted image demonstrates bilateral hemispheric cerebellar restricted diffusion cause by edema (Fig. 8.4).

Case 2: Traumatic Head Injury

Susana Calle Restrepo

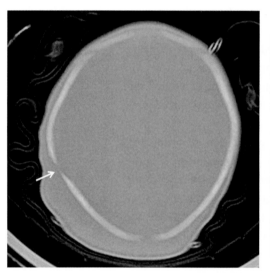

Fig. 8.5

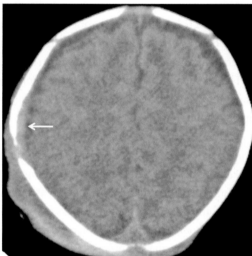

Fig. 8.6

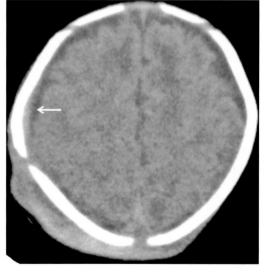

Fig. 8.7

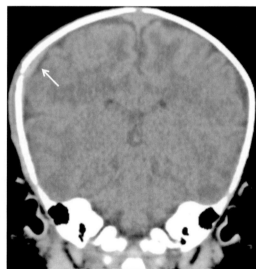

Fig. 8.8

A 40-day-old infant is brought by his mother after having sustained mild trauma to the head without loss of consciousness.

Head trauma constitutes a leading cause of morbidity and mortality in childhood. A large head, weak neck musculature, and soft and thin calvarium place children at greater risk for sustaining this type of injury, particularly those under the age of 5 years. Traditionally, loss of consciousness and altered mental status were thought to be adequate screening indicators for CT scanning in children. Nevertheless, a liberal imaging policy is warranted in patients with significant trauma, despite normal neurological status.

At present, CT is the modality of choice for imaging acute head injury due to its wide availability, relatively low cost, and ability to accommodate to monitoring devices and life-support equipment in the emergency department setting. Furthermore, it is highly sensitive in the detection of pneumocephalus, hemorrhage, and skull fractures. Linear fractures are the most common type of skull fracture in children. They are usually detected as lucent linear defects on CT but may be missed if the fracture line is parallel to the scanning plane.

Acute extra-axial hemorrhages present as hyperdense fluid collections that displace the adjacent brain parenchyma. Epidural hematomas, caused by rupture of the middle meningeal artery or by venous lacerations, are characteristically lentiform in shape and do not cross suture lines. Subdural hematomas, more common in this age group, are frequently bilateral, generated by injury to bridging cortical veins and present as crescentic fluid collections that may cross suture lines, but do not cross the midline. On the other hand, subarachnoid hemorrhage, most commonly visualized at the Sylvian fissure and interpeduncular cistern, is usually secondary to leptomeningeal or cerebral surface vessel injury and appears as increased attenuation in the subarachnoid space rather than as a true fluid collection.

Comments

Axial bone-window head CT shows a linear, nondisplaced fracture of the right parietal bone (*arrow*) with an associated subgaleal hematoma and soft tissue edema (Fig. 8.5). Axial (Figs. 8.6 and 8.7) and coronal images (Fig. 8.8) in brain window demonstrate a crescent-shaped hyperdense collection (*arrows*) located adjacent to the described fracture, at the lateral aspect of the right parietal region, consistent with a small subdural hematoma, which generates mild displacement of the adjacent brain parenchyma.

Imaging Findings

Case 3: Pediatric Ischemic Stroke

Natalia Aguilar Pérez and María I. Martínez-León

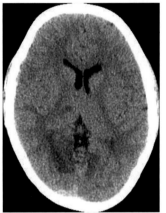

Fig. 8.9

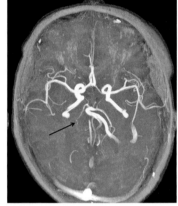

Fig. 8.11

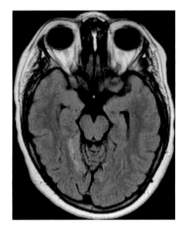

Fig. 8.12

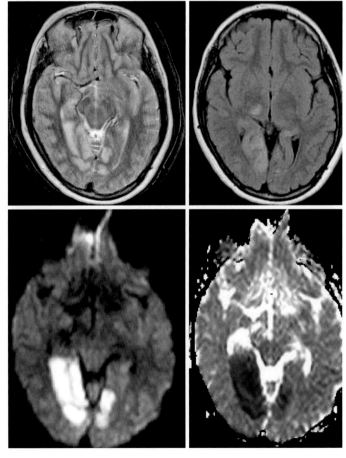

Fig. 8.10

A 12-year-old boy with left hemiparesis, left arm tremor, and dysmetria, with 24-h onset.

Comments

Stroke can be defined as a clinical syndrome characterized by a neurological deficit related to the perfusion territory of a cerebral artery with neuroradiological evidence of an ischemic lesion. This means that a stroke is a clinical diagnosis, but radiology is required for the initial diagnosis and on subsequent follow-up.

Stroke is a relatively rare disease in childhood, but it represents one of the most common causes of death, with very high morbidity and long-term outcome. Its management requires urgent multidisciplinary competence and approach.

Strokes are primarily ischemic or hemorrhagic. While adult strokes are predominantly ischemic and secondary to atherosclerosis, in childhood, up to 45% of strokes are hemorrhagic and are associated with a wide spectrum of risk factors.

Arterial ischemic stroke (AIS) is defined as ischemia, infarction, or encephalomalacia in a vascular arterial territory. A risk factor is present in almost half of the children at the time of stroke. The most frequently reported risk factors for AIS in childhood are: congenital or acquired heart disease, hematologic disorders such as sickle cell disease, metabolic disorders, vasculitis and vasculopathies, and various prothrombotic conditions. Recent studies emphasize the important role of infection because it seems that at least one-third of cases of pediatric stroke occur in that context.

Noncontrast computed tomography (CT) can be performed urgently to exclude hemorrhagic stroke or parenchymal abnormalities with a mass effect and may reveal a low-density lesion in case of arterial ischemic stroke. However, CT is usually normal in the first 12 h after the onset of symptoms.

MRI should be considered as the first diagnostic step because it provides a complete diagnostic set of information. Diffusion-weighted sequences are very useful to identify regions of early ischemia and infarction.

Imaging Findings

Initial CT showed bilateral hypodense lesions in both occipital lobes and thalamus, with greater involvement on the right side; there was no hemorrhagic lesion (Fig. 8.9). MRI shows hyperintense lesions in T2-WI and FLAIR-WI, with severe restriction in diffusion and ADC map in vascular territories of both posterior cerebral arteries (Fig. 8.10). Axial reconstruction of the MRI study of the circle of Willis identifies both posterior cerebral arteries with a kink in the right one, which is smaller in diameter (*arrow*) (Fig. 8.11). We can see the evolution of the lesions in MRI FLAIR sequences 2 months after the acute event (Fig. 8.12). A genetic study showed that the patient had a gene mutation for hyperhomocysteinemia.

Case 4: Nonneonatal Hypoxic-Ischemic Encephalopathy (HIE)

Cristina Serrano García and Ernesto Doménech Abellán

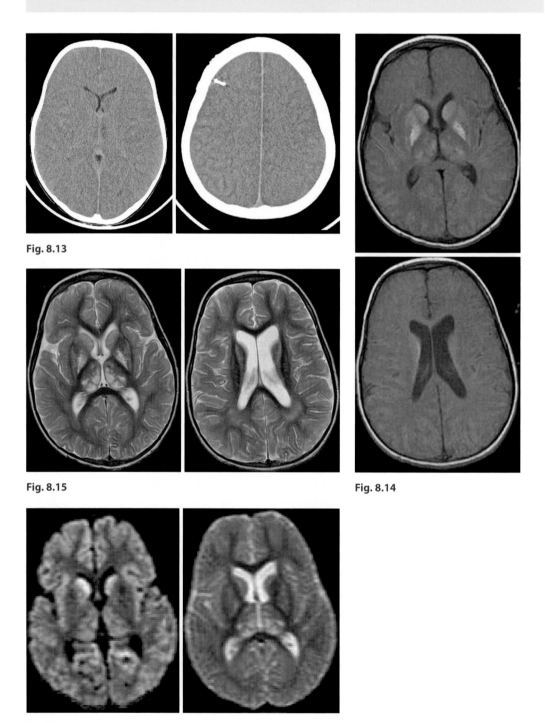

Fig. 8.13

Fig. 8.15

Fig. 8.14

Fig. 8.16

A 2-year-old patient with hypoxic-ischemic encephalopathy secondary to cardiac arrest.

Hypoxic-ischemic encephalopathy (HIE) is a devastating entity that frequently results in death or profound long-term neurological disability. HIE in infants and young children is usually the result of drowning, choking, or nonaccidental trauma.

The common underlying physiological processes that result in HIE are diminished cerebral blood flow (ischemia) and reduced blood oxygenation (hypoxemia).

For the prediction of outcome in HIE patients, several clinical and laboratory findings have been reported to be useful. Neuroimaging can play an important role early in the postanoxic state since magnetic resonance (MR) imaging with diffusion-weighted (DW) imaging is useful in revealing acute findings. Treatment consists of supportive care; new neuroprotective strategies designed to limit the extent of brain injury are still under investigation. Many of these treatment strategies have a limited scope of effectiveness, making the early detection of injury critically important.

Imaging findings in HIE depend on factors such as brain maturity, severity and duration of insult, and type and timing of imaging studies. Once ultrasound (US) is no longer feasible, computer tomography (CT) becomes the initial imaging study of choice. If the study is positive, no additional imaging is usually necessary, although delayed MR should be performed to assess the overall extent of injury. A negative CT study should prompt further evaluation with MR imaging because CT is relatively insensitive for detecting injury in the acute setting.

Early CT performed within 24 h of an HIE may be negative. Subsequent CT will demonstrate diffuse basal ganglia abnormalities along with diffuse cerebral edema.

MR with DW imaging is the earliest imaging modality to become positive within the first few hours and pseudonormalize by the end of the first week. DW images demonstrate bright signal intensity of the basal ganglia and the cortex. Conventional MR T1- and T2-weighted images obtained in the first 24 h are often normal. By 48 h, images will demonstrate diffuse basal ganglia and cortical signal intensity abnormality that represents edema. MR spectroscopy is very sensitive and indicative of the severity of injury in the first 24 h.

Nonenhanced cranial CT performed 72 h after the episode reveals signs of cerebral edema with cortical hypoattenuation and poor gray-white matter differentiation (Fig. 8.13). MRI with T1 (Fig. 8.14) and T2 (Fig. 8.15) sequences shows involvement of basal ganglia and signs of cortical edema. Diffusion sequences and apparent diffusion coefficient (ADC) map (Fig. 8.16) demonstrate basal ganglia injury due to hypoxic-ischemic damage.

Case 5: Orbital Cellulitis

Víctor Pérez Candela and Alberto Acosta Mendoza

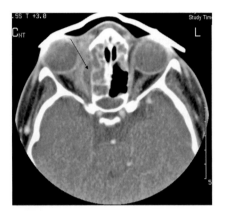

Fig. 8.17

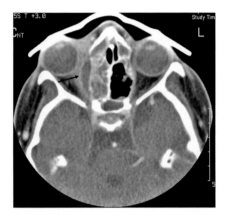

Fig. 8.18

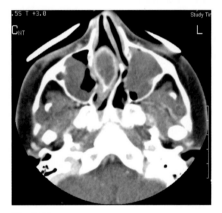

Fig. 8.19

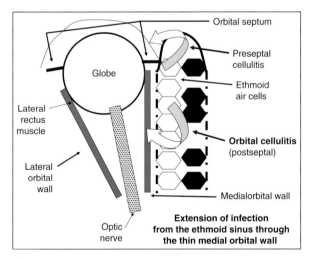

Fig. 8.20

A 12-year-old girl with a right eyelid edema and erythema of the periorbital tissue, with pain upon eye movement.

Postseptal orbital cellulitis is used to describe infectious involvement of the soft tissues posterior to the orbital septum, including the fat and muscle within the bony orbit. Preseptal cellulitis, in contrast, characterizes a cellulitis of the tissues localized anterior to the orbital septum. This distinction is important, as orbital cellulitis may be associated with significant visual and life-threatening sequelae, including optic neuropathy, encephalomeningitis, cavernous sinus thrombosis, sepsis, and intracranial abscess formation.

Comments

The orbital septum is part of the anterior orbital connective tissue framework and provides the mechanical function of containing orbital fat.

The medial orbital wall that separates the orbit from the ethmoid sinus is very thin, particularly in childhood, and several perforations exist through which valveless blood vessels and nerves travel. This combination of thin bone, perforations, and loosely adherent periorbita allows for communication of infectious and inflammatory processes between the ethmoidal air cells and the medial orbit. For these reasons, the medial wall is a common location for the development of subperiosteal abscesses.

Orbital cellulitis is an emergency that requires immediate treatment with intravenous antibiotic coverage. Surgical intervention should be considered in patients who fail to respond and deteriorate on medical therapy.

Enhanced axial CT scan shows the low-density area with an enhancing margin tapering to the bone (*arrow*) by a subperiosteal abscess, with ethmoid and sphenoid sinusitis and postseptal cellulitis, and a tiny preseptal cellulitis (Fig. 8.17). Enhanced axial CT scan at a lower level shows the subperiosteal abscess (*arrow*) much better, with ethmoid and sphenoid sinusitis and the increased attenuation in the preseptal and postseptal fat, a finding consistent with inflammation (Fig. 8.18). An enhanced axial CT scan at the level of maxillary sinuses shows a nasal septal deviation to the left side, the maxillary sinuses with soft tissue opacification, and a right concha bullosae involving the inferior turbinate with soft-tissue opacification (Fig. 8.19).

Imaging Findings

(Fig. 8.20). A diagram of the right orbit with the orbital septum as the border between preseptal cellulitis and orbital cellulitis (postseptal) for inflammatory processes, from the ethmoid sinus through the medial orbital wall.

Case 6: Retropharyngeal Infections in Children

María Isabel Martínez Marín

A 2-year-old patient presented with 4 days of fever, neck stiffness, and rejection of any oral intake. Physical examination revealed edematous pharynx, cervical lymphadenopa-

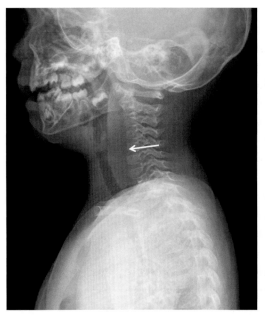

Fig. 8.21

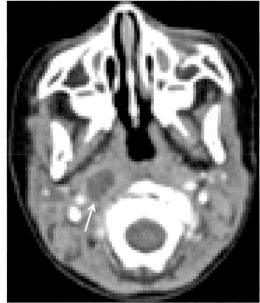

Fig. 8.22

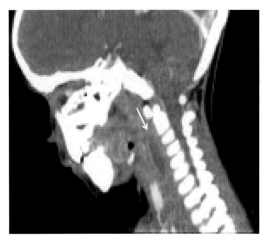

Fig. 8.23

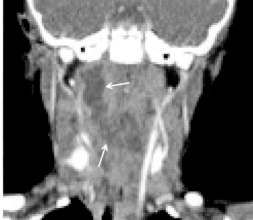

Fig. 8.24

thy, and wryneck. Laboratory analyses revealed bacteremia. The patient was treated with intravenous antibiotics therapy, with good initial control of the fever and overall improvement. Persistence of wryneck and the appearance of speech disturbances required a computed tomography (CT) scan of the neck.

Comments

Retropharyngeal abscess (RPA) is a potentially serious deep space neck infection. The retropharyngeal space (RS) extends from the base of the skull to the posterior mediastinum. It is generally caused by infection of the upper respiratory tract, producing adenitis of the retropharyngeal lymphatic nodules, which may evolve through suppuration and abscess formation. RPA is more frequent in infants and young children because these lymph nodes spontaneously regress by early childhood.

Its diagnosis is based on clinical suspicion, supported by imaging studies. RPA clinical display is often faint, and its variety of symptoms depends on the developmental stage of the disease. Generally, children show moderate fever, dysphagia, odynophagia, wryneck, dysphonia, and cervical lymphadenopathy. In addition, respiratory difficulty develops as the disease progresses.

Radiological evaluation of retropharyngeal infection includes lateral neck radiograph and contrast-enhanced CT. The choice of the imaging technique depends on the clinical condition of the child and on the degree of suspected retropharyngeal infection. If there are no signs of airway compromise, the initial radiological study must be carried out using lateral neck radiographs. CT is the best tool to identify abscesses in the RS and the eventual spreading of an abscess to contiguous spaces in the neck or the mediastinum.

Empiric antibiotics therapy should be initiated as soon as possible. Immediate surgical drainage is necessary in patients with airway compromise. If RPA is in its early stage, antibiotic therapy can prevent the progression of the infection. Some experts recommend this option in patients with a small abscess (diameter smaller than 2 cm), while surgical drainage in addition to antibiotic therapy should be applied in the case of a larger abscess. When no medical complications appear, expectations for complete healing are generally high. However, mortality can reach 40–50% when serious complications appear. Expected complications include airway obstruction, aspiration pneumonia, spread of infection to other spaces and the mediastinum, sepsis, internal jugular vein thrombophlebitis, carotid artery rupture, atlantoaxial dislocation, or hypoglossal nerve palsy.

Imaging Findings

(Fig. 8.21). Lateral neck radiograph demonstrating widening of the retropharyngeal space (*arrow*) and loss of the cervical lordosis. The retropharyngeal space is considered widened if it is greater than 7 mm at C2 or 14 mm at C6. Axial (Fig. 8.22), sagittal, and coronal (Figs. 8.23 and 8.24) CT reconstructions demonstrate prevertebral space abscess extending from the right high parapharyngeal space to prevertebral space and upper mediastinum (*arrows*). After the administration of contrast material, the abscess presents a hypodense center and the walls are enhanced after contrast administration.

Case 7: Acute Bacterial Sinusitis

Cristina Segovia Verjel and María I. Martínez-León

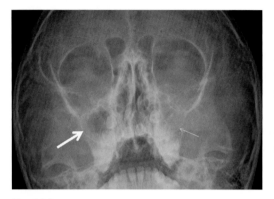

Fig. 8.25

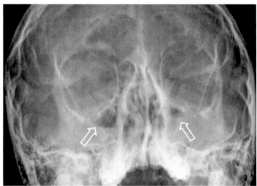

Fig. 8.26

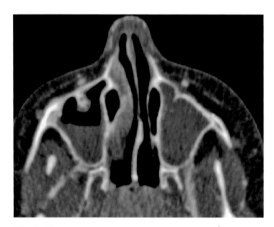

Fig. 8.27

Symptoms and Signs of ABS	
Persistent	Severe
• >10 days	• High fever > 39°C
• No appreciable improvement	• Purulent nasal discharge
• Nasal discharge of any quality	• Present for at least 3–4 days
• Cough (must be present during day)	• Headaches may be present
• Malodorous breath	• Periorbital swelling occasionally
• Facial pain and headache are rare	
• If fever then low grade	
• May not appear very ill	

Fig. 8.28

The ethmoid and maxillary sinuses are present at birth and expand rapidly by 4 years of age. The sphenoid sinuses are typically pneumatized by 5 years of age and attain their permanent size by age 12. The frontal sinuses can be distinguished at 6–8 years, but they do not complete their development until 14–16 years of age.

Acute sinusitis results from infection of one or more of the paranasal sinuses. A viral infection associated with the common cold is the most frequent etiology of acute sinusitis, which is usually solved without treatment in 7–10 days. Approximately 10% of episodes of viral rhinosinusitis in children are complicated by acute bacterial sinusitis (ABS).

Viral upper respiratory infection and allergic rhinitis are the most frequent predisposing factors for ABS in children. The clinical and radiographic manifestations of ABS in children are similar to those of uncomplicated viral rhinosinusitis. The clinical course, particularly the persistence and severity of symptoms, helps to differentiate between the two conditions. Distinguishing between acute viral rhinosinusitis and ABS is important so that antibiotics can be reserved for the patients in whom they are likely to be effective. The diagnosis of ABS can be made clinically in children with nasal symptoms (discharge, obstruction, and/or congestion) and/or daytime cough that have persisted for >10 and <30 days without improvement. A clinical diagnosis of ABS can also be made in children with "severe" or "worsening" symptoms. The examination should focus on signs of orbital or intracranial complications of ABS. Sinus radiography (occipitomental or Waters view) should be obtained in children who have failed to improve after appropriate medical therapy if radiograph was not performed before therapy was initiated. The findings include complete opacification, mucosal thickening of at least 4 mm, and air-fluid level. Abnormal X-rays cannot distinguish between bacterial, viral, or other causes of sinusitis and must always be interpreted in the context of clinical findings. Contrast-enhanced computed tomography is recommended in children with potential orbital and intracranial complications.

Sinus X-rays (*Waters view*). Complete opacification of the left maxillary sinus (*thin arrow*), mucosal thickening of the right maxillary sinus (*thick arrow*) (Fig. 8.25), and bilateral air-fluid level in maxillary sinus (*hollow arrows*) (Fig. 8.26): both figures are suggestive of acute sinusitis. Well-ventilated frontal buds (Fig. 8.25) and more developed frontal sinus in an older patient (Fig. 8.26). Skull base CT (*bone window*) was done due to sinusitis complications, showing fluid level content in right maxillary sinus and total occupation of the left maxillar sinus (Fig. 8.27). Unfortunately, the images do not inform us about the etiology of the inflammation (viral, bacterial, allergic, or other). Symptoms and signs of ABS (Fig. 8.28). When viral rhinosinusitis is complicated by ABS, there are three potential clinical presentations: persistent symptoms, severe symptoms, or worsening symptoms.

Case 8: Palm Tree Thorn Foreign Body Injury at the Knee

Víctor Pérez Candela and Rafael Avila Suárez

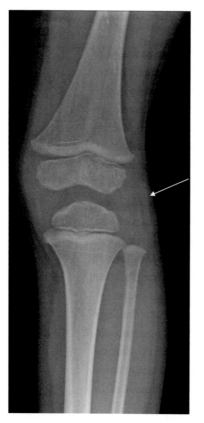

Fig. 8.29

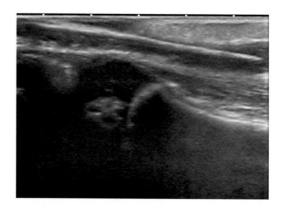

Fig. 8.31

Fig. 8.32

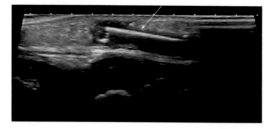

Fig. 8.30

A 4-year-old boy with a painful swollen left knee was referred to the Radiology department by his pediatrician for a knee X-Ray.

Injuries in which palm tree thorns become embedded in soft tissues, leaving no external evidence of their presence, sometimes present a baffling diagnostic problem. A child at play falls on a palm tree and a cone-shaped thorn penetrates the skin, usually at the knee, and breaks off. A pediatrician examining the wound may not see the thorn. A few days later, there may be swelling at the site of injury and the child may limp and complain of pain. There will be no fever, no leukocytosis, no acceleration of the erythrocyte sedimentation rate, and at this stage no abnormality observable in X-ray films. Ultrasound of the soft tissues is the best imaging modality for the diagnosis of palm tree thorn foreign body injury because you can see it.

Bone changes caused by palm tree thorns usually manifest in the form of inflammation, which appears some time after the injury. Bone scan demonstrates a localized increased uptake.

Thorns have been shown to cause foreign body cysts, bursitis, tenosynovitis, synovitis, and bony reaction.

Treatment should be aimed at surgical exploration and debridement with appropriate antibiotics.

The X-ray of the left knee shows a mild soft tissue enlargement and a faint linear image (*arrow*) that looks like a radiolucent foreign body, the thorn, in the fibular side (Fig. 8.29). A longitudinal panoramic view of an ultrasound exam of the soft tissues of the knee at the fibular side shows the foreign body (*arrow*) as an echogenic linear structure. The surrounding hypoechoic area represents edema (Fig. 8.30). Another longitudinal view of the same ultrasound exam shows the palm tree thorn embedded in granulation tissue forming a small abscess (*arrow*) (Fig. 8.31). Another longitudinal view of the ultrasound exam shows the relationship of the thorn with the knee (Fig. 8.32).

Case 9: Ovarian Torsion

Anabel Doblado López and María I. Martínez-León

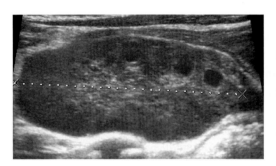

Fig. 8.33

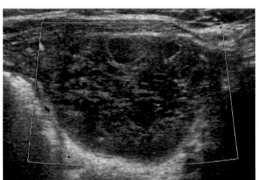

Fig. 8.35

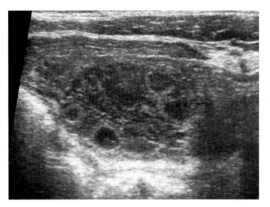

Fig. 8.34

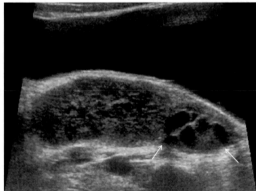

Fig. 8.36

A 4-year-old girl with a 6-day history of lower colicky abdominal pain.

Ovarian torsion is defined as partial or complete rotation of the ovarian vascular pedicle that causes obstruction of venous outflow and arterial inflow.

Torsion may occur in normal ovaries because of a markedly mobile mesosalpinx but is usually associated with a cyst or tumor. These masses may act as a fulcrum to potentiate torsion of the ovary and fallopian tube.

Symptoms are often nonspecific, making it difficult to differentiate from other causes of acute abdominal pain. The classic presentation includes localized right or left lower abdominal pain, tenderness with a palpable abdominal mass, and peritoneal signs. Nausea and vomiting as well as pyrexia have been observed.

Ultrasonography (US) is the primary imaging modality for evaluation of ovarian torsion. US features include:

1. A unilateral enlarged ovary (>4 cm).
2. Uniform peripheral cystic structures "string of pearls sign."
3. Possibility of a coexistent mass within the affected ovary.
4. Lack of arterial or venous flow. The presence of flow in the ovary at color Doppler imaging does not allow exclusion of torsion but instead suggests that the ovary may be viable, especially if flow is present centrally.
5. A twisted vascular pedicle. Absence of flow in the twisted vascular pedicle may indicate that the ovary is not viable.
6. Free pelvic fluid.

The treatment of choice is untwisting the vascular pedicle. If needed, a second surgery may perform an oophorectomy. When a conservative approach is undertaken, an ultrasound should be performed about 2–3 weeks postoperatively to exclude a tumor. Oophoropexy of the detorsed adnexa or the contralateral ovary may be appropriate, especially in children and adolescents who have previously suffered from adnexal torsion.

Longitudinal sonogram shows an enlarged 6-cm ovary (*between cursors*) with some peripheral cysts. There is no coexistent mass within the twisted ovary (Fig. 8.33). Six days later, after detorsion surgery, the ovary has less volume and has more heterogeneous echogenicity with increase of the peripheral cysts (Fig. 8.34). Power Doppler US shows flow only in the periphery and not within the parenchyma (Fig. 8.35). Three weeks later, the ovary is somewhat smaller, but it continues to enlarge and with heterogeneous echogenicity. The left ovary (*between arrows*) is normal (Fig. 8.36).

Case 10: The Limping Child: A Systematic Approach to Diagnosis

María Dolores Domínguez-Pinos and María I. Martínez-León

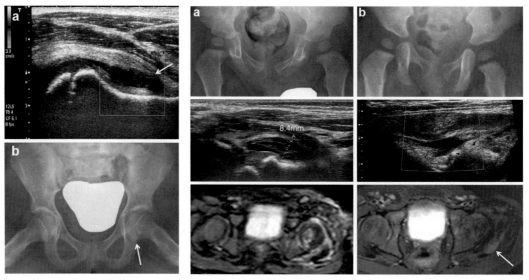

Fig. 8.37

Fig. 8.38

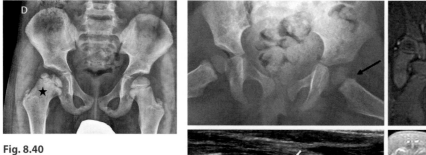

Fig. 8.40

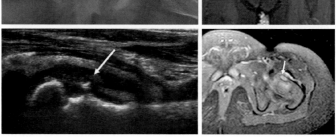

Fig. 8.39

(Fig. 8.37). (a) A 6 year-old boy with a 2-day history of pain and lameness after catarrhal process. Normal exploration. (b) Obese 10-year-old girl. Hip pain and limp after mild trauma 24 h ago. Pain on passive abduction and flexion of the hip.

(Fig. 8.38). (a) An 11-month-old infant with 6-day hip pain and 48 h of fever. (b) 13-month-old infant, lameness of 2 weeks duration. Fever in the last 48 h. Left hip with flexion posture and painful to rotation.

(Fig. 8.39). A 19-month-old infant, lameness of more than 1 month without fever.

(Fig. 8.40). A 6-year-old child, left lameness of long duration, normal exploration.

Comments

History of trauma and overuse should be investigated. In case of a positive history, X-ray should be performed to rule out fractures. In case of a negative traumatic history, systemic disease should be assessed. In negative systemic disease, radiographs should be done to detect femoral head injury. In case of systemic symptoms, a complete study with X-ray, CBC (complete blood count), and CRP (C-reactive protein) should be done. Ultrasound must be done in case of a positive study. Intra-articular fluid puncture must be done in suspected septic arthritis. MRI must be performed in doubtful cases or for complementary study.

Imaging Findings

(Fig. 8.37). (a) Transient synovitis: Thickening of the anterior recess of the hip (*arrow*), more than 3 mm on ultrasound. (b) Epiphysiolysis: Axial projection of hip X-ray showing the backward and downward displacement of the left femoral epiphysis in relation to the neck (*arrow*).

(Fig. 8.38). (a) Septic arthritis: Hip radiograph with left hip flexion and lateral deviation of the left femoral head. Ultrasound shows bulging capsule with internal linear echoes. Synovial uptake after administration of gadolinium on MRI. (b) Pyomyositis: Hip radiograph with obscuring of fat lines of left hip. Hypoechoic area in thickening gluteus on ultrasound. MRI with collection between gluteus medius and minimus (*arrow*).

(Fig. 8.39). Osteomyelitis: Hip radiograph with lytic lesion of the left femoral metaphysic (*black arrow*). Ultrasound shows synovial thickening, small amount of fluid in the anterior recess, and the lytic metaphyseal lesion (*long arrow*). Lytic lesion (*short arrow*) with bone edema (*asterisk*) on MRI.

(Fig. 8.40). Legg-Calve-Perthes disease: Hip X-ray with alteration of the morphology of the right proximal epiphyseal nucleus, irregularity, height loss, fragmentation, and sclerosis. Widening of the femoral neck and coxa magna (*asterisk*).

Further Reading

Case 1: Acute Cerebellitis

Book

Osborn AG (2004) Diagnostic imaging: brain. Amirsys, Salt Lake City, pp I-8–I-49

Web Link

http://sumerdoc.blogspot.com/2010/11/acute-cerebellitis-mri.html

Articles

Bruecker Y, Claus F, Demaerel P, Ballaux F, Sciot R, Lagae L (2004) MRI findings in acute cerebellitis. Eur Radiol 14:1478–1483

Brunberg JA (2008) Ataxia. AJNR Am J Neuroradiol 29:1420–1422

Cijhlich-Ratmann C, Wallot M, Baethmann M, Scharper J, Roggendorf M, Roll C (1998) Acute cerebellitis with near-fatal cerebellar swelling and benign outcome under conservative treatment with high dose steroids. Eur J Paediatr Neurol 2:157–162

Hayakawa H, Katoh T (1995) Severe cerebellar atrophy following acute cerebellitis. Pediatr Neurol 12:159–161

Kamate M, Chetal V, Hattiholi V (2009) Fulminant cerebellitis: a fatal, clinically isolated syndrome. Pediatr Neurol 41:220–222

Komatsu H, Kuroki S, Shimizu Y, Takada H, Takeuchi Y (1998) *Mycoplasma pneumoniae* meningoencephalitis and cerebellitis with antiganglioside antibodies. Pediatr Neurol 18:160–164

Martínez-León M, Díaz-Martí T, Ros B, López-Ruiz P (2005) Pediatric hemicerebellitis: a case report. Radiologia 47(5):283–286

Montenegro MA, Santos S, Li LM, Cendes F (2002) Neuroimaging of acute cerebellitis. J Neuroimaging 12:72–74

Shkalim V, Amir J, Kornreich L, Scheuerman O, Straussberg R (2009) Acute cerebellitis presenting as tonsillar herniation and hydrocephalus. Pediatr Neurol 41:200–203

Xu F, Ren SQ, Liu JY (2008) Acute cerebellitis in identical twins. Pediatr Neurol 39:432–434

Case 2: Traumatic Head Injury

Book

Latchaw R, Kucharczyk J, Mosely M (eds) (2004) Imaging of the nervous system: diagnostic and therapeutic applications. Mosby, St. Louis

Web Link

Stock A (2011) Pediatric head trauma. Medscape reference. http://emedicine.medscape.com/article/1137207-overview. Updated: 1 Nov 2011

Articles

Bernardi B, Zimmerman RA, Bilaniuk LT (1993) Neuroradiologic evaluation of pediatric craniocerebral trauma. Top Magn Reson Imaging 5(3):161–173

Cakmakci H (2009) Essentials of trauma: head and spine. Pediatr Radiol 39:S391–S405

Hymel KP, Hall CA (2005) Diagnosing pediatric head trauma. Pediatr Ann 34:358–370

Parkin PC, Maguire JL (2009) Clinically important head injuries after head trauma in children. Lancet 374:1127–1129

Poussaint TY, Moeller KK (2002) Imaging of pediatric head trauma. Neuroimaging Clin N Am 12:271–294

Savitsky EA, Votey SR (2000) Current controversies in the management of minor pediatric head injuries. Am J Emerg Med 18:96–101

Simon B, Letorneau P, Vitorino E, McCall J (2001) Pediatric minor head trauma: indications for computed tomographic scanning revisited. J Trauma 51:231–238

Tang PH, Lim CC (2009) Imaging of accidental paediatric head trauma. Pediatr Radiol 39:438–446

Tung GA, Kumar M, Richardson RC, Jenny C, Brown WD (2006) Comparison of accidental and non accidental traumatic head injury in children on non contrast computed tomography. Pediatrics 118:626–633

Woodcock RJ, Davis PC, Hopkins KL (2001) Imaging of head trauma in infancy and childhood. Semin Ultrasound CT MR 22:162–182

Case 3: Pediatric Ischemic Stroke

Book

Ganesan V, Chong K et al (2004) Stroke in childhood. Clinical guidelines for the diagnosis, management and rehabilitation. Paediatric Stroke Working Group, Royal College of Physicians. IBSN 1 86016 236 3

Web Link

http://www.stroke.org/site/PageServer?pagename=PEDSTROKE

Articles

Danchaivijitr N, Cox TC, Saunders DE, Ganesan V (2006) Evolution of cerebral arteriopathies in childhood arterial ischemic stroke. Ann Neurol 59:620–626

Ganesan V, Savvy L, Chong WK, Kirkham FJ (1999) Conventional cerebral angiography in children with ischaemic stroke. Pediatr Neurol 20:38–42

Ganesan V, Prengler M, Mc Shane M, Wade A, Kirkham FJ, Chri B (2003) Investigation of risk factors in children with arterial ischaemic stroke. Ann Neurol 53:167–173

Lanni G, Catalucci A, Conti L, Di Sibio A, Paonessa A, Gallucci M (2011) Pediatric stroke: clinical findings and radiological approach. Stroke Res Treat 2011:172168, Epub 2011 Apr 19

Mackay MT, Wiznitzer M, Benedict SL, Lee KJ, Deveber GA, Ganesan V, International Pediatric Stroke Study Group (2011) Arterial ischemic stroke risk factors: the International Pediatric Stroke Study. Ann Neurol 69:130–140

Martínez-Martínez M, Cazorla-García R, Rodríguez de Antonio LA, Martínez-Sánchez P, Fuentes B, Diez-Tejedor E (2010) Estados de hipercoagulabilidad e ictus isquémico en pacientes jóvenes. Neurologia 25:343–348

Roach ES, DeVeber GA, Kirkham FJ (2000) Knowledge of consequences: understanding stroke in children. J Child Neurol 15:277–278

Sébire G, Fullerton H, Riou E, DeVeber G (2004) Toward the definition of cerebral arteriopathies of childhood. Curr Opin Pediatr 16:617–622

Sträter R, Becker S, von Eckardstein A, Heinecke A, Gutsche S, Junker R et al (2002) Prospective assessment of risk factors for recurrent stroke during childhood – a 5-year follow-up study. Lancet 360: 1540–1545

Trenor CC 3rd, Michelson AD (2010) Thrombophilia and pediatric stroke. Circulation 121:1795–1797

Beltz EE, Mullins ME (2010) Radiological reasoning: hyperintensity of the basal ganglia and cortex on FLAIR and diffusion-weighted imaging. AJR Am J Roentgenol 195:S1–S8

Biagas K (1999) Hypoxic-ischemic brain injury: advancements in understanding of mechanisms and potential avenues for therapy. Curr Opin Pediatr 11:223–228

Christophe C, Fonteyne C, Ziereisen F, Christiaens F, Deltenre P, De Maertelaer V et al (2002) Value of MR imaging of the brain in children with hypoxic coma. AJNR Am J Neuroradiol 23:716–723

Dubowitz DJ, Bluml S, Arcinue E, Dietrich RB (1998) MR of hypoxic encephalopathy in children after near drowning: correlation with quantitative proton MR spectroscopy and clinical outcome. AJNR Am J Neuroradiol 19:1617–1627

Gutierrez LG, Rovira A, Portela LA, Leite Cda C, Lucato LT (2010) CT and MR in non-neonatal hypoxic-ischemic encephalopathy: radiological findings with pathophysiological correlations. Neuroradiology 52:949–976

Huang BY, Castillo M (2008) Hypoxic-ischemic brain injury: imaging findings from birth to adulthood. Radiographics 28:417–439

McKinney AM, Teksam M, Felice R, Casey SO, Cranford R, Truwit CL et al (2004) Diffusion-weighted imaging in the setting of diffuse cortical laminar necrosis and hypoxic-ischemic encephalopathy. AJNR Am J Neuroradiol 25:1659–1665

Topcuoglu MA, Oguz KK, Buyukserbetci G, Bulut E (2009) Prognostic value of magnetic resonance imaging in post-resuscitation encephalopathy. Intern Med 48:1635–1645

Case 4: Non-neonatal Hypoxic-Ischemic Encephalopathy (HIE)

Book

Barkovich AJ (2000) Brain pediatric neuroimaging, 4th edn. Lippincott-Raven, Philadelphia

Web Link

http://radiopaedia.org/articles/hypoxic-ischaemic-injury-in-older-children-and-adults

Articles

Arbelaez A, Castillo M, Mukherji S (1999) Diffusion weighted MR imaging of global cerebral anoxia. AJNR Am J Neuroradiol 20:999–1007

Barkovich AJ (1992) MR and CT evaluation of profound neonatal and infantile asphyxia. AJNR Am J Neuroradiol 13:959–972

Case 5: Orbital Cellulitis

Book

Ric Harnsberger H (1995) Handbook of head and neck imaging, 2nd edn. Mosby, St. Louis

Web Link

http://www.merckmanuals.com/professional/eye_disorders/orbital_diseases/preseptal_and_orbital_cellulitis.html

Articles

Capps EF, Kinsella JJ, Gupta M, Bhatki AM, Opatowsky MJ (2010) Emergency imaging assessment of acute, nontraumatic conditions of the head and neck. Radiographics 30:1335–1352

Chung EM, Smirniotopoulos JG, Specht CS, Schoroeder JW, Cube R (2007) Pediatric orbit tumors and tumor-like lesions:nonosseous lesions of the extraocular orbit. From the archives of the AFIP. Radiographics 27:1777–1799

Curtin HD, Rabinov JD (1998) Extension to the orbit from paraorbital disease. The sinuses. Radiol Clin North Am 36:1201–1213

Hopper KD, Sherman JL, Boal DK, Eggli KD (1992) CT and MR imaging of the pediatric orbit. Radiographics 12:485–503

Khanna G, Sato Y, Smith RJ, Baumen NM, Nerad J (2006) Causes of facial swelling in pediatric patients: correlation of clinical and radiological findings. Radiographics 26:157–171

LeBedis CA, Sakai O (2008) Nontraumatic orbital conditions: diagnosis with CT and MR imaging in the emergent setting. Radiographics 28:1741–1753

Lee S, Yen MT (2011) Management of preseptal and orbit cellulitis. Saudi J Ophthalmol 25:21–29

Ludwig BJ, Foster BR, Saito N, Nadgir RN, Castro-Aragón I, Sakai O (2010) Diagnostic imaging in nontraumatic pediatric head and neck emergencies. Radiographics 30:781–799

Towbin R, Han BK, Kaufman RA, Burke M (1986) Postseptal cellulitis: CT in diagnosis and management. Radiology 158:735–737

Wells RG, Sty JR, Gonnering RS (1989) Imaging of the pediatric eye and orbit. Radiographics 9:1023–1044

Case 6: Retropharyngeal Infections in Children

Book

Long SS, Pickering LK, Prober CG (eds) (2008) Principles and practice of pediatric infectious diseases, 3rd edn. Elsevier, Philadelphia, pp 213–221

Web Link

http://www.uptodate.com

Articles

Bakshi RB, Grover GG (2009) Retroharyngeal with mediastinal extension in an infant-still existing? Pediatr Emerg Care 25:181–183

Craig FW, Schunk JE (2003) Retropharyngeal abscess in children: clinical presentation, utility of imaging, and management. Pediatrics 6:1394–1398

Croche Santander B, Prieto del Prado A, Madrid Castillo O, Obando Santaella I (2011) Abscesos retrofaringeo y parafaríngeo: experiencia en un hospital terciario de Sevilla durante la última década. An Pediatr 75:266–272

Courtney MJ, Mahadevan M, Miteff A (2007) Management of paediatric retropharyngeal infection: non surgical versus surgical. ANZ J Surg 77:985

Daya H, Lo S, Papsin BC (2005) Retropharyngeal and parapharyngeal infections in children: the Toronto experience. Int J Pediatr Otorhinolaryngol 69:81–86

Grisaru-Soen G, Komisar O, Aizenstein O, Soudack M, Schartz D (2010) Retropharyngeal and parapharyngeal abscess in children – epidemiology, clinical features and treatment. Int J Pediatr Otorhinolaryngol 74:1016–1020

Hon KL, Chu WC, Sung JKK (2010) Retropharyngeal abscess in a young child due to ingestion of eel vertebrae. Pediatr Emerg Care 26:439–441

Marín Campagne E, del Castillo Martín F, Martínez López MM, BorquedeAndrés C, José de Gómez M, García de Miguel MJ, Baquero Artigao F (2006) Abscesos periamigdalino y retrofaringeo: estudio de 13 años. An Pediatr 65:32–36

Morrison JE Jr, Pashley NR (1998) Retropharyngeal abscesses in children: a 10-year review. Pediatr Emerg Care 4:9

Propst EJ, Prager JD, Shott SR, Koch B, Mortensen JE, Greinwald JH (2011) Resolution of hypoglossal nerve palsy associated with retropharyngeal abscess prompt medical and surgical treatment. Int J Pediatr Otorhinolaryngol 6:74–77

Case 7: Acute Bacterial Sinusitis

Book

Cherry JD, Shapiro NL (2009) Sinusitis. In: Feigin RD, Cherry JD, Demmler-Harrison GJ, Kaplan SL (eds) Feign and Cherry's textbook of pediatric infectious diseases, 6th edn. Saunders, Philadelphia, p 20116

Web Link

http://www.uptodate.com/contents/acute-bacterial-sinusitis-in-children

Articles

American Academy of Pediatrics (2001) Subcommittee on management of sinusitis and committee on quality improvement. Clinical practice guideline: management of sinusitis. Pediatrics 108:798–808

Arruda LK, Mimica IM, Solé D et al (1990) Abnormal maxillary sinus radiographs in children: do they represent bacterial infection? Pediatrics 85:553–558

Diament MJ (1992) The diagnosis of sinusitis in infants and children: x-ray, computed tomography, and magnetic resonance imaging. Diagnostic imaging of pediatric sinusitis. J Allergy Clin Immunol 90:442–444

Goytia VK, Giannoni CM, Edwards MS (2011) Intraorbital and intracranial extension of sinusitis: comparative morbidity. J Pediatr 158:486–491

Lindbaek M, Hjortdahl P, Johnsen UL (1996) Use of symptoms, signs, and blood tests to diagnose acute sinus infections in primary care: comparison with computed tomography. Fam Med 28:183–188

Meltzer EO, Hamilos DL, Hadley JA et al (2004) Rhinosinusitis: establishing definitions for clinical research and patient care. J Allergy Clin Immunol 114:155–212

Revai K, Dobbs LA, Nair S et al (2007) Incidence of acute otitis media and sinusitis complicating upper respiratory tract infection: the effect of age. Pediatrics 119:e1408–e1412

Slavin RG, Spector SL, Bernstein IL et al (2005) The diagnosis and management of sinusitis: a practice parameter update. J Allergy Clin Immunol 116:S13–S47

Wald ER (1998) Sinusitis. Pediatr Ann 27:811–818

Wolf G, Anderhuber W, Kuhn F (1993) Development of the paranasal sinuses in children: implications for paranasal sinus surgery. Ann Otol Rhinol Laryngol 102:705–711

Case 8: Palm Tree Thorn Foreign Body Injury at the Knee

Book

Siegel MJ, Coley BD (2006) Pediatric imaging. Lippincott Williams & Wilkins, Philadelphia

Web Link

http://www.botanical-dermatology-database.info/BotDermFolder/PALM.html

Articles

Banee B, Das RK (1991) Sonographic detection of foreign bodies of the extremities. Br J Radiol 64:107–112

Clarke JD, McCeffrey DD (2007) Thorn injury mimicking a septic arthritis of the knee. Ulster Med J 76:164–165

Cozen L, Fonda M (1953) Palm thorn injuries. Difficulty in diagnosis of late sequelae. Calif Med 79:40–41

Gerle RD (1971) Thorn induced pseudo-tumors of bone. Br J Radiol 44:642–645

Karshner RG, Hanafee W (1953) Palm thorns as a cause of joint effusion in children. Radiology 60:592–595

Klein B, McGahan JP (1985) Thorn synovitis CT diagnosis. J Comput Assist Tomogr 6:1135–1136

Kratz A, Greenberg D, Barki Y, Cohen E, Lifshitz M (2003) *Pantoea agglomerans* as a cause of septic arthritis after palm tree thorn injury; a case report and literature review. Arch Dis Child 88:542–544

Pai VS, Tan E, Matheson JA (2004) Box thorn embedded in the cartilaginous distal femur. Injury Extra 35:45–47

Southgate GW, Murray RO (1982) Thorn-induced synovitis. Skeletal Radiol 8:79–80

Vega Curiel A, Villaverde Romon M, Carrillo Lucia F, RuizdelPortal B, Carranza M, Bencano A (2001) Injuries from palm tree thorn simulating tumoral or pseudotumoral bone lesions. Acta Orthop Belg 67:279–282

Case 9: Ovarian Torsion

Book

Siegel M (2004) Pediatric sonography, 2nd edn. Marban, Madrid, pp 551–554

Web Link

http://imaging.consult.com/imageSearch?query=ovarian+torsion&global_search=Search&modality=+&anatomicRegion=

Articles

Anders J, Powell E (2005) Urgency of evaluation and outcome of acute ovarian torsion in pediatric patients. Arch Pediatr Adolesc Med 159:532–535

Chang H, Bhatt S, Dogra V (2008) Pearls and pitfalls in diagnosis of ovarian torsion. Radiographics 28:1355–1368

Garel L, Dubois J, Grignon A, Filiatrault D, Van Vliet G (2001) US of the pediatric female pelvis: a clinical perspective. Radiographics 21:1393–1407

Linam LE, Darolia R, Naffaa LN, Breech LL, O'Hara SM, Hillard PJ et al (2007) US findings of adnexal torsion in children and adolescents: size really does matter. Pediatr Radiol 37:1013–1019

Meyer JS, Harmon CM, Harty MP, Markowitz RI, Hubbard AM, Bellah RD (1995) Ovarian torsion: clinical and imaging presentation in children. J Pediatr Surg 30:1433–1436

Oelsner G, Shashar D (2006) Adnexal torsion. Clin Obstet Gynecol 49:459–463

Rody A, Jackish C, Klockenbush W (2002) The conservative management of adnexal torsion: a case report and review of the literature. Eur J Obstet Gynecol Reprod Biol 101:83–86

Servaes S, Zurakowski D, Laufer M, Feins N, Chow J (2007) Sonographic findings of ovarian torsion in children. Pediatr Radiol 37:446–451

Siegel M, Stark J (1994) Ovarian torsion in prepubertal and pubertal girls: sonographic findings. AJR Am J Roentgenol 163:1479–1482

Sung T, Callahan M, Taylor G (2006) Clinical and imaging mimickers of acute appendicitis in the pediatric population. AJR Am J Roentgenol 186:67–74

Case 10: The Limping Child: A Systematic Approach to Diagnosis

Book

Fleisher Gary R, Stephen Ludwig et al (2010) Textbook of pediatric emergency medicine. Wolters Kluwer/ Lippincott Williams & Wilkins Health, Philadelphia. ISBN 9781605471594 1605471593

Web Link

http://www.acr.org/SecondaryMainMenuCategories/ quality_safety/app_criteria/pdf/ExpertPanelon PediatricImaging/LimpingChildUpdateinProgress Doc6.aspx

Articles

Abbassian A (2007) The limping child: a clinical approach to diagnosis. Br J Hosp Med (Lond) 68:246–250

Barkin RM, Barkin SZ, Barkin AZ (2000) The limping child. J Emerg Med 18:331–339

Dabney KW, Lipton G (1995) Evaluation of limp in children. Curr Opin Pediatr 7:88–94

Fabry G (2010) Clinical practice: the hip from birth to adolescence. Eur J Pediatr 169:143–148

Leet AI, Skaggs DL (2000) Evaluation of the acutely limping child. Am Fam Physician 61:1011–1018

Leung AK, Lemay JF (2004) The limping child. J Pediatr Health Care 18:219–223

MacEwen GD, Dehne R (1991) The limping child. Pediatr Rev 12:268–274

Sawyer JR, Kapoor M (2009) The limping child: a systematic approach to diagnosis. Am Fam Physician 79:215–224

Swischuk LE (2007) The limping infant: imaging and clinical evaluation of trauma. Emerg Radiol 14:219–226

Taekema HC, Landham PR, Maconochie I (2009) Towards evidence based medicine for paediatricians. Distinguishing between transient synovitis and septic arthritis in the limping child: how useful are clinical prediction tools? Arch Dis Child 94:167–168

CRISTINA BRAVO BRAVO

Contents

M.I. Martínez-León et al., *Imaging for Pediatricians*, Imaging for Clinicians,
DOI 10.1007/978-3-642-28629-2_9, © Springer-Verlag Berlin Heidelberg 2012

Case 1: Developmental Dysplasia of the Hip

María I. Martínez-León and Antonio Martínez-Valverde

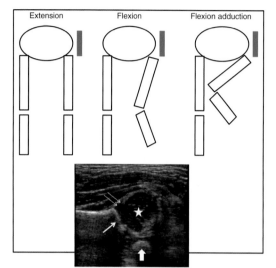

Fig. 9.1

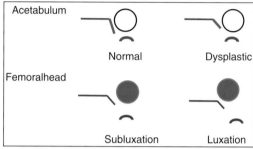

Fig. 9.4

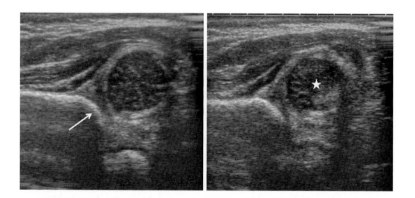

Fig. 9.2

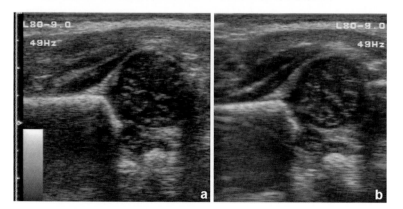

Fig. 9.3

Female neonate with breech presentation and positive Ortolani and Barlow maneuvers.

Developmental dysplasia of the hip (DDH) comprises a spectrum of disorders affecting the proximal femur and acetabulum that leads to alteration in the position of the femoral head in the coxofemoral joint, based on ligament and joint instability. Early diagnosis and treatment is important because failure to diagnose DDH in neonates and young infants can result in significant morbidity.

Ortolani and Barlow maneuvers, among others, are the most generalized clinical tests for detecting the DDH.

Ultrasonography (US) is the preferred radiological modality for evaluating the hip in infants who are approximately 6 months or younger. US enables direct imaging of the cartilaginous portions of the hip that cannot be seen on plain radiographs. Furthermore, US permits a dynamic approach of the hip with different stress maneuvering.

A dynamic study should be performed at rest with stress maneuvers on the hip; hips that are morphologically normal and stable in dynamic study are considered to be "sonographically normal." Different pathological situations are defined as:

1. Instability of the hip: this is the subluxation or dislocation of the hip with the hip stress positions of the hip.
2. Subluxation: it is incomplete contact between the articular surfaces of the proximal femoral epiphysis and the acetabulum.
3. Luxation: this is related to complete loss of contact between the femoral head and the acetabulum. Generally, this kind of pathology is associated to acetabular dysplasia or "dysplastic hip." It consists in the shortening or rectification of the acetabulum.

This entire pathological hip spectrum is called DDH, and the different treatments that each one requires should be studied and followed by sequential hip US.

(Fig. 9.1). Dynamic study of the hip in extension, flexion, and flexion with adduction, scheme, and correlate US figures. In red, the coronal position of the high frequency transducer. Normal hip in extension, acetabulum (*arrow*), femoral head without ossification center (*asterisk*), labrum (*double arrow*), pubis (*thick arrow*). (Fig. 9.2). Severe acetabular dysplasia (*arrow*) with secondary luxation of the femoral head (*asterisk*). (Fig. 9.3). Unstable hips, normal sonography in extension (a) and subluxation in the stress study (b). (Fig. 9.4). Scheme of different types of DDH related to the acetabulum (*blue line*) and the femoral head (*blue circle*).

Case 2: Asphyxiating Thoracic Dysplasia

Anabel Doblado López and Cristina Bravo Bravo

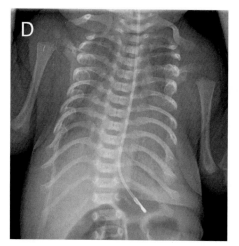

Fig. 9.5

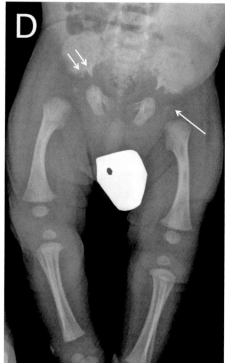

Fig. 9.7

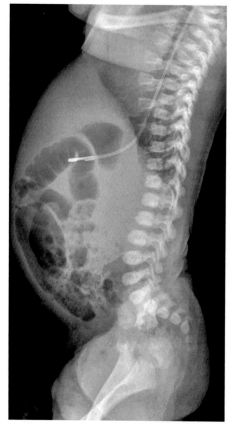

Fig. 9.6

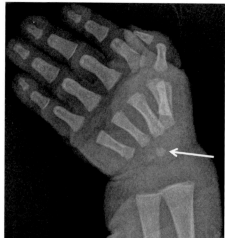

Fig. 9.8

A 10-day-old newborn was admitted to our hospital with severe respiratory distress. He was referred from another hospital where prenatal ultrasound suspected a skeletal dysplasia.

Asphyxiating thoracic dysplasia (ATD), also known as Jeune syndrome, is a rare autosomal recessive skeletal dysplasia characterized by a small thorax, short-limbed dwarfism, and renal and hepatic anomalies. ATD has a wide phenotypic variability, from severe and lethal forms to dormant presentations.

The diagnosis is based on clinical and radiographic findings.

The most striking clinical feature is a small and narrow chest that results in respiratory distress. Patient is prone to asphyxia and recurrent lung infections due to the thoracic malformation and resulting lung hypoplasia. Other clinical findings are variable limb shortness and polydactyly. Patients surviving infancy may develop chronic cystic renal disease and hepatic disease later in life.

Radiological findings include a narrow, bell-shaped thorax with short, horizontally oriented ribs and irregular bulbous costochondral junctions. Iliac bones are shortened in the cephalocaudal diameter and acetabula have a typical trident appearance. Long bones of the limbs are shorter and wider, causing slight rhizomelic dwarfism; metaphyses are irregular and there is premature ossification of proximal femoral and humeral epiphyses. Polydactyly is occasionally encountered.

The main differential diagnosis is Ellis-van Creveld chondroectodermal dysplasia, an autosomal recessive dysplasia with similar radiological features, but often with cardiac anomalies.

The poor prognosis of the disease is due to the severity of chest deformity, and most patients die in their first year because of respiratory failure.

Thorax is small in both anteroposterior and transverse dimensions, ribs are very short, and costochondral junctions are bulbous (Figs. 9.5 and 9.6). The spine is normal. Pelvis (Fig. 9.7) has a trident appearance (*short arrows*), with small flattened iliac. There is premature epiphyseal ossification of the femoral heads (*large arrow*). Hand radiograph (Fig. 9.8) shows premature ossification of the carpal bones (*arrow*).

Case 3: Neonatal Pneumonia

Roberto Llorens Salvador and Amparo Moreno Flores

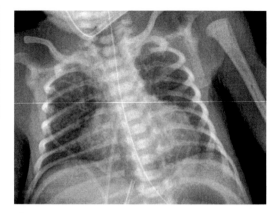

Fig. 9.9

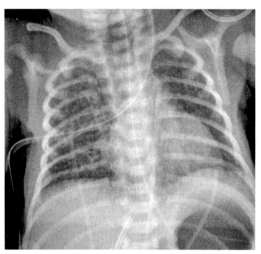

Fig. 9.10

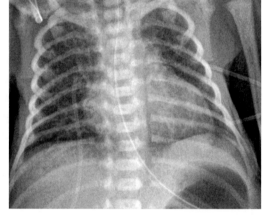

Fig. 9.11

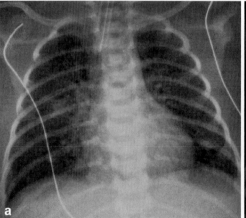

Fig. 9.12

A 31-week-old preterm is born after prolonged rupture of the fetal membranes and presents respiratory distress. Ureaplasma urealyticum is isolated in tracheal aspirate.

Neonatal pneumonia (NP) is the lung infection affecting neonates within the first 28 days of life. It is the most common cause of sepsis in neonates and despite recent advances in therapy, NP remains a principal cause of death in newborn. Risk factors are prolonged rupture of the fetal membranes, maternal amnionitis, premature delivery, maternal intrapartum fever, perinatal asphyxia, and postnatal assisted ventilation. NP can be acquired by several routes, the most common being an ascending vaginal infection, aspiration of infected amniotic fluid during delivery, or nosocomial infection after birth. Bacterial pathogens are the most common cause of NP, especially Group B streptococcus and gram-negative bacteria. However, a large number of viral or fungal pathogens can cause NP.

The clinical picture can range from an early-onset NP with severe respiratory distress and respiratory failure within 24 h to late-onset NP, which develops during hospitalization or after discharge by organisms acquired nosocomially. Early diagnosis requires identification of pathogenic organisms in blood cultures or in gastric or tracheal aspirate.

Recognition of the wide range of nonspecific radiographic changes and their correlation with the clinical features can aid in the diagnosis of NP. Serial chest radiographs are used to detect bilateral coarse pattern of perihilar reticular densities or interstitial diffuse reticulonodular pattern. Frank consolidation is unusual in neonates. NP may be difficult to distinguish from surfactant deficiency disease in preterm infants, transient tachypnea of the newborn, or meconium aspiration syndrome. NP usually presents with pleural effusion and normal lung volume.

Empirical antibiotic therapy such as ampicillin plus gentamicin should be started when NP is suspected or there is high risk of neonatal infection.

Chest X-ray on day two after birth (Fig. 9.9) shows interstitial reticular pattern in upper right lobe that is more evident in chest radiographs on day four (Fig. 9.10) and seven (Fig. 9.11) showing a coarse interstitial diffuse reticular pattern. Figures show other NP radiographic patterns in patients with confirmed Streptococcal NP (Fig. 9.12a) and congenital NP by Listeria (Fig. 9.12b).

Case 4: Pyogenic Liver Abscess in Neonates

Cristina Bravo Bravo and María Gracia Espinosa Fernández

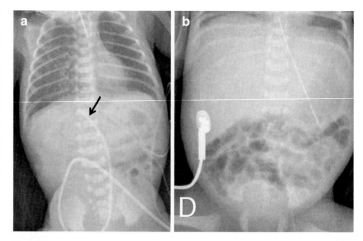

Fig. 9.13

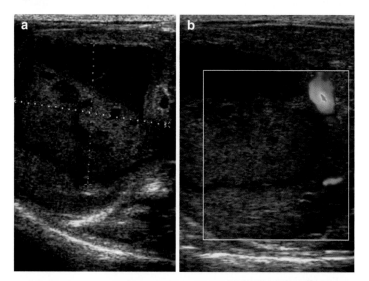

Fig. 9.14

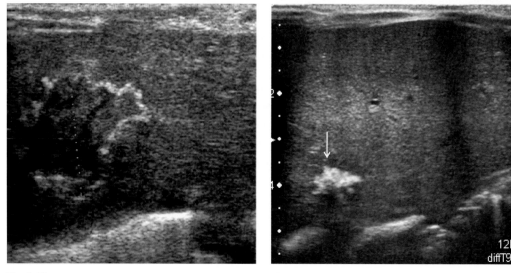

Fig. 9.15

Fig. 9.16

On the 21st day of life, an extremely low-birthweight female neonate with ongoing sepsis developed abdominal distension. Inflammatory markers remained elevated despite adequate antimicrobial therapy.

Liver abscess in the neonatal period is a rare but serious disorder. Clinical signs are unspecified and a high degree of suspicion is required to make an early diagnosis and prompt treatment. It should be considered in any neonate with persistent elevated inflammatory markers in spite of treatment with appropriate antibiotics, especially when signs of abdominal infection are present.

Risk factors for liver abscesses are umbilical venous catheterization, prematurity, sepsis, necrotizing enterocolitis, and abdominal surgery. The abscesses can be solitary or multiple. Solitary pyogenic abscesses comprise 30% of reported neonatal liver abscesses. Most of them are found in the right hepatic lobe and are usually associated to a misplaced umbilical vein. *Staphylococcus* spp. and gram-negative enteric bacteria are the most commonly isolated organisms.

Abdominal X-ray may be normal or show a malpositioned umbilical line, hepatomegaly, pleural effusion, elevated diaphragm, or radiolucency over liver shadow.

Ultrasound (US) is the best diagnostic tool: it is useful for diagnosis, percutaneous drainage, and monitoring the therapy. Usually liver abscess appears as a hypoechoic round lesion with well-defined echogenic rim, central coarse debris, low level echos or fluid debris level. After treatment, serial US shows progressive decrease in size and dystrophic calcifications at the site of the abscess.

CT or MR must be kept for complications.

Conservative treatment with antibiotics can be successful in some cases, but early US-guided aspiration or drainage is recommended if abscess does not resolves to obtain microbiological diagnosis, speed up resolution, reduce thAe length of intravenous antibiotic course, and prevent complications.

Abdominal X-rays show a malpositioned umbilical vein line on first day of life (*arrow*) (Fig. 9.13a) and hepatomegaly on 21st day of life (Fig. 9.13b). High-resolution US reveals a right hepatic lobe heterogeneous mass with well defined wall, fluid debris level (Fig. 9.14a), and without internal flow (Fig. 9.14b). After image-guided percutaneous drainage and long-term antibiotic therapy, follow-up sonograms show progressive decrease in size and dystrophic calcifications (*arrow*) at previous abscess site (Figs. 9.15 and 9.16).

Case 5: Inspissated Bile Syndrome

Cristina Bravo Bravo and Pascual García-Herrera Taillefer

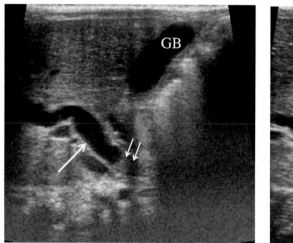

Fig. 9.17

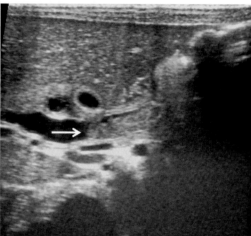

Fig. 9.19

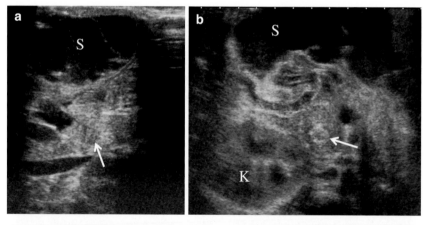

Fig. 9.18

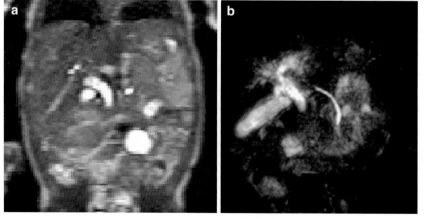

Fig. 9.20

A 7-week-old male infant was admitted with jaundice and acholic stools. He was born at normal gestational age and his perinatal history was uncomplicated. Laboratory data showed conjugated hyperbilirubinemia and elevated gamma-glutamyl transferase (GGT).

Comments

Inspissated bile syndrome (IBS) or bile-plug syndrome is defined as extrahepatic obstruction of the bile ducts by biliary sludge without anatomic abnormalities. It is an uncommon cause of obstructive cholestasis jaundice in neonates, caused by a difficult clearance of bile.

The clinical presentation is similar to other conditions, such as biliary atresia and neonatal hepatitis, with jaundice, weight stagnation, acholic stools, and hepatomegaly. Predisposing factors are prematurity, sepsis, hemolysis, hemorrhage, delayed enteral feeding and total parenteral nutrition, cystic fibrosis, and drugs (ceftriaxona). Up to 43% of cases are idiopathic.

The diagnosis of IBS is based on imaging. Ultrasound (US) should be the first imaging modality in the study of conjugated hyperbilirubinemia, providing information about the appearance of the liver and biliary tree. US shows a dilatated extrahepatic duct filled with echogenic material. So the diagnosis of biliary atresia is discarded, but differentiation of choledochal malformation can be more difficult. In most cases, US obviates the need for other imaging studies and prevents unnecessary interventional procedures or surgery.

Cholangio-MR imaging can provide more complete imaging of the biliary tree and aid to confirm the absence of choledochal malformation.

IBS can resolve spontaneously or with oral ursodeoxycholic acid treatment. In refractory cases, flushing the biliary ducts with saline o mucolytic agents (N-acetylcysteine) may be necessary. This treatment can be performed by percutaneous transhepatic cholangiography, by cholecystostomy, or by choledochotomy. Sometimes, it may require endoscopic retrograde cholangiopancreatographic sphincterotomy.

Imaging Findings

High-resolution US (Fig. 9.17) shows a large gall bladder (GB) and dilatated extrahepatic biliary ducts (*large arrow*), with sludge in common biliary duct (*short arrows*). Longitudinal image of the choledochal duct (Fig. 9.18a) shows a dilated duct filled with echogenic material without shadow (*arrow*). In axial plane (Fig. 9.18b) the choledochal duct is seen at the pancreatic head (*arrow*) with highly echogenic content. S, stomach; K, kidney. Some days later (Fig. 9.19), after oral treatment, a sludge mold is seen in the dilated duct (*arrow*). Coronal hepatic MR (Fig. 9.20a) and 3D cholangio-MR (Fig. 9.20b) show the complete biliary tree and confirm the US findings.

Case 6: Hirschsprung Disease

Almudena Pérez Lara and Pascual García-Herrera Taillefer

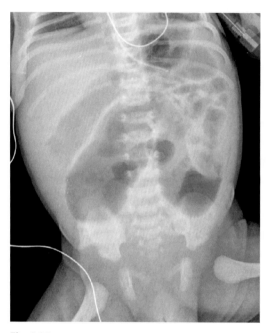

Fig. 9.21

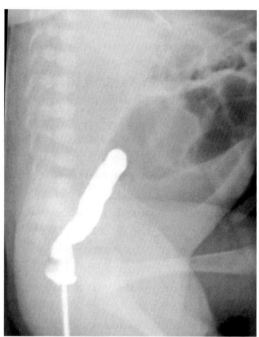

Fig. 9.22

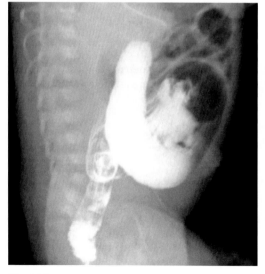

Fig. 9.23

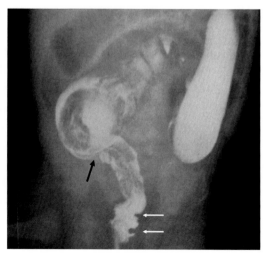

Fig. 9.24

A 3-day-old term neonate who presented bilious vomiting and failure to pass meconium.

Hirschsprung disease is the congenital absence of normal myenteric ganglion cells in a segment, or in all of the colon, which results in the failure of the distal intestine to relax normally. It is the most common hereditary cause of intestinal obstruction. The aganglionosis area varies in length but always extends proximally from the anal canal, and the rectosigmoid area is involved in 80% of cases. Most patients are term neonates, and it is more frequent in males. Twenty percent of patients have associated abnormalities.

In most cases, the diagnosis of Hirschsprung disease is made in the newborn period. Abdominal distention, constipation, delay in passage of meconium, and bilious vomiting are the predominant signs and symptoms of obstruction appear within a few days after birth. Some patients are diagnosed later in infancy or in adulthood with severe constipation and chronic abdominal distention.

Three basic tests are available in the diagnostic work-up of Hirschsprung disease: contrast enema, anorectal manometry, and rectal suction biopsy.

1. Water-soluble contrast enema is the imaging method to be performed when a low-grade obstruction is suspected in a neonate. The best diagnostic clue is a rectosigmoid ratio <1 (rectum smaller than sigmoid). A transition zone (TZ) between the narrow and dilated portions of the colon, in the shape of an inverted cone, is a characteristic radiologic finding, but it is only seen in 50% of neonates during the first week of life. Abnormal peristaltic activity of the aganglionic portion of the colon may be a useful indicator of the disease, although the findings are nonspecific.
2. Anorectal manometry is frequently used as an adjunct to help diagnose HD or for complementary study, but it is not routinely necessary.
3. A rectal suction biopsy is the gold standard for the diagnosis of Hirschsprung disease.

Children who have Hirschsprung disease require surgery to remove the area of the aganglionosis, usually with an endorectal pull-through technique using a transanal approach.

Abdominal X-ray (Fig. 9.21) shows a severe dilation of multiple bowel loops consistent with distal obstruction. Lateral views of water-soluble contrast enema demonstrate patency of the rectum (Fig. 9.22) and distal colon (Fig. 9.23). Anteroposterior view (Fig. 9.24) shows a transitional zone (*black arrow*) between the narrow rectum and dilated sigmoid colon and abnormal rectal contractions (*white arrows*).

Case 7: Neonatal Renal Vein Thrombosis

Inmaculada González Almendros and Cristina Bravo Bravo

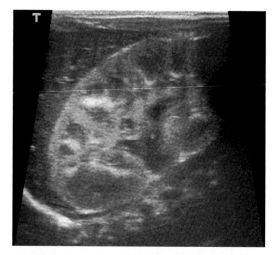

Fig. 9.25

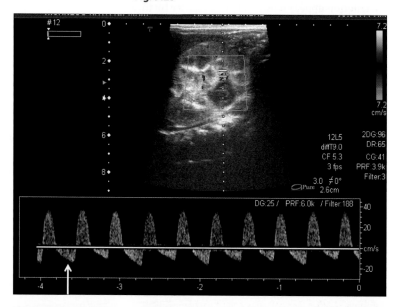

Fig. 9.26

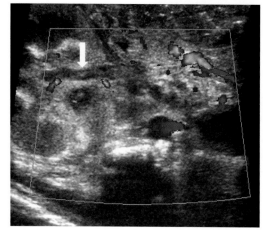

Fig. 9.27

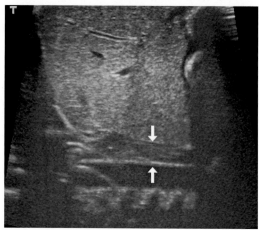

Fig. 9.28

On the first day of life, a newborn is admitted to NICU with suspicion of vertical sepsis. Physical examination revealed a right abdominal palpable mass.

Renal vein thrombosis (RVT) is the most common non-catheter venous thromboembolic event in newborns.

Risk factors include coagulopathy and prothrombotic hereditary conditions, dehydration, neonatal infection, sepsis, birth asphyxia, and maternal diabetes. Although 80% of all VRT present within the first month, within the first week of life some neonates may have prenatal onset of RVT.

RVT shows a slight male predominance. Usually, RVT is unilateral (70%), more prevalent in the left side, and is associated with adrenal hemorrhage.

The classic clinical presentation of a palpable flank mass, hematuria, and thrombocytopenia is only seen in a minority of patients.

Ultrasound (US) is the imaging test of choice for diagnosis. Sonographic findings vary with the time of onset, severity, and extent of thrombus. During the first week, US shows a generalized renal enlargement, with increased echogenicity, loss of corticomedullary differentiation, and echogenic interlobular streaking. The appearance of thrombus in the renal vein or IVC may range from echopoor to highly echogenic. Duplex and color Doppler US show absent renal venous flow and decreased or reversed diastolic arterial flow. In the second week, the renal appearance is more heterogeneous. Later, the kidney usually decreases to become atrophic.

There are no characteristic gray-scale or Doppler prognostic features to predict the outcome of neonatal RVT, and follow-up of these neonates is required.

There is very little consensus regarding the management of RVT in newborn infants: conservative treatment, anticoagulation therapy, or fibrinolytic treatment. Evidence-based recommendations for the optimal treatment of neonatal RVT are not currently possible.

Enlarged right kidney (6.5 cm) on longitudinal ultrasound with echopoor medullary pyramids (Fig. 9.25). Color and spectral Doppler sonogram of the right kidney (Fig. 9.26) reveals reversed end-diastolic flow in the main renal artery (*arrow*). Color Doppler transversal renal sonogram shows absence of color signal in the main renal vein (*arrow*), indicative of occlusive thrombus (Fig. 9.27). Longitudinal Doppler sonogram through the IVC shows the thrombus (*arrows*) (Fig. 9.28).

Case 8: Posterior Urethral Valves

Celestino Gómez Rebollo and
Pascual García-Herrera Taillefer

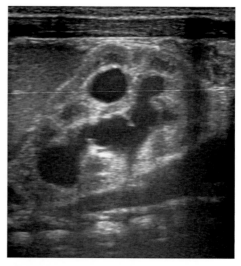

Fig. 9.29

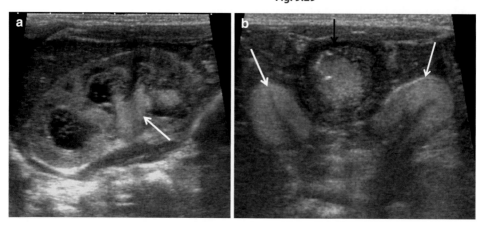

Fig. 9.30

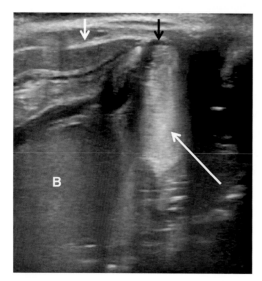

Fig. 9.31

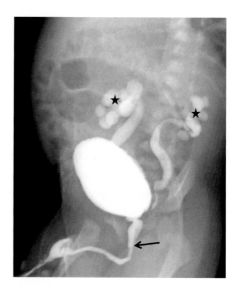

Fig. 9.32

A male newborn with hydronephrosis detected in prenatal ultrasound and poor urinary stream after birth.

Posterior urethral valves are the most common cause of lower urinary tract obstruction in males and occur in one of every 4,000–8,000 infants. There is an elevated incidence in African-Americans and children with Down's syndrome.

The embryologic defect leading to the development of posterior urethral valves is not known. Many authors believe the anomaly is caused by abnormal integration of the Wolffian ducts into the urethra, while others consider it to be a result of persistence of the cloacal membrane.

The valves are composed of connective tissue interspersed with smooth muscle, similar to the tissue encasing the ejaculatory ducts, and are lined with stratified squamous epithelium rather than the transitional epithelium that lines the posterior urethra.

According to the Young classification, type I valves are the most common (95%). This type arises from the verumontanum and extends distally to attach to the lateral walls of the urethra.

The consequences of posterior urethral valves are bilateral renal obstruction, bladder dysfunction, vesicoureteral reflux, hydronephrosis, and, finally, renal damage.

Ultrasonography is the initial imaging modality, revealing a thick bladder wall, dilatation of posterior urethra, and bilateral but asymmetric hydronephrosis. Good corticomedullary differentiation and cortical thickness are signs of preserved renal function and good prognosis (Fig. 9.29).

Contrast-enhanced voiding urosonography (VUS) (Fig. 9.30a, b) shows bilateral vesicoureteral (*thick white arrows*) and pelvicalicial (*thin white arrow*) reflux and thick bladder wall (*black arrow*).

Transperineal approach (Fig. 9.31) reveals dilatation of the posterior urethra (*large white arrow*) and normal caliber of the anterior urethra (*short white arrow*). In this case, the valve is seen as a hypoechoic lineal structure (*short black arrow*). B: bladder.

Voiding cystourethrography (VUCG) (Fig. 9.32) shows bilateral reflux (*asterisks*), spiculated wall bladder, posterior urethra dilatation, and the valves (*black arrow*).

Case 9: Cerebellar Hemorrhage in Preterm Infants

Pascual García-Herrera Taillefer
and Alejandro Aranda Mora

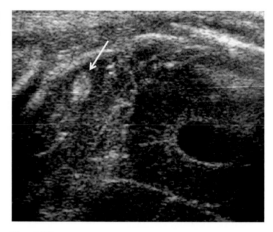

Fig. 9.35

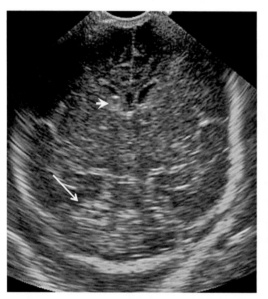

Fig. 9.33

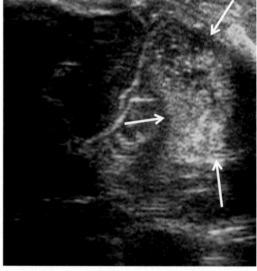

Fig. 9.34

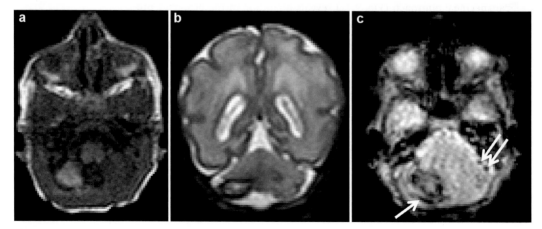

Fig. 9.36

A 27-week preterm infant, 800-g weight, with motor agitation and thrombocytopenia on seventh day of life.

Cerebellar hemorrhage (CBH) is more common than clinically appreciated at present, with a prevalence of up to 25% in neuropathologic studies in very low-birthweight infants. It is not always concomitant with extensive supratentorial bleed and constitutes one of the causes of cerebellar damage in preterm neonates.

CBH originates in the germinal matrix in the subependymal layer of the fourth ventricle roof or in the subpial external granule cell layer, which is thickest at 25 weeks of gestation.

Sometimes it is preceded by motor agitation or discovered after an unexplained ventriculomegaly in routine ultrasound (US) scanning. The use of mastoid or posterolateral fontanelle, especially with high-frequency probes, can detect them as hyperechoic change in hemisphere, vermis, or subarachnoid layer. Magnetic resonance imaging (MRI) can confirm the diagnosis and evaluate associated lesions.

The late consequences of cerebellar lesions are motor impairment (hypotonia, gait abnormalities), impaired language, cognitive, and socialization-behavioral deficits.

US in coronal plane through anterior fontanelle (Fig. 9.33) and right mastoid fontanelle (Fig. 9.34) shows a focal hyperechoic lesion in right cerebellar hemisphere (*large arrows*), corresponding to a hemorrhage. A little subependymal right hemorrhage (*short arrow*) is also seen through anterior fontanelle (Fig. 9.33). Left mastoid fontanelle view shows a folial hemorrhagic focus in the left cerebellar hemisphere (*arrow*) (Fig. 9.35).

MRI shows hemorrhagic foci, hyperintense in axial TSE T1-weighted image (Fig. 9.36a) and with different signals in coronal TSE T2-weighted images (Fig. 9.36b). The axial susceptibility-weighted MRI (Fig. 9.36c) detects hemosiderin residue in the right cerebellar hemisphere (*single arrow*) and in the superficial left hemisphere (*double arrows*).

Case 10: Neonatal Brain Abscesses

Fátima Nagib Raya and Cristina Bravo Bravo

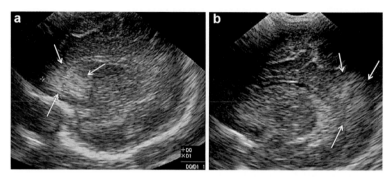

Fig. 9.37

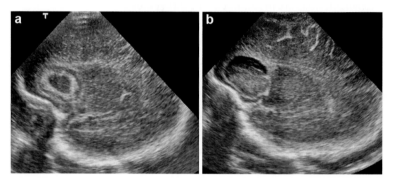

Fig. 9.38

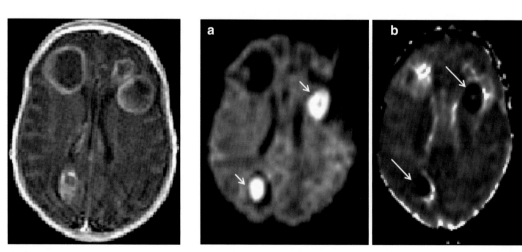

Fig. 9.39   Fig. 9.40

Preterm neonate with ongoing sepsis. Brain US on fifth day of life showed two intraparenchymal echogenic foci. Follow-up US showed new lesions and their progression to abscesses. Blood culture showed growth of Klebsiella pneumoniae.

Brain abscess is rare in children and extremely rare in neonates. It is an inflammatory lesion characterized by the collection of pus in the brain parenchyma that is potentially fatal. **Comments**

Neonatal brain abscess is most commonly caused by virulent gram-negative bacteria, such as Citrobacter and Proteus. Klebsiella is an uncommon cause because of its inability to cause necrotizing lesions.

Abscesses can be caused by continuity, hematogenous spread, or direct inoculation. In neonates, they are characteristically relatively large, with poorly developed capsules, and show preferential periventricular location.

The imaging features vary with the stage of infection: early cerebritis, late cerebritis, early capsule formation, and late capsule formation.

At US, early suppuration may only show a mildly hyper- or hypoechoic area, while a frankly purulent abscess appears as a cystic cavity with fluid of varying echogenicity.

At MRI, the cerebritis appears as an ill-defined hyperintense area on T2-weighted images and as a hypointense region within poorly delineated enhancing foci on contrast-enhanced T1-weighted images. In the later stages, the abscess capsule appears as a well-delineated hyperintense ring on contrast-enhanced images that is hypointense on T2-weighted sequences. Diffusion-weighted image (DWI) is a diagnostic clue in cases of a cerebral ring-enhancing mass. Pyogenic brain abscesses typically show restricted diffusion (related to the presence of pus) and thus have markedly increased signal intensity on DWI and low ADC values on ADC maps.

Treatment of neonatal brain abscess includes prolonged antibiotic therapy and sometimes also requires neurosurgical drainage. US, MRI, and specially DWI are used to follow up and to monitor the therapy.

US parasagittal images through anterior fontanelle show ill-defined hyperechoic areas (*arrows*) in right frontal (Fig. 9.37a) and occipital lobes (Fig. 9.37b). Follow-up ultrasounds (Fig. 9.38) display the right frontal abscess formation, from a mass with a target appearance (Fig. 9.38a) to a well-circumscribed hypoechogenic mass with debris in the dependent portion (Fig. 9.38b). Axial contrast-enhanced T1-weighted image shows multiple ring-enhancing lesions (Fig. 9.39). Restricted diffusion due to pyogenic content of the abscess is seen on DWI (Fig. 9.40a) and ADC map (Fig. 9.40b), with high signal on diffusion (*short arrow*) and correlated low values on ADC map (*long arrow*). **Imaging Findings**

Further Reading

Case 1: Developmental Dysplasia of the Hip

Book

De Bruyn R (2010) The musculoskeletal system. In: de Bruyn R (ed) Pediatric ultrasound. How, why and when, 2nd edn. Churchill Livingstone, Elsevier, Edinburg, pp 319–330

Web Link

Norton KI (2011) Imaging in developmental dysplasia of the hip. eMedicine http://emedicine.medscape.com/article/408225-overview. Updated May 25, 2011

Articles

(2000) Clinical practice guideline: early detection of developmental dysplasia of the hip. Committee on Quality Improvement, Subcommittee on Developmental Dysplasia of the Hip. American Academy of Pediatrics. Pediatrics 105:896–905

(2009) AIUM practice guideline for the performance of an ultrasound examination for detection and assessment of developmental dysplasia of the hip. J Ultrasound Med 28:114–119

Delaney LR, Karmazyn B (2011) Developmental dysplasia of the hip: background and the utility of ultrasound. Semin Ultrasound CT MR 32:151–156

Dogruel H, Atalar H, Yavuz OY, Sayh U (2008) Clinical examination versus ultrasonography in detecting developmental dysplasia of the hip. Int Orthop 32:415–419

Donaldson JS, Feinstein KA (1997) Imaging of developmental dysplasia of the hip. Pediatr Radiol 44:591–614

Finne PH, Dalen I, Ikonomou N, Ulimoen G, Hansen TW (2008) Diagnosis of congenital hip dysplasia in the newborn. Acta Orthop 79:313–320

Graf R (2007) The use of ultrasonography in developmental dysplasia of the hip. Acta Orthop Traumatol Turc 41(Suppl 1):6–13

Kosar P, Ergun E, Unlübay D, Kosar U (2009) Comparison of morphologic and dynamic US methods in examination of the newborn hip. Diagn Interv Radiol 15:284–289

Mahan ST, Katz JN, Kim YJ (2009) To screen or not to screen? A decision analysis of the utility of screening for developmental dysplasia of the hip. J Bone Joint Surg Am 91:1705–1719

Synder M, Harcke HT, Domzalski M (2006) Role of ultrasound in the diagnosis and management of developmental dysplasia of the hip: an international perspective. Orthop Clin North Am 37:141–147

Ultrasound in Medicine; American College of Radiology (2009) AIUM practice guideline for the performance of an ultrasound examination for detection and assessment of developmental dysplasia of the hip. J Ultrasound Med 28:114–119

Case 2: Asphyxiating Thoracic Dysplasia

Book

Murray RO, Jacobson HG (1982) Radiología de los trastornos esqueléticos, 1st edn. Salvat, Barcelona, p 1950

Web Link

http://www.omim.org/entry/208500

Articles

Chen CP, Lin SP, Liu FF, Jan SW, Lin SY, Lan CC (1996) Prenatal diagnosis of asphyxiating thoracic dysplasia (Jeune syndrome). Am J Perinatol 13:495–498

Glass BJ, Norton K, Mitre S, Kang E (2002) Pediatrics ribs: a spectrum of abnormalities. Radiographics 22:87–104

Langer L (1968) Thoracic pelvic phalangeal dystrophy. Radiology 91:447–456

Pirnar T, Neuhauser EBD (1966) Asphyxiating thoracic dystrophy of the newborn. AJR Am J Roentgenol 98:358–364

Poggiani C, Gasparoni MC, Mangili G, Colombo A (2000) Asphyxiating thoracic displasia in a lethal form: radiological and sonographic findings. Minerva Pediatr 52(1–2):63–67

Rodriguez E, Jiménez E, Muro JM, González A, Rodríguez C, Fernández F (1990) Distrofia torácica asfixiante o enfermedad de Jeune. Bol Pediatr 31:135–139

Spirt BA, Oliphant M, Gottlieb RH, Gordon LP (1990) Prenatal sonographic evaluation of short-limbed dwarfism: an algorithmic approach. Radiographics 10:217–236

Tongsong T, Chanprapaph P, Thongpadungroj T (1999) Prenatal sonographic findings associated with asphyxiating thoracic dystrophy (Jeune syndrome). J Ultrasound Med 18:573–576

Tüysüz B, Baris S, Aksoy F, Madazli R, Ungür S, Sever L (2009) Clinical variability of asphyxiating thoracic dystrophy: evaluation and classification of 13 patients. Am J Med Genet A 149:1727–1733

Vries J, Yntema JL, Van Die CE, Crama N, Cornelissen E, Hamel BCJ (2010) Jeune syndrome: description of the 13 cases and a proposal for follow-up protocol. Eur J Pediatr 169:77–88

Case 3: Neonatal Pneumonia

Book

Swischuk LE (2003) Imaging of the newborn, infant and young child, 5th edn. Lippincott Williams & Wilkins, Philadelphia, pp 43–46

Web Link

ME (2011) Neonatal pneumonia. http://www.uptodate. com/contents/neonatal-pneumonia. Accessed Oct 2011

Articles

Abzug MJ, Levin MJ (1991) Neonatal adenovirus infection: four patients and review of the literature. Pediatrics 87:890–896

Apisarnthanarak A, Holzmann-Pazgal G, Hamvas A, Olsen MA, Fraser VJ (2003) Ventilator-associated pneumonia in extremely preterm neonates in a neonatal intensive care unit: characteristics, risk factors and outcomes. Pediatrics 112:1283–1289

Belady JE, Farkouh LJ, Gibbs RS (1997) Intra-amniotic infection and premature rupture of the membranes. Clin Perinatol 24:43–57

Crouse DT, Odrezin GT, Cutter GR et al (1993) Radiographic changes associated with tracheal isolation of ureaplasma urealyticum from neonates. Clin Infect Dis 17(Suppl 1):S122–S130

Davies HD, Wang EE, Manson D, Babyn P, Shuckett B (1996) Reliability of the chest radiograph in the diagnosis of lower respiratory infections in young children. Pediatr Infect Dis J 15:600–604

Dennehy PH (1987) Respiratory infections in the newborn. Clin Perinatol 14:667–682

Duke T (2005) Neonatal pneumonia in developing countries. Arch Dis Child Fetal Neonatal Ed 90(3):F211c–F219c

Engle WD, Jackson GL, Sendelbach D, Ford D, Olesen B, Burton KM et al (2000) Neonatal pneumonia: comparison of 4 vs. 7 days of antibiotic therapy in term and near-term infants. J Perinatol 20:421–426

Haney PJ, Bohlman M, Chen-Chih JS (1984) Radiographic findings in neonatal pneumonia. AJR Am J Roentgenol 143:23–26

Webber S, Wilkinson AR, Lindsell D, Hope PL, Dobson SRM, Isaacs D (1990) Neonatal pneumonia. Arch Dis Child 65:207–211

Case 4: Pyogenic Liver Abscess in Neonates

Book

Swischuk LE (2005) Absceso hepático. Tracto alimentario. In: Swischuk LE (ed) Radiología en el niño y en el recién nacido. Edición en español de Imaging of the newborn, infant, and young child. Marbán Libros SL, Madrid, pp 520–523

Web Link

Peralta R (2011) http://emedicine.com/MED/topic1316. htm. Updated November 30, 2011

Articles

Aggarwal S, Mathur NB, Garg A (2003) Portal vein thrombosis complicating neonatal hepatic abscess. Indian Pediatr 40:997–1001

Bustos R, Cordero L (2001) Absceso hepático piógeno: complicación del cateterismo venoso umbilical en un paciente prematuro. Rev Chil Pediatr 72:449–453

Lee SH, Tomlinson Ch, Temple M, Amaral J, Connolly B (2008) Imaging-guided percutaneous needle aspiration or catheter drainage of neonatal liver abscesses: 14-year experience. AJR Am J Roentgenol 190:616–622

Mannan K, Tadros Sh, Patel K, Aladangady N (2009) Liver abscess within the first week of life in a very low birthweight infant. BMJ Case Reports 2009; doi:10.1136/bcr.05.2009.1874

Moens E, Dooy JD, Jansens H, Lammens C, Op de Beeck B, Mahieu L (2003) Hepatic abscesses associated with umbilical catheterisation in two neonates. Eur J Pediatr 162:406–409

Ravishankaran P, Rajamani G (2010) Liver abscesses with pyopericardium: laparoscopic management in a preterm neonate. J Indian Assoc Pediatr Surg 15:72–73

Sharma Sh, Mohta A, Sharma P (2007) Hepatic abscess in a preterm neonate. Indian Pediatr 44:226–228

Simeunovic E, Arnold M, Sidler D, Moore SW (2009) Liver abscess in neonates. Pediatr Surg Int 25:153–156

Tan NWH, Sriram B, Tan-Kendrick APA (2005) Neonatal hepatic abscess in preterm infants: a rare entity? Ann Acad Med Singapore 34:558–564

Vade A, Sajous Ch, Anderson B, Challaplli M (1998) Neonatal hepatic abscess. Comput Med Imaging Graph 22:357–359

Case 5: Inspissated Bile Syndrome

Book

Swischuk LE (2005) Síndrome del tapón de bilis. Tracto alimentario. In: Swischuk LE (ed) Radiología en el niño y en el recién nacido. Edición en español de Imaging of the newborn, infant, and young child. Marbán Libros SL, Madrid, pp 498

Web Link

Abrams S, Shulman R (2010) Causes of neonatal cholestasis. http://www.uptodate.com/contents/causes-of-neonatal-cholestasis. Last literature review version 19.3: Sept 2011. This topic last updated: 1 Sept 2010

Articles

Bernstein J, Braylan R, Brough AJ (1969) Bile-plug syndrome: a correctable cause of obstructive jaundice in infants. Pediatrics 43:273–276

Brown D (1990) Bile plug syndrome. Successful management with a mucolytic agent. J Pediatr Surg 25:351–352

Davenport M, Betalli P, D'Antiga L, Cheeseman P, Mieli-Vergani G, Howard ER (2003) The spectrum of surgical Jaundice in infancy. J Pediatr Surg 38:1471–1479

Gubernick JA, Rosenberg HK, Ilaslan H, Kessler A (2000) US approach to jaundice in infants and children. Radiographics 20:173–195

Gunnarsdóttir A, Holmqvist P, Arnbjörnsson E, Kullendorff CM (2008) Laparoscopic aided cholecystostomy as a treatment of inspissated bile syndrome. J Pediatr Surg 43:33–35

Lang EV, Pinckney LE (1995) Spontaneous resolution of bile-plug syndrome. AJR Am J Roentgenol 156:1225–1226

Mahr MA, Hugosson C, Nazer HM, Saad SA, Ali MA (1988) Bile-plug syndrome. Pediatr Radiol 19:61–64

Metreweli C, So NMC, Chu WCW, Lam WWM (2004) Magnetic resonance cholangiography in children. Br J Radiol 77:1059–1064

Miloh T, Rosenberg HK, Kochin I, Kerkar N (2009) Inspissated bile syndrome in a neonate treated with cefotaxime. Sonographic aid to diagnosis, management, and follow-up. J Ultrasound Med 28:541–544

Pfeiffer WR, Robinson LH, Balsara VJ (1986) Sonographic feature of bile plug syndrome. J Ultrasound Med 5:161–163

Case 6: Hirschsprung Disease

Book

Swischuk LE (2005) Enfermedad de Hirschprung (aganglionosis del colon). In: Swischuk LE (ed) Radiología en el niño y en el recién nacido. Edición en español de Imaging of the newborn, infant and young child. Marbán Libros SL, Madrid, pp 445–454

Web Link

Yoshida C, Lin EC (2011) Hirschsprung disease imaging. http://emedicine.medscape.com/article/409150-overview. Accessed 24 Sept 2011

Articles

Amiel J, Lyonnet S (2008) Hirschsprung disease, associated syndromes and genetics: a review. J Med Genet 45:1–14

Berrocal T, Lamas M, Gutierrez J, Torres I, Prieto C, Del Hoyo ML (1999) Congenital anomalies of the small intestine, colon, and rectum. Radiographics 19:1219–1236

Das Narla L, Hingsbergen E (2000) Case 22: total colonic aganglionosis. Long-segment hirschsprung disease. Radiology 215:391–394

De Lorijn F, Kremer LC, Reitsma JB, Benninga MA (2006) Diagnostic tests in hirschsprung disease: a systematic review. J Pediatr Gastroenterol Nutr 42:496–505

Diamond I, Casadiego G, Traubici J, Langer JC, Wales PW (2007) The contrast enema for Hirschsprung disease: predictors of a false-positive result. J Pediatr Surg 42:792–795

Granero Cendón R, Moya Jiménez MJ, Cabrera García R, Tuduri Limousin I, Hernández Orgaz A, De Agustín Asensio JC et al (2010) Relación entre la longitud radiológica del enema opaco y la longitud aganglónica de la pieza en la enfermedad de Hirschsprung. Cir Pediatr 23:53–56

Martucciello G, Prato AP, Puri P, Holschneider AM, Meier-Ruge W, Jasonni V, Tovar JA, Grosfeld JL (2005) Controversies concerning diagnostic guidelines for anomalies of the enteric nervous system: a report from the fourth international symposium on Hirschsprung's disease and related neurocristopathies. J Pediatr Surg 40:1527–1531

O'Donovan A, Habra G, Somers S, Malone DE, Rees A, Winthrop AL (1996) Diagnosis of Hirschsprung's disease. AJR Am J Roentgenol 167:517–520

Reid JR, Buonomo C, Moreira C, Kozakevich H, Nurko SJ (2000) The barium enema in constipation: comparison with rectal manometry and biopsy to exclude Hirschsprung's disease after the neonatal period. Pediatr Radiol 30:681–684

Suita S, Taguchi T, Kamimura T, Yanai K (1997) Total colonic aganglionosis with or without small bowel involvement: a changing profile. J Pediatr Surg 32:1537–1541

Case 7: Neonatal Renal Vein Thrombosis

Book

Swischuk LE (2005) Aparato genitourinario y glándulas suprarrenales. In: Swischuk LE (ed) Radiología en el niño y en el recién nacido. Edición en español de Imaging of the newborn, infant, and Young child. Marbán Libros SL, Madrid, pp 611–612

Web Link

http://www.uptodate.com/contents/pathogenesis-clinical-features-and-diagnosis-of-thrombosis-in-the-newborn. Last literature review version 19.3: septiembre 2011. This topic last updated: 15 diciembre 2010

Articles

Brandao LR, Simpson EA, Lau KK (2011) Neonatal renal vein trombosis. Semin Fetal Neonatal Med 16:323–328

Elsaify WM (2008) Neonatal renal vein thrombosis: grey-scale and Doppler ultrasonic features. Abdom Imaging 34:413–418

Hibbert J, Howlett DC, Greenwood KL, MacDonald LM, Saunders AJ (1997) The ultrasound appearances of neonatal renal vein thrombosis. Br J Radiol 70:1191–1194

Hilario Barrio A, Gallego Herrero C, Miralles Molina M, Medina López C, Rasero Ponferrada M, del Pozo García G et al (2009) Trombosis Venosa renal neonatal: diagnóstico precoz en ecografía Doppler y secuelas a largo plazo. Radiologia 51:583–590

Hoppe C, Matsunaga A (2002) Pediatric thrombosis. Pediatr Clin North Am 49:1257–1283

Kraft J, Brandao L, Navarro O (2011) Sonography of renal venous thrombosis in neonates and infants: can we predict outcome? Pediatr Radiol 41:299–307

Marks SD, Massicotte MP, Steel BT, Matsell DG, Filler G, Shah PS et al (2005) Neonatal renal venous thrombosis: clinical outcomes and prevalence of prothrombotic disorders. J Pediatr 146:811–816

Wilkinson AG, Murphy AV, Stewart G (2001) Renal venous thrombosis with calcification and preservation of renal function. Pediatr Radiol 31:140–143

Case 8: Posterior Urethral Valves

Book

Swischuk LE et al (2005) Valvas uretrales posteriores. Aparato genitourinario y glándulas suprarrenales. In: Swischuk LE (ed) Radiología en el niño y en el recién nacido. Edición en español de Imaging of the newborn, infant and young child. Marbán Libros SL, Madrid, pp 659–661

Web Link

Holmes N (2011) http://www.uptodate.com/contents/clinical-presentation-and-diagnosis-of-posterior-urethral-valves. Last literature review version 19.3: septiembre 2011. This topic last updated: 7 junio 2011

Articles

Berrocal T, Lopez-Pereira P, Arjonilla A et al (2002) Anomalies of the distal ureter, bladder, and urethra in children: embryologic, radiologic, and pathologic features. Radiographics 22:1139–1164

Berrocal T, Gaya F, Arjonilla A (2005) Vesicoureteral reflux: can the urethra be adequately assessed by using contrast-enhanced voiding US of the bladder? Radiology 234:235–241

Bosio M (2002) Role of ultrasound in the imaging of posterior urethral valves. Rays 27:135–139

Darge K (2010) Voiding urosonography with US contrast agent for the diagnosis of vesicoureteric reflux in children: an update. Pediatr Radiol 40:956–962

Duran C, Valera A, Alguersuari A, Ballesteros E, Riera L, Martin C et al (2009) Voiding urosonography: the study of the urethra is no longer a limitation of the technique. Pediatr Radiol 39:124–131

Hodges SJ, Patel B, McLorie G et al (2009) Posterior urethral valves. Scientific World Journal 9:1119–1126

Mercado-Deane MG, Beeson JE, John SD (2002) US of renal insufficiency in neonates. Radiographics 22:1429–1438

Riccabona M (2006) Imaging of the neonatal genito-urinary tract. Eur Radiol 60:187–198

Taskinen S, Heikkilä J, Rintala R (2009) Posterior urethral valves: primary voiding pressures and kidney function in infants. J Urol 182:699

Terry LL, Bokyung H, Brent PL (2007) Congenital anomalies of male urethra. Pediatr Radiol 37:851–862

Case 9: Cerebellar Hemorrhage in Preterm Infants

Book

Barkovich JA (2005) Brain and spine injuries in infancy and childhood. Cerebellar injury in premature neonates. In: Pediatric neuroimaging, 4th edn. Lippincott Williams & Wilkins, Philadelphia, pp 221–222

Web Link

http://www.slideshare.net/yassermetwally/topic-of-the-month-cerebellar-hemorrhage-in-extremely-low-birth-weight-infants-presentation

Articles

Di Salvo DN (2001) A New view of the neonatal brain: clinical utility of supplemental neurologic US imaging windows. Radiographics 21:943–955

Ecury-Goosen GM, Dudink J, Lequin M, Feijen-Roon M, Horsch S, Govaert P (2010) The clinical presentation of preterm cerebellar haemorrhage. Eur J Pediatr 169:1249–1253

Enriquez G, Correa F, Aso C, Carreño JC, González R, Padilla N, Vázquez E (2006) Mastoid fontanelle approach for sonographic imaging of the neonatal brain. Pediatr Radiol 36:532–540

Limperopoulos C, Benson CB, Bassan H, Disalvo DN, Kinnamon D, Moore M et al (2005) Cerebellar hemorrhage in the preterm infant: ultrasonographic finding and risk factors. Pediatrics 116:717–724

Limperopoulos C, Bassan H, Gauvreau K, Robertson RL, Sullivan NR, Benson CB et al (2007) Does cerebellar injury in premature infants contribute to the high prevalence of long-term cognitive, learning, and behavioral disability in survivors? Pediatrics 120:584–593

Limperopoulos C, Robertson RL, Sullivan NR, Bassas H, du Plessis AJ (2009) Cerebellar injury in term infants: clinical characteristics, magnetic resonance imaging findings, and outcome. Pediatr Neurol 41:1–8

Merrill JD, Piecuch RE, Sean CF, Barkovich J, Goldstein RB (1988) A new pattern of cerebellar hemorrhages in preterm infants. Pediatrics 102:E62

Müller H, Beedgen B, Schenk JP, Tröger J, Linderkamp O (2007) Intracerebellar hemorrhage in premature infants: sonographic detection and outcome. J Perinat Med 35:67–70

Steggerda SJ, Leijser LM, Wiggers-de Bruïne FT, van der Grond J, Walther FJ, van Wezel-Meijler G (2009) Cerebellar injury in preterm infants: incidence and findings on US and MR images. Radiology 252:190–199

Volpe JJ (2009) Cerebellum of the premature infant: rapidly developing, vulnerable, clinically important. J Child Neurol 24:1085–1104

Case 10: Neonatal Brain Abscesses

Book

Barkovich JA (2005) Infections of the nervous system. Brain abscess. In: Pediatric neuroimaging, 4th edn. Lippincott Williams & Wilkins, Philadelphia, pp 221–222

Web Link

Edwars MS, Baker CJ (2011) Neurologic complications of bacterial meningitis in neonates. http://www.uptodate.com/contents/neurologic-complications-of-bacterial-meningitis-in-the-neonate This topic last updated: jun 6, 2011

Articles

Azrak MA, D'Agustini M, Fernandez Z, Peruffo MV (2009) Absceso cerebral por Citrobacter Koseri en lactantes. Presentación de un caso y revisión de la bibliografía. Arch Argent Pediatr 107(6):542–556

Basu S, Mukherjee KK, Poddar B, Goraya JS, Chawla K, Parmar VR (2001) An unusual case of neonatal brain abscess following klebsiella pneumoniae septicemia. Infection 29(5):283–285

Cartes-Zumelzu FW, Stavrou I, Castillo M, Eisenhuber E, Knosp E, Thurnher MM (2004) Diffusion-weighted imaging in the assessment of brain abscesses therapy. AJNR Am J Neuroradiol 25:1310–1317

de Oliveira RS, Ferreira Pinho V, Gurjao Madureira JF, Rubens Machado H (2007) Brain abscess in a neonate: an unusual presentation. Childs Nerv Syst 23:139–142

Epelman M, Daneman A, Blaser SI, Ortiz-Neira C, Konen O, Jarrín J et al (2006) Differential diagnosis of intracranial cystic lesions at head US: correlation with CT and MR imaging. Radiographics 26:173–196

Pant P, Banerjee S, Ganguly S (2008) Klebsiella pneumoniae brain abscess in two neonates. Indian Pediatr 45:693–694

Qureshi UA, Wani NA, Charoo BA, Kosar T, Qurieshi MA, Altaf U (2011) Klebsiella brain abscess in a neonate. Arch Dis Child Fetal Neonatal Ed 96:F19

Smirniotopoulos JG, Murphy FM, Rushing EJ, Rees JH, Schroeder JW (2007) Patterns of contrast enhancement in the brain and meninges. Radiographics 27:525–551

Stadnik TW, Demaerel P, Luypaert RR, Chaskis C, Van Rompaey KL, Michotte A et al (2003) Imaging tutorial: differential diagnosis of bright lesions on diffusion-weighted MR images. Radiographics 23:e7

Sundaram V, Agrawal S, Chacham S, Mukhopadhyay K, Dutta S, Kumar P (2010) Klebsiella pneumoniae brain abscess in neonates: a report of 2 cases. J Child Neurol 25:370–382

María I. Martínez-León

Contents

M.I. Martínez-León et al., *Imaging for Pediatricians*, Imaging for Clinicians,
DOI 10.1007/978-3-642-28629-2_10, © Springer-Verlag Berlin Heidelberg 2012

Case 1: Fetal Microlissencephaly

Élida Vázquez Méndez and Ignacio Delgado Álvarez

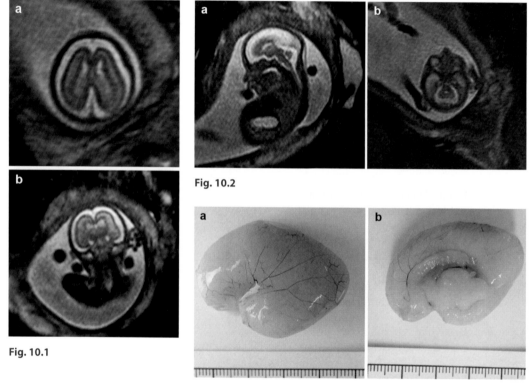

Fig. 10.1

Fig. 10.2

Fig. 10.3

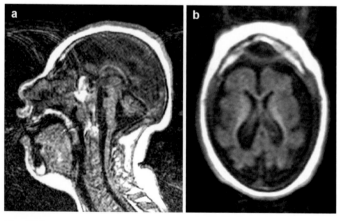

Fig. 10.4

A 20-week gestation fetus was found to have severe microcephaly on ultrasound study. Family history documented in our hospital included a 2-year-old sister with microcephaly and severe developmental delay. In view of the extremely unfavorable prognosis, pregnancy was interrupted.

Comments

Microlissencephaly is characterized by severe microcephaly and abnormal sulcation. Affected patients present with congenital microcephaly (head circumference <3 SD) without recognizable in utero injury. This disorder results from either decreased cell production or increased apoptosis in the germinal zone of the cerebral cortex, caused by the gene involved in neuronal and glial proliferation in the ventricular zone and in tangential neuronal migration from the ganglionic eminence; most cases show an autosomal recessive inheritance.

Two main types are recognized: Type A (previously called the Norman-Roberts syndrome with no infratentorial anomalies) and Type B (or Barth syndrome) which is associated with severe hypoplasia of the cerebellum and corpus callosum.

Affected fetuses can have dysmorphic features consistent with the fetal akinesia/hypokinesia sequence. Postnatally, infants who survive suffer developmental delay, intellectual disability, neurological deficits, and epilepsy.

The condition has been mainly described postnatally with a genetic origin for some familial forms (autosomal recessive transmission); prenatal diagnosis is quite uncommon and MRI is required in fetuses with microcephaly to achieve the definitive diagnosis of microlissencephaly.

On imaging, microlissencephaly is characterized by a smooth cortical surface with a simplified gyral pattern, hypoplasia of bilateral cerebral hemispheres with a reduction in gray and white matter volumes, and enlarged extra-axial spaces and lateral ventricles.

Imaging Findings

(Fig. 10.1). (a) Axial and (b) coronal HASTE images show extremely small skull, enlarged subarachnoid spaces, diminished cerebral parenchyma, and absence of primary sulcal formation. (Fig. 10.2). (a) Sagittal and (b) axial HASTE images demonstrate presence of corpus callosum and normal appearing cerebellum. (Fig. 10.3). Fetopsy specimen with (a) lateral and (b) medial views confirms the small agyric brain. (Fig. 10.4). MR imaging obtained from our files of a 2-year-old sister examined because of microcephaly and severe developmental delay. (a) Sagittal and (b) axial MPGR images displayed similar findings with the fetus, including microcephaly, enlarged subarachnoid spaces, poor myelination, and very simplified gyral pattern

Case 2: Alobar Holoprosencephaly

Elena Pastor-Pons and María Culiáñez-Casas

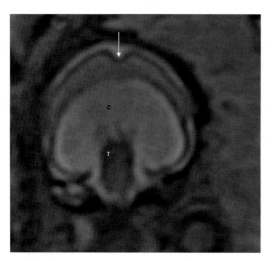

Fig. 10.5

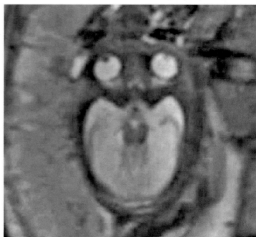

Fig. 10.7

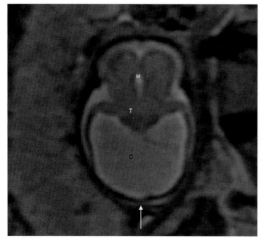

Fig. 10.6

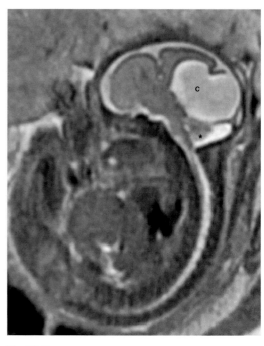

Fig. 10.8

A 26-year-old primipara underwent routine ultrasound scan at 28 weeks of gestation which revealed ventriculomegaly and cerebral malformation. Fetal MRI was performed.

Holoprosencephaly (HPE) represents a failure of the forebrain to bifurcate into two hemispheres with lack of cleavage of midline structures. It is classified, in descending order of severity, as alobar, semilobar, lobar, and middle interhemispheric (MIH) fusion variant or syntelencephaly. These types of holoprosencephaly are usually diagnosed by ultrasound. When the sonographic diagnosis is uncertain, MR imaging can be helpful. Fetal MR imaging is particularly helpful in distinguishing holoprosencephaly from agenesis of the corpus callosum with large midline clefts or cysts.

In alobar HPE, there is a cerebral holosphere, like a pancake mass of anterior cerebral tissue, with a monoventricle that communicates with a dorsal cyst. The falx cerebri, interhemispheric fissure, and corpus callosum are totally absent. The thalami are fused with absence of the third ventricle. Midline craniofacial malformations are often present.

In semilobar HPE, the anterior hemispheres remain fused and small, while some portions of the posterior interhemispheric fissure, falx cerebri, and splenium of the corpus callosum can be identified. The thalami are partially separated, resulting in a small third ventricle. The frontal horns of the lateral ventricles are absent, but posterior horns and trigones are present, although the hippocampus is incompletely formed. The septum pellucidum is absent. Facial malformations are usually mild or absent.

In lobar HPE, the cerebral hemispheres are fairly well separated. The interhemispheric fissure and falx cerebri are present anteriorly, although they are hypoplastic owing to the frontal lobe fusion. There are rudimentary frontal horns, and the third ventricle is fully formed. The thalamic nuclei are separated. The splenium and posterior body of the corpus callosum are present.

In the middle interhemispheric variant (syntelencephaly), the interhemispheric fissure is formed in the anterior frontal and occipital lobes, while the posterior frontal and parietal lobes are fused. The genu and splenium of the corpus callosum are normal, but the callosal body is absent.

Alobar holoprosencephaly at 28 weeks gestational age. Oblique coronal (Fig. 10.5), oblique axial (Figs. 10.6 and 10.7), and sagittal (Fig. 10.8) T2-SSFSE-weighted images show that interhemispheric fissure is totally absent (*arrow*), fused thalami (T), monoventricle (M), and large dorsal cyst (c). The head is small, with hypotelorism, and protuberant orbits. The cerebellum is compressed but normal (*). Anhydramnios is associated.

Case 3: Fetal Arachnoid Cyst

César Martín Martínez
and Conxita Escofet Soteras

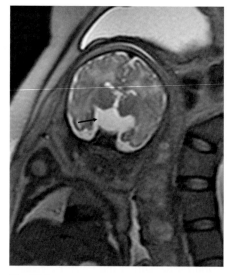

Fig. 10.9

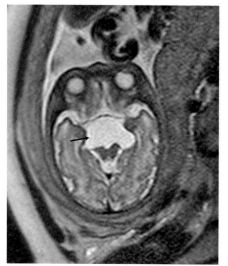

Fig. 10.10

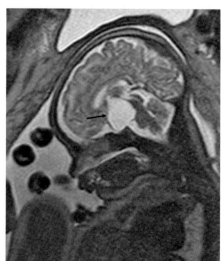

Fig. 10.11

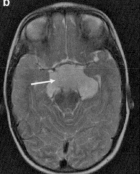

Fig. 10.12

Fetal MRI was used to study a cystic intracranial lesion detected at sonography at 33 weeks' gestation. Born at term, the boy underwent neonatal cerebral sonography and MRI when he was 3 years old. At 5 years of age, he remains asymptomatic after conservative treatment consisting of clinical follow-up and watchful waiting.

Arachnoid cysts (AC) are accumulations of a fluid resembling cerebrospinal fluid in the subarachnoid space. They can occur between the pia mater and the arachnoid membrane (subarachnoid cyst), between the two leaves of the arachnoid membrane (intra-arachnoid cyst), or between the exterior arachnoid membrane and the dura mater. AC are rare, accounting for approximately 1% of all intracranial masses in fetuses; they can be primary (congenital) or secondary (acquired). Primary AC are thought to develop from the malformation of the leptomeninges; they do not usually communicate with the subarachnoid space. Secondary AC develop as a result of hemorrhage, trauma, or infection; they usually communicate with the subarachnoid space. AC most commonly occur on the surface of the cerebral hemispheres, especially in the major fissures, the region of the sella turcica, and the posterior fossa. The diagnosis is reached by obstetric sonography and fetal MRI. Both techniques show a space-occupying cystic lesion with well-defined margins.

The differential diagnosis should include porencephalic cysts, schizencephaly, ventriculomegaly, Dandy-Walker complex, and rare cystic intracerebral tumors. AC are not usually associated with other anomalies, although large cysts can cause obstructive hydrocephalus. On rare occasions, AC have been reported in association with absence of the septum pellucidum, agenesis of the corpus callosum, cervical syringomyelia, and Chiari type I malformation. Isolated AC have a good prognosis and no intrauterine treatment is usually necessary. Karyotyping is rarely recommended. If the size of the head is normal, the time and mode of delivery need not be changed. After birth, most patients are asymptomatic; however, AC can cause epilepsy and motor and/or sensory anomalies. Depending on the size and location of the cyst and the symptoms, the treatment is watchful waiting, surgical resection, or shunting.

Coronal, axial, and sagittal (Figs. 10.9, 10.10, and 10.11) HASTE images show extra-axial fluid collection in the region of the sella turcica (*arrows*); the adjacent cerebral parenchyma is distorted, but there is no ventricular dilation. Postnatal sonogram (Fig. 10.12a) shows the same findings (*black arrow*). MRI at 3 years (Fig. 10.12b, c) shows a suprasellar cystic lesion measuring 50 × 30 × 30 mm outside the parenchyma (*white arrows*), distortion of the optic chiasm, posterior displacement of the brainstem, and compression of the hypothalamic region and of the floor of the third ventricle.

Case 4: Dandy-Walker Malformation

Elena Pastor-Pons and María Culiáñez-Casas

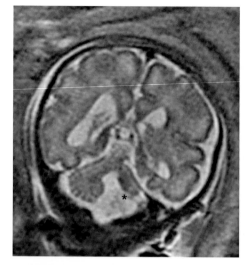

Fig. 10.14

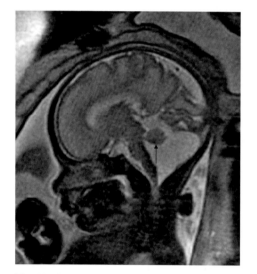

Fig. 10.13

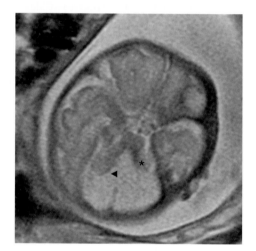

Fig. 10.15

	DWM	DWV	BPC	MCM
Posterior fossa size	Enlarged	Normal	Normal	Normal or enlarged
Vermis	Agenesia or hypoplasia	Hypoplasia	Normal	Normal
Fourth ventricle	Cystic dilatation	Cystic dilatation	Normal	Normal
Torcular-lambdoid inversion	Yes	No	No	No
Hydrocephalus	75%	25%	Rare	Rare
Cerebellum hemipheres hypoplasia	Yes	Rare	No	No
Supratentorial anomalies	Frequent	Infrequent	Rare	Rare
Prognosis	Bad	Good	Good	Good

Fig. 10.16

A 36-year-old woman underwent routine ultrasound scan at 32 + 2 weeks of gestation which revealed an enlarged posterior fossa with vermian hypoplasia. Fetal MRI confirmed these findings and showed left cerebellar hypoplasia, not identified in ultrasound.

Comments

Dandy-Walker complex represents a spectrum of cystic posterior fossa anomalies which includes, in descending order of severity, "classic" Dandy-Walker malformation (DWM), Dandy-Walker variant (DWV), persistent Blake pouch cyst (BPC), and mega cisterna magna (MCM) (Fig. 10.16).

The features of classic DWM are enlarged posterior fossa with cranial displacement of the tentorium cerebelli and the torcular herophili (torcular-lambdoid inversion), cystic dilatation of the fourth ventricle communicating with the posterior fossa, and vermian agenesis or severe hypoplasia with cranial and anterior rotation of the remaining vermis (Fig. 10.13). The cerebellar hemispheres may be hypoplastic (Fig. 10.14) and in extreme cases are compressed laterally to the wall of the posterior fossa. DWM is often associated with other central nervous system abnormalities, their most critical prognostic factors, or systemic anomalies. It is important to consider the gestational age at diagnosis as the vermis is completely formed by the end of the 18th week.

The DWV consists of variable vermian hypoplasia with cystic dilatation of the fourth ventricle that communicates with the cisterna magna but without enlargement of the posterior fossa. It has higher survival rates than the DWM, and there are cases of living patients without any symptoms. The BPC is thought to be secondary to failure of perforation of the foramen of Magendie with ballooning of the fourth ventricular roof during development resulting in a cyst of the posterior fossa, inferior and posterior to the vermis. It is associated with rotated but normal appearing vermis.

The MCM consists of an enlarged posterior fossa secondary to an enlarged cisterna magna >10 mm with normally formed vermis and fourth ventricle. It can be found incidentally in adults and children as a normal variant.

Imaging Findings

Dandy-Walker malformation at 32 weeks gestational age. Sagittal (Fig. 10.13), oblique coronal (Fig. 10.14), and oblique axial (Fig. 10.15) T2-SSFSE-weighted images show an enlarged posterior fossa, hypoplasia of the vermis (*arrow*) elevated above the large fourth ventricle which is in continuity with a large posterior fossa cyst, and an abnormal midline communication between the fourth ventricle and the cistern magna, bordered on both sides by cerebellar hemispheres (*arrow head*). It is associated with unilateral cerebellar hypoplasia (*). (Fig. 10.16). Dandy-Walker spectrum and differential diagnosis. DWM: "classic" Dandy-Walker malformation; DWV: Dandy-Walker variant; BPC: persistent Blake pouch cyst; MCM: mega cisterna magna.

Case 5: Vein of Galen Aneurysmal Malformation

Roberto Llorens Salvador and Ana María Viegas Sainz

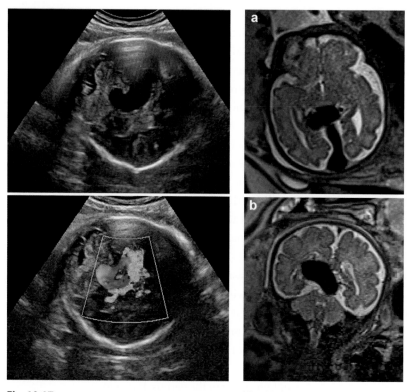

Fig. 10.17   Fig. 10.18

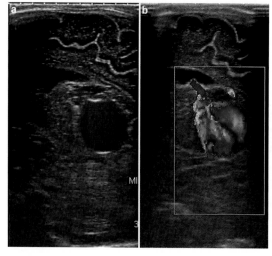

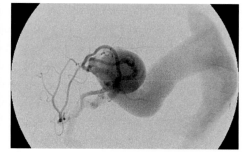

Fig. 10.19   Fig. 10.20

A brain vascular malformation is found in a 20-week-old fetus by prenatal ultrasound. Fetal MRI was performed at 32 weeks of gestation.

Vein of Galen aneurysmal malformation (VGAM) is a rare congenital arteriovenous fistula between deep choroidal arteries and the embryonal median prosencephalic vein. It is usually diagnosed at the end of the second trimester by prenatal ultrasound (US) as an echogenic elongated midline lesion. Doppler imaging is necessary to confirm its vascular nature and differentiate it from a midline intracranial cyst. As a VGAM can receive multiple arterial feeders, the impact of the shunt on fetal heart function must be systematically evaluated as it is the main prognostic factor. When in a prenatal US, fetal cardiomegaly or nonimmune hydrops are found; the fetal brain must be thoroughly studied with Doppler imaging to detect an undiagnosed VGAM. Fetal MRI allows a detailed study of the angioarchitecture of the VGAM depicting high-flow fistulae, bad prognosis malformations with multiple arterial feeders, or complications like cerebral ischemia or hydrocephalus, as well as other possible brain vascular malformations.

In the neonatal period, VGAM may present as a high-output congestive heart failure in a newborn with a structurally normal heart. In benign forms, the patients are normal at birth, although in the first postnatal months they develop progressive hydrocephalus. Neonatal imaging must start with a brain Doppler US to control the VGAM and chest X-ray and echocardiography to evaluate the heart function. Brain MR-angiography or contrast enhanced-CT are other imaging techniques used in these patients. Provided there is no destruction of brain tissue or early heart failure that does not respond to medical treatment, endovascular occlusion is usually the preferred treatment of VGAM, if possible after 6 months, because early embolization in the perinatal period carries a poorer prognosis.

Fetal brain US showing a tubular-shaped hypoechogenic process in cerebellar tentorium (Fig. 10.17a) whose vascular nature is demonstrated by Doppler imaging (Fig. 10.17b). Axial T2- (Fig. 10.18a) and coronal T2-weighted (Fig. 10.18b) images of fetal MRI show homogenous low signal intensity midline varix. The aneurysmal sac in the region of the vein of Galen is depicted by postnatal brain B-mode (Fig. 10.19a) and Doppler US (Fig. 10.19b). Finally, lateral projection of a right carotid angiogram demonstrating a venous sac with multiple choroidal feeders is seen in Fig. 10.20.

Case 6: Fetal Cerebral Ventriculomegaly

Yolanda Ruiz Martín
and Carlos Marín

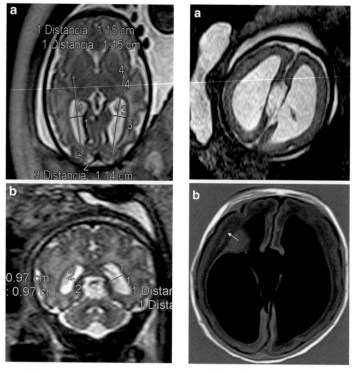

Fig. 10.21

Fig. 10.23

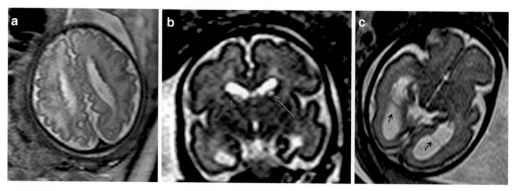

Fig. 10.22

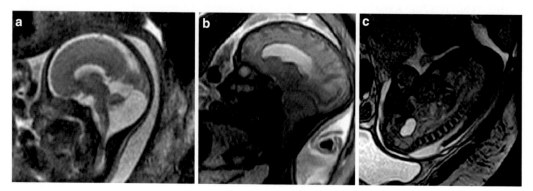

Fig. 10.24

Fetal ventriculomegaly (VM) seen at US can be the "tip of the iceberg" of different underlying abnormalities that magnetic resonance imaging (MRI) can help to identify.

VM is important for its high prevalence and high risk of association to other brain abnormalities. MRI helps to differentiate, better than ultrasound (US), between isolated VM and VM with an underlying pathology, which increases the probability of poor neurologic and/or developmental outcome. The prognosis of VM also depends on the scale of the dilatation.

The first step is to confirm the diagnostic by finding an atrium width ≥10 mm in an adequate axial plane, using the US reference method.

A coronal plane can also be used for the measurement, with close agreement with US measurement. The VM is classified as mild (10–12 mm), moderate (12–15 mm), and severe (>15 mm). The second step is to look for other anatomic or signal intensity anomalies that can give us clue regarding the VM etiology. Three major processes can be the cause of VM: malformative, destructive, and abnormal turnover of cerebrospinal fluid.

In order to find these associated anomalies, a careful examination must be performed of the margins of the lateral ventricles (LV) looking for nodularity or hemorrhage of the ventricular content, the white matter, the cortex looking for polymicrogyria or lissencephaly, the midline structures looking for callosal malformations or holoprosencephaly, and the posterior fossa (PF).

(Fig. 10.21a). It shows the adequate axial plane to make the measurement at the level of cavum septi pellucidi and ambient cistern. The calipers must be placed at the inner edges of the ventricular walls, perpendicular to the long axis of the LV at the level of the internal parieto-occipital sulcus. (Fig. 10.21b). It shows the coronal measurement at the mid-height of the LV. (Fig. 10.22a). Axial SSH-TSE T2-WI of a 35 gestational week (GW) fetus shows multiple hypointense nodules along the margins of both LV corresponding to periventricular nodular heterotopia. (Fig. 10.22b–c). Subependymal pseudocysts (*red arrows*) and linear synechiae within the LV (*black arrows*) were noted in a 31 GW fetus with VM at US due to cytomegalovirus infection. (Fig. 10.23a). It shows a 32 GW fetus with a smooth brain and absence of the expected sulci plus complete callosal agenesis. (Fig. 10.23b). Postnatal control confirms the classical lissencephaly with arrested migration of neurons (*arrow*). (Fig. 10.24a). Dandy-Walker malformation and tight PF syndrome (Fig. 10.24b) with lumbar myelomeningocele (Fig. 10.24c) are some of the PF anomalies that can be found in a patient referred for VM.

Case 7: Bronchial Atresia

Lina Cadavid Álvarez and
Amparo Castellote Alonso

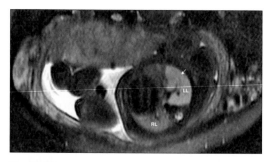

Fig. 10.25

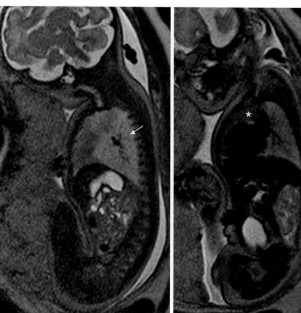

Fig. 10.26

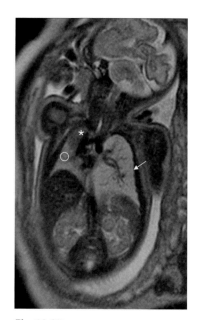

Fig. 10.27

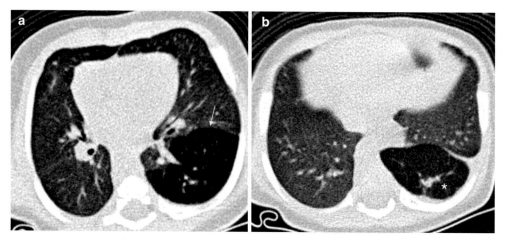

Fig. 10.28

A 31-year-old primipara underwent routine ultrasound scan at 20 + 5 weeks of gestation which revealed a left congenital pulmonary airway malformation. Fetal MRI was performed at 31 weeks of gestation.

Comments

Ultrasound remains the imaging modality of choice to study pulmonary malformations. However, maternal obesity, oligo- or anhydramnios, fetal pelvic position, or specific chest malformations may cause unfavorable acoustic windows and therefore seriously affect ultrasound diagnostic potential. In this context, magnetic resonance imaging (MRI) is a potentially valuable complementary diagnostic tool.

Fetal MRI may aid the characterization of congenital pulmonary airway malformations, since it permits the analysis of signal intensity of fetal lung tissue and complete three-dimensional lung volume, thereby helping to narrow down the differential diagnosis.

In this case, the right lung has a size, volume, and normal signal intensity for gestational age. The left lung has two different intensities: the anterior one similar to the contralateral lung and the posterior one more homogeneously intense, which is pathological. This is consistent with a left bronchial atresia (BA). BA is a condition secondary to focal obliteration of a segmental or subsegmental bronchus. The post-stenotic bronchus is filled with mucus to form a bronchocele, and the alveoli distal to the stenosis are ventilated by collateral airways. BA most commonly manifests as a focal pulmonary mass with homogeneously high-signal intensity at T2-weighted MRI. The areas most frequently involved are the apical and posterior segments of the left upper lobe. The differential diagnosis includes congenital cystic adenomatoid malformation and bronchopulmonary sequestration. These malformations may occur simultaneously and are currently considered to form part of a spectrum termed congenital pulmonary airway malformation.

Imaging Findings

(Fig. 10.25). Axial HASTE in this 31-week gestational age fetus shows a left lung with two different intensities: one posterior, homogeneously hyperintense (*arrow*) compromising an entire segment without cysts inside or anomalous vasculature, and the other anterior with similar signal intensity to the right lung. The right lung has normal intensity and volume for gestational age. RL: right lung. LL: left lung. (Fig. 10.26). Sagittal HASTE shows (a) left lung with two different intensities: one posterior, triangular in shape, homogeneously hyperintense (*arrow*), compromising the posterior lower lobe, and the other anterior with similar signal intensity to the right lung. (b). The right lung is normal, thymus (*). (Fig. 10.27). Coronal HASTE shows a BA (*arrow*) compromising left posterior lower lobe causing mass effect with contralateral mediastinal deviation, thymus (*) and RL (circle) (Fig. 10.28a, b). Postnatal CT scan (low-dose high-resolution axial protocol) shows mucoid impaction (*) just distal to the bronchial atresia in the left lower lobe. Distal air trapping is also noted (*arrow*).

Case 8: Fetal Sacrococcygeal Teratoma

María I. Martínez-León
and Luisa Ceres-Ruiz

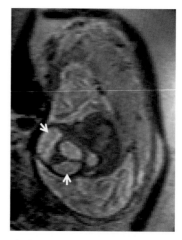

Fig. 10.31

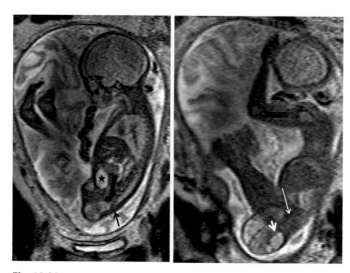

Fig. 10.29

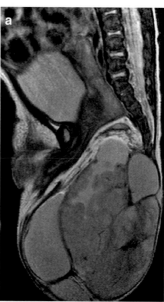

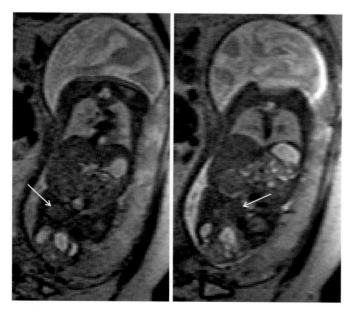

Fig. 10.30

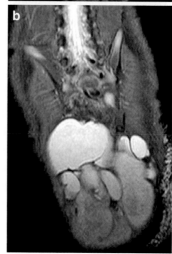

Fig. 10.32

A 27-week gestation fetus with mixed solid and cystic lesion studied with ultrasound.

Teratomas occur along the midline of the body from the coccyx to the pineal gland. The sacrococcygeal region is the most common site for teratomas, with 70–80% of all teratomas being located in this location.

Teratomas are composed of all three germ cell layers (ectoderm, mesoderm, and endoderm). Some of the histologic features of fetal teratomas are unique, compared with teratomas seen later in life, for example, the ectodermal components, especially neural tissues, are a dominant feature of fetal teratomas and the mesodermal tissues (fat, bone, smooth muscle, and cartilage) are also common.

Sacrococcygeal teratomas (SCTs) are classified into four types based on the proportion of mass located internally and externally. Type I SCT, the mass is external with minimal or no internal components. Type II is predominantly an external mass with internal extension into the presacral space (our case). Type III is an external and internal mass with extension into the abdominal cavity. Type IV is an entirely internal mass with no external component. This system of classification has important prognostic implications because pediatric SCT with an undiagnosed internal component are more likely to undergo malignant transformation.

The location, size, extension, and content of the mass are far more important than the histologic grade (mature or immature) for predicting outcome. Fully resectable, immature teratomas in the newborn have a generally favorable prognosis. Fetuses with predominantly solid and highly vascularized masses have a poorer prognosis than fetuses with tumors that are mainly cystic and avascular in appearance.

(Figs. 10.29, 10.30, and 10.31). Sagittal, coronal, and axial SSh T2-weighted fetal MRI show a heterogeneous mixed mass, with a predominantly septated cystic component (*short arrows*) but also with a solid component (*long arrows*). The SCT extends into the presacral space. The urinary bladder (*asterisk*) is slightly displaced anteriorly and cranially. There is no hydrops which portends a better outcome. There is no relation with the spinal canal (*black arrow*) and the fetal spine is normal, therefore, the primary differential diagnosis, myelomeningocele, is excluded.

(Fig. 10.32). Sagittal TSE T2 weighted and coronal T2 weighted with fat suppression of the newborn accurately characterized the presacral and intrapelvic extent of the mixed tumor, providing more information about relation of adjacent organs and improving preoperative planning for surgical resection.

Case 9: Fetal Ureterocele

Luisa Ceres-Ruiz and María Vidal Denis

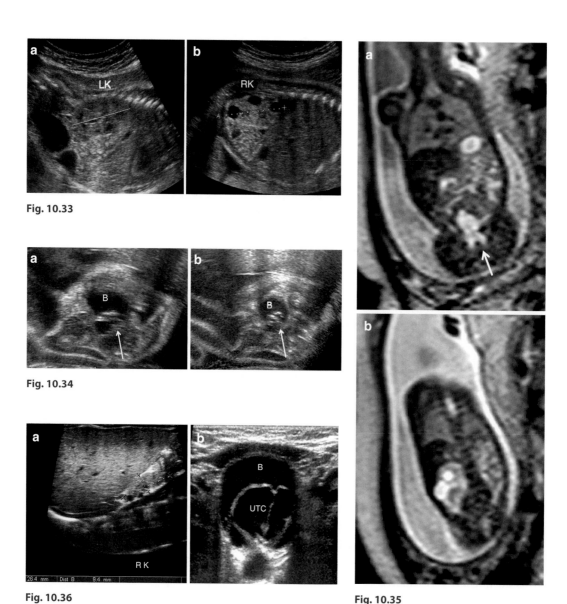

Fig. 10.33

Fig. 10.34

Fig. 10.36

Fig. 10.35

A 33-year-old pregnant woman, 20 weeks of gestation, referred for ultrasound examination.

The ureterocele (UTC) is a congenital cystiform dilatation of the terminal submucosal ureter, occurring with single or duplicated collecting systems. Simple UTC drains in the bladder and ectopic UTC in the bladder neck or proximal urethra. It is more common in girls (ratio 4:1) and in association with ureteral duplication (80%). UTC is most often associated with obstruction of the upper pole of a duplicated collecting system, and ultrasound shows unilateral upper pole hydroureteronephrosis with little or absent parenchyma. When the UTC is large or has a cecoureterocele, it may obstruct the bladder outlet.

Increasingly, UTC is detected on prenatal ultrasound (US) assessment, as early as 16–17 weeks of gestation. When a UTC is identified on prenatal US, serial US studies should be conducted to assess the volume of amniotic fluid, bladder volume, degree of hydronephrosis, and echogenicity of the kidneys (increased echogenicity with cysts is associated with dysplasia secondary to obstruction). In utero surgical interventions are designed to decompress the UTC and restore bladder emptying and the volume of amniotic fluid. However, in utero treatment is controversial, as it does not seem to improve the function of the upper pole. Prenatal diagnosis has allowed early indication of prophy-lactic antibiotics and decreased the incidence of UTIs from 60% to 70%. The postnatal surgical procedure depends on the function of the ipsilateral upper and lower pole, as well as the contralateral kidney, and the presence of reflux or obstruction.

(Fig. 10.33a). Normal fetal left kidney with good cortico-medullary differentiation. (Fig. 10.33b). Fetal right kidney with cortical cysts, increased parenchyma echogenicity and poor cortico-medullary differentiation. (Fig. 10.34a, b). Fetal bladder with multiple cystic images in the trigone area (*arrow*) that corresponds to a refolding or septet UTC "pseudoseptated fetal bladder," from a single system. (Fig. 10.35). MRI SSH-TSE, coronal plane, focused on the bladder, the remarkable degree of bladder filling with two small well-defined cystic lesions located in the bladder base (Fig. 10.35a), which is associated with septate UTC (*arrow*). (Fig. 10.35b). Both kidneys, the left is normal and the right one has two cystic images located in the upper pole and interpolar region, in relation to dysplastic kidney. US of the newborn: (Fig. 10.36a). Longitudinal section of right kidney showing a small dysplastic kidney, 26 mm long, with loss of cortico-medullary differentiation. (Fig. 10.36b). Bladder with a low filling degree and presence of folding UTC.

Case 10: Persistent Urachus and Allantoid Cyst

María I. Martínez-León and Isidoro Narbona Arias

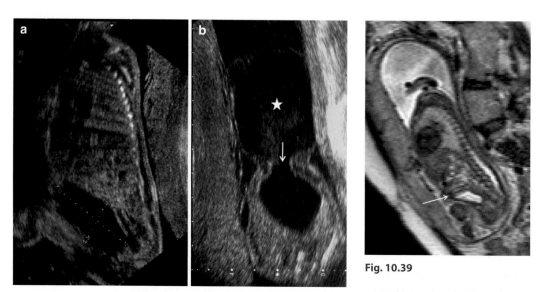

Fig. 10.37

Fig. 10.39

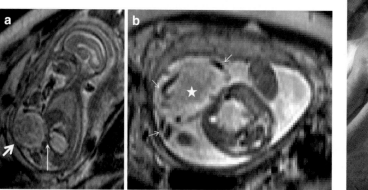

Fig. 10.38

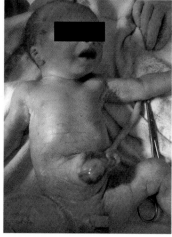

Fig. 10.40

A 33-year-old woman referred to the prenatal diagnosis center at 21 weeks of gestation because of bladder anomalies and an umbilical cyst in a routine screening ultrasound. The patient underwent subsequent US examinations as well as a fetal MRI.

Comments

The urachus is an embryological canal connecting the urinary bladder with the allantois, a structure that contributes to the formation of the umbilical cord. The lumen of the urachus is obliterated during the course of embryonic development. The urachus lies between the transversalis fascia anteriorly and the peritoneum posteriorly. Persistent urachus is a tubular connection between the dome of the bladder and the umbilicus. Persistence of the urachus may be partial, giving rise to urachal cyst, vesicourachal diverticulum, umbilical-urachal sinus, or totally patent urachus (complete persistence, allowing communication with the bladder). Careful fetal evaluation to rule out associated anomalies (especially urogenital anomalies) is indicated when patent urachus is diagnosed in utero. Prognosis is excellent when no significant associated anomalies are present. Surgical excision at birth is recommended.

The differential diagnosis of persistent urachus includes anterior abdominal wall defects, bladder exstrophy, omphalocele, vascular lesions of the umbilical cord, and allantoic or omphalomesenteric cysts.

A patent urachus can present as an allantoic cyst in the umbilical cord antenatally. An allantoic cyst is a rare swelling formed at the base of the umbilicus associated with a patent urachus which results from an allantoic remnant. Our reported case corresponds to a patent urachus with an allantoic cyst diagnosed via US and fetal MR imaging. Early detection allowed for appropriate counseling and corrective surgery after birth.

(Fig. 10.37a, b). Sagittal US revealed a mega urinary bladder (between cursors) with anterosuperior traction of the dome. Axial US shows an umbilical cyst (*asterisk*) corresponding to an allantoid cyst in communication with the dome of the bladder through a small channel (*arrow*). (Fig. 10.38a, b). Sagittal and axial fetal MRI shows the allantoids cyst (*asterisk*) located between the vessels (*short arrows*); the cyst is located on the abdominal wall near the cord insertion. The true cyst has a thin wall (*thick arrow*). There is a large, deformed bladder in connection with the cyst (*long arrow*). There are no other associated anomalies. (Fig. 10.39). Parasagittal fetal MRI a month later shows the persistence of the dome deformity of the bladder (*arrow*), now without dilatation due to the connection with the patent urachus. The allantoids cyst is smaller (not shown). (Fig. 10.40). Postnatally, an unusually thick umbilical cord with a yellow fluid-filled cyst was noted. Normal external genital organs. The fluid from the cyst was confirmed as urine.

Further Reading

Case 1: Fetal Microlissencephaly

Book

Garel C (2004) MRI of the fetal brain: normal development and cerebral pathologies, 1st edn. Springer, Berlin/Heidelberg

Web Link

http://imaging.consult.com/imageSearch?query=lissencephaly&global_search=Search&modality=+&anatomicRegion=

Articles

Abdel Razek AA, Kandell AY, Elsorogy LG, Elmongy A, Basett AA (2009) Disorders of cortical formation: MR imaging features. AJNR Am J Neuroradiol 30:4–11

Barkovich J, Raybaud C (2004) Neuroimaging in disorders of cortical development. Neuroimaging Clin N Am 14:231–254

Barkovich AJ, Ferriero DM, Barr RM et al (1998) Microlissencephaly: a heterogeneous malformation of cortical development. Neuropediatrics 29:113–119

Dobyns WB, Truwit CL, Ross ME et al (1999) Differences in the gyral pattern distinguish chromosome 17-linked and X-liked lissencephaly. Neurology 53:270–277

Gadadoia A, Gupta P, Sharma R, Kumar S (2011) Prenatal diagnosis of lissencephaly: a case report. J Clin Ultrasound 39:91–92

Gaitanis J, Walsh C (2004) Genetics of disorders of cortical development. Neuroimaging Clin N Am 14:219–229

Ghai S, Fong K, Tai A, et al (2006) Prenatal US and MR imaging findings of lissencephaly: review of fetal cerebral sulcal development. Radiographics 26:389–406

Hirose M, Haginoya K, Yokoyama H et al (2011) Progressive atrophy of the cerebrum in 2 Japanese sisters with microcephaly with simplified gyri and enlarged extraaxial space. Neuropediatrics 42(4):163–166

Sztriha L, Al-Gazali LI, Várady E et al (1999) Autosomal recessive micrencephaly with simplified gyral pattern, abnormal myelination and arthrogryposis. Neuropediatrics 30:141–145

Sztriha L, Dawodu A, Gururaj A et al (2004) Microcephaly associated with abnormal gyral pattern. Neuropediatrics 35:346–352

Case 2: Alobar Holoprosencephaly

Book

Barkovich AJ (2005) Congenital malformations of the brain and skull. In: Barkovich AJ (ed) Pediatric neuroimaging. Lippincott Williams & Wilkins, Philadelphia, pp 291–439

Web Link

http://www.casesjournal.com/content/3/1/35

Articles

Dill P, Poretti A, Boltshauser E, Huisman T (2009) Fetal magnetic resonance imaging in midline malformations of the central nervous system and review of the literature. J Neuroradiol 36:138–146

Hahn JS, Barnes PD (2010) Neuroimaging advances in holoprosencephaly: refining the spectrum of the midline malformation. Am J Med Genet C Semin Med Genet 154C:120–132

Hsieh TY, Yu CH, Kuo PL, Chang FM (2006) Prenatal diagnosis of alobar holoprosencephaly with cystic hygroma. Taiwan J Obstet Gynecol 45:146–149

Malinger G, Lev D, Kidron D, Heredia F, Hershkovitz R, Lerman-Sagie T (2005) Differential diagnosis in fetuses with absent septum pellucidum. Ultrasound Obstet Gynecol 25:42–49

Marcorelles P, Laquerriere A (2010) Neuropathology of holoprosencephaly. Am J Med Genet C Semin Med Genet 154C:109–119

Pulitzer SB, Simon EM, Crombleholme TM, Golden JA (2004) Prenatal MR findings of the middle interhemispheric variant of holoprosencephaly. AJNR Am J Neuroradiol 25:1034–1036

Sawhney S, Machado L, Jain R (2008) Prenatal MRI image of a fetus with semilobar holoprosencephaly. Sultan Qaboos Univ Med J 8:93–94

Simon EM, Barkovich AJ (2001) Holoprosencephaly: new concepts. Magn Reson Imaging Clin N Am 9:149–164

Volpe P, Campobasso G, De Robertis V, Rembouskos G (2009) Disorders of prosencephalic development. Prenat Diagn 29:340–354

Wong A, Bilaniuk LT, Ng KK, Chang YL, Chao AS (2005) Lobar holoprosencephaly: prenatal MR diagnosis with postnatal MR correlation. Prenat Diagn 25:296–299

Case 3: Fetal Arachnoid Cyst

Book

McGahan JP, Pilu G, Nyberg DA (2003) Cerebral malformations. In: Nyberg DA, McGahan JP, Pretorius DH, Pilu G (eds) Diagnostic imaging of fetal anomalies. Lippincott Williams & Wilkins, Philadelphia, pp 381–420

Web Link

http://www.sonoworld.com/Fetus/Home.aspx

Articles

Al-Holou WN, Yew Ay, Boomsaad ZE, Garton HJ, Murasko KM, Maher CO (2010) Prevalence and natural history of arachnoid cysts in children. J Neurosurg Pediatr 5:578–585

Booth TN, Timmons C, Shapiro K, Rollins NK (2004) Pre- and postnatal MR imaging of hypothalamic hamartomas associated with arachnoid cysts. AJNR Am J Neuroradiol 25(7):1283–1285

El-Ghandour NMF (2011) Endoscopic treatment of suprasellar arachnoid cysts in children. J Neurosurg Pediatr 8:6–14

Gelabert M (2004) Intracranial arachnoid cysts [in Spanish]. Rev Neurol 39(12):1161–1166

Girard N, Raybaud C, Gambarelli D, Figarella-Branger D (2001) Fetal brain MR imaging. Magn Reson Imaging Clin N Am 9:19–56

Hosny IA, Elghawabi HS (2010) Ultrafast MRI of the fetus: an increasingly important tool in prenatal diagnosis of congenital anomalies. Magn Reson Imaging 28(10):1431–1439

Osborn AG, Preece MT (2006) Intracranial cysts: radiologic-pathologic correlation and imaging approach. Radiology 239:650–664

Prayer D, Brugger PC, Prayer L (2004) Fetal MRI: techniques and protocols. Pediatr Radiol 34:685–693

Shim KW, Lee YH, Park EK, Park YS, Choi JU, Kim DS (2009) Treatment options for arachnoid cysts. Childs Nerv Syst 25:1459–1466

Woodward PJ, Sohaey R, Kennedy A, Koeller KK (2005) From the archives of the AFIP: a comprehensive review of fetal tumors with pathologic correlation. Radiographics 25(1):215–241

Case 4: Dandy-Walker Malformation

Book

Blaser SI (2007) Dandy Walker spectrum. In: Barkovich AJ (ed) Diagnostic imaging: pediatric neuroradiology. Amirsys, Salt Lake City, pp 22–25, Section I:4

Web Link

http://radiopaedia.org/articles/dandy-walker-continuum

Articles

Adamsbaum C (2005) MRI of the fetal posterior fossa. Pediatr Radiol 35:124–140

Bernard JP, Moscoso G, Renier D, Ville Y (2001) Cystic malformations of the posterior fossa. Prenat Diagn 21:1064–1069

Calabrò F, Arcuri T, Jinkins JR (2000) Blake's pouch cyst: an entity within the Dandy-Walker continuum. Neuroradiology 42:290–295

Epelman M, Daneman A, Blaser SI, Ortiz-Neira C, Konen O (2006) Differential diagnosis of intracranial cystic lesions at head US: correlation with CT and MR imaging. Radiographics 26:173–196

Guibaud L (2004) Practical approach to prenatal posterior fossa abnormalities using MRI. Pediatr Radiol 34:700–711

Klein O, Pierre-Kahn A, Boddaert N, Parisot D, Brunelle F (2003) Dandy-Walker malformation: prenatal diagnosis and prognosis. Childs Nerv Syst 19:484–489

Lavanya T, Cohen M, Gandhi SV, Farrell T, Whitby EH (2008) Case report: Dandy-Walker variant: a multidisciplinary approach for accurate diagnosis. Br J Radiol 81:242–245

Sanz-Cortes M, Raga F, Leon JL, Sniderman A, Bonilla-Musoles F (2007) MRI and multiplanar 3D ultrasound compared in the prenatal assessment of enlarged posterior fossa. J Perinat Med 35:422–424

Sasaki-Adams D, Elbabaa SK, Jewells V, Carter L, Campbell JW, Ritter AM (2008) The Dandy–Walker variant: a case series of 24 pediatric patients and evaluation of associated anomalies, incidence of hydrocephalus, and developmental outcomes. J Neurosurg Pediatr 2:194–199

Wong AM, Bilaniuk LT, Zimmerman RA, Liu PL (2012) Prenatal MR imaging of Dandy-Walker complex: midline sagittal area analysis. Eur J Radiol 81(1):e26–e30. doi:10.1016/j.ejrad.2010.11.003

Case 5: Vein of Galein Aneurysmal Malformation

Book

Lasjaunias P (1997) Vascular diseases in neonates, infants and children. Vein of Galen Aneurysmal malformation. Springer, Berlin/Heidelberg, pp 67–202

Web Link

Sheth RD (2010) Vein of Galen malformation. http://emedicine.medscape.com/article/1179888. Accessed 2 Oct 2011

Articles

Chen M-Y, Liu H-M, Weng W-C (2010) Neonate with severe heart failure related to vein of Galen malformation. Pediatr Neonatol 51:245–248

De Koning TJ, Gooskens R, Veenhoven R, Meijboom EJ, Jansen GH, Lasjaunias P et al (1997) Arteriovenous malformation of the vein of Galen in three neonates: emphasis on associated early ischaemic brain damage. Eur J Pediatr 156:228–229

Golombek SG, Ally S, Woolf PK (2004) A newborn with cardiac failure secondary to a large vein of Galen malformation. South Med J 97:516–518

Hoang S, Choudhri O, Edwards M, Guzman R (2009) Vein of Galen malformation. Neurosurg Focus 27:E8

Huisman TAGM, Singhi S (2010) Non-invasive imaging of intracranial pediatric vascular lesions. Childs Nerv Syst 26:1275–1995

Kalra V, Malhotra A (2010) Fetal MR diagnosis of vein of Galen aneurysmal malformation. Pediatr Radiol 40(Suppl 1):S155

Lasjaunias PL, Cheng SM, Sachet M, Alvarez H, Rodesch G, Garcia-Monaco R (2006) The management of vein of Galen aneurysmal malformations. Neurosurgery 59:S184–S194; discussion S3–S13

Lylyk P, Vinuela F, Dion JE, Duckwiler G, Guglielmi G, Peacock W et al (1993) Therapeutic alternatives for vein of Galen vascular malformations. J Neurosurg 78:438–445

Raybaud CA, Strother CM, Hald JK (1989) Aneurysms of the vein of Galen: embryonic considerations and anatomical features relating to the pathogenesis of the malformation. Neuroradiology 31:109–128

Squires LA, Thomas S, Betz BW, Cottingham S (1998) Vein of Galen malformation with diencephalic syndrome: a clinical pathologic report. J Child Neurol 13:575–577

Case 6: Fetal Cerebral Ventriculomegaly

Book

Sohaey R, Filipek MS (2005) Mild ventriculomegaly. In: Woodward PJ, Kennedy A, Sohaey R, Byrne JLB, Oh KY, Puchalsk MD (eds) Diagnostic imaging obstetric, 1st edn. Amirsys Inc., Salt Lake City, pp 2–26

Web Link

http://eradiology.bidmc.harvard.edu/LearningLab/genito/McLeod.pdf

Articles

Almog B, Gamzu R, Achiron R, Fainaru O, Zalel Y (2003) Fetal lateral ventricular width: what should be its upper limits? A prospective cohort study and reanalysis of the current and previous data. J Ultrasound Med 22:39–43

Cardoza JD, Goldstein RB, Filly RA (1988) Exclusion of fetal ventriculomegaly with a single measurement: the width of the lateral ventricular atrium. Radiology 169:711–714

Gaglioti P, Oberto M, Todros T (2009) The significance of fetal ventriculomegaly: etiology, short- and long-term outcomes. Prenat Diagn 29:381–388

Garel C, Alberti C (2006) Coronal measurement of the fetal lateral ventricles: comparison between ultrasonography and magnetic resonance imaging. Ultrasound Obstet Gynecol 27:23–27

Ghai S, Fong KW, Toi A, Chitayat D, Pantazi S, Blaser S (2006) Prenatal US and MR imaging findings of lissencephaly: review of fetal cerebral sulcal development. Radiographics 26:389–405

Glenn OA (2010) MR of fetal brain. Pediatr Radiol 40:68–81

Guibaud L (2009) Contribution of fetal cerebral MRI for diagnosis of structural anomalies. Prenat Diagn 29:420–433

ISUOG (2007) Sonographic examination of the fetal central nervous system: guidelines for performing the 'basic examination' and the 'fetal neurosonogram'. Ultrasound Obstet Gynecol 29:109–116

Jaspan T (2008) New concepts on posterior fossa malformations. Pediatr Radiol 38(Suppl 3):S409–S414, 98

Salomon LJ, Garel C (2007) Magnetic resonance imaging examination of fetal brain. Ultrasound Obstet Gynecol 30:1019–1032

Case 7: Bronchial Atresia

Book

Prayer D (2011) Fetal MRI, 1st edn. Springer, New York/ London

Web Link

http://www.casesjournal.com/content/2/1/17

Articles

Biyyam DR, Chapman T, Ferguson MR, Deutsch G, Dighe MK (2010) Congenital lung abnormalities: embryologic features, prenatal diagnosis, and postnatal radiologic pathologic correlation. Radiographics 30:1721–1738

Cannie M, Jani J, De Keyzer F, Van Kerkhove F, Meersschaert J, Lewi L et al (2008) Magnetic resonance imaging of the fetal lung: a pictorial essay. Eur Radiol 18:1364–1374

Coakley FV, Lopoo JB, Lu Y et al (2000) Volumetric assessment of normal and hypoplastic lungs by prenatal single-shot RARE MR imaging. Radiology 216:107–111

Daltro P, Werner H, Gasparetto TD, Cortes R, Rodrigues L, Marchiori E et al (2010) Congenital chest malformations: a multimodality approach with emphasis on fetal MR imaging. Radiographics 30:385–395

Dhingsa R, Coakley FV, Albanese CT, Filly RA, Goldstein R (2003) Prenatal sonography and MR imaging of pulmonary sequestration. AJR Am J Roentgenol 180:433–437

Keller TM, Rake A, Michel SCA, Seifert B, Wisser J, Marincek B et al (2004) MR assessment of fetal lung development using lung volumes and signal intensities. Eur Radiol 14:984–989

Kocao lu M, Frush DP, U urel MS, Somuncu I (2010) Bronchopulmonary foregut malformations presenting as mass lesions in children: spectrum of imaging findings. Diagn Interv Radiol 16:153–161

Levine D, Barnewolt CE, Mehta TS, Trop I, Estroff J, Wong G (2003) Fetal thoracic abnormalities: MR imaging. Radiology 228:379–388

Newman B (2006) Congenital bronchopulmonary foregut malformations: concepts and controversies. Pediatr Radiol 36:773–779

Victoria T, Johnson AM, Chauvin NA, Kramer SS, Epelman M (2011) Fetal MRI of common non-CNS abnormalities: a review. Appl Radiol 40:8–17

Case 8: Fetal Sacrococcygeal Teratoma

Book

Flake AW (2000) The fetus with sacrococcygeal teratoma. In: Harrison MR, Evans MI, Adzick NS, Holzgreve W (eds) The unborn patient, 3rd edn. WB Saunders, Philadelphia, pp 315–323

Web Link

http://www.chw.org/display/PPF/DocID/35571/Nav/1/router.asp

Articles

Avni FE, Guibaud L, Robert Y et al (2002) MR imaging of fetal sacrococcygeal teratoma: diagnosis and assessment. AJR Am J Roentgenol 178:179–183

Brace V, Grant SR, Brackley KJ, Kilby MD, Whittle MJ (2000) Prenatal diagnosis and outcome in sacrococcygeal teratoma: a review of cases between 1992 and 1998. Prenat Diagn 20:51–55

Chisholm CA, Heider AL, Kuller JA, von Allmen D, McMahon MJ, Chestcheir NC (1998) Prenatal diagnosis and perinatal management of fetal sacrococcygeal teratoma. Am J Perinatol 15:503–505

Danzer E, Hubbard AM, Hedrick HL, Hohnson MO, Wilson RD, Howell LJ et al (2006) Diagnosis and characterization of fetal sacrococcygeal teratoma with prenatal MRI. AJR Am J Roentgenol 187:350–356

Flake AW (1993) Fetal sacrococcygeal teratoma. Semin Pediatr Surg 2:113–120

Hedrick HL, Flake AW, Crombleholme TM, Howell LJ, Johnson MP, Wilson RD et al (2004) Sacrococcygeal teratoma: prenatal assessment, fetal intervention, and outcome. J Pediatr Surg 39:430–438

Kocaoglu M, Frush DP (2006) Pediatric presacral masses. Radiographics 26:833–857

Ueno T, Tanaka YO, Nagata M, Tsunoda H, Anno I, Ishikawa S et al (2004) Spectrum of germ cell tumors: from head to toe. Radiographics 24:387–404

Westerburg B, Feldstein VA, Sandberg PL, Lopoo JB, Harrison MR, Albanese CT (2000) Sonographic prognostic factors in fetuses with sacrococcygeal teratoma. J Pediatr Surg 35:322–325

Woodward PJ, Sohaey R, Kennedy A, Koeller KK (2005) From the archives of the AFIP: a comprehensive review of fetal tumors with pathologic correlation. Radiographics 25:215–242

Case 9: Fetal Ureterocele

Book

Fleisher AC, Romero R, Manning FA et al (1999) The principles and practice of ultrasonography in obstetrics and gynecology. Appleton & Lange, Norwalk, pp 266–267

Web Link

www.sonoworld.com/fetus/page.aspx?id=561

Articles

Adiego B, Martinez-Ten P, Perez-Pedregosa J, Illescas T, Barron E, Wong AE et al (2011) Antenatally diagnosed renal duplex anomalies: sonographic features and long-term postnatal outcome. J Ultrasound Med 30:809–815

Avni FE, Nicaise N, Hall M et al (2001) The role of MR imaging for the assessment of complicated duplex kidneys in children: preliminary report. Pediatr Radiol 31:215–223

Chertin B, Rabinowitz R, Pollack A, Koulikov D, Fridmans A, Hadas-Halpern I et al (2005) Does prenatal diagnosis influence the morbidity associated with left in situ nonfunctioning or poorly functioning renal moiety after endoscopic puncture of ureterocele? J Urol 173:1349–1352

Jeffrey RB, Laing FC, Wing VW, Hoddick W (1984) Sonography of the fetal duplex kidney. Radiology 153:123–124

Merlini E, Lelli Chiesa P (2004) Obstructive ureterocele, an ongoing challenge. World J Urol 22:107–114

Pohl HG (2011) Recent advances in the management of ureteroceles in infants and children: why less may be more. Curr Opin Urol 21:322–327

Quintero RA, Homsy Y, Bornick PW et al (2001) In-utero treatment of fetal bladder outlet obstruction by a ureterocele. Lancet 357:1947–1948

Sepúlveda W, Campana C, Carstens E, Rodriguez J (2003) Prenatal sonographic diagnosis of bilateral ureteroceles: the pseudoseptated fetal bladder. J Ultrasound Med 22:841–844

Soothill PW, Bartha JL, Tizard J (2003) Ultrasound guided laser treatment for fetal bladder outlet obstruction resulting from ureterocele. Am J Obstet Gynecol 188:1107–1108

Sozubir S, Lorenzo AJ, Twickler DM, Baker LA, Ewalt DH (2003) Prenatal diagnosis of a prolapsed ureterocele with magnetic resonance imaging. Urology 62:144

Case 10: Persistent Urachus and Allantoid Cyst

Book

Moore KL (1982) The urogenital system. In: Moore KL (ed) The developing human, 3rd edn. WB Saunders, Philadelphia, pp 255–297

Web Link

Prenatal diagnosis of a patent urachus cyst with the use of 2D, 3D, 4D ultrasound and fetal MRI. SonoWorld. http://www.sonoworld.com/Client/ModuleContent/ModuleContent.aspx?ModuleId=5&ContentId=1942

Articles

Bunch PT, Kline-fath BM, Imhoff SC, Calvo-García MA, Crombleholme TM, Donnelly LF (2006) Allantoic cyst: a prenatal clue to patent urachus. Case report. Pediatr Radiol 36:1090–1095

Cilento BG Jr, Bauer SB, Retik AB, Peters CA, Atala A (1998) Urachal anomalies: defining the best diagnostic modality. Urology 52:120–122

Costakos DT, Williams AC, Love LA, Wood BP (1992) Patent urachal duct. Am J Dis Child 146:951–952

DiSantis DJ, Siegel MJ, Katz ME (1991) Simplified approach to umbilical remnant abnormalities. Radiographics 11:59–66

Frazier HA, Guerrieri JP, Thomas RL, Christenson PJ (1992) The detection of patent urachus and allantoic cyst of the umbilical cord on prenatal ultrasonography. J Ultrasound Med 11:117–120

Mesrobian HGO, Zacharias A, Balcom AH, Cohen RD (1997) Ten years of experience with isolated urachal anomalies in children. J Urol 158:1316–1318

Nix JT, Menville JG, Albert M, Wendt DL (1957) Congenital patent urachus. J Urol 79:264–273

Persutte WH, Lenke RR (1990) Disappearing fetal umbilical cord masses. Are these findings suggestive of urachal anomalies? J Ultrasound Med 9:547–551

Tolaymat LL, Maher GE, Stalnaker R, Kea K, Walker A (1997) Persistent patent urachus with allantoic cyst: a case report. Ultrasound Obstet Gynecol 10:366–368

Yu JS, Kim KW, Lee HJ, Lee YJ, Yoon CS, Kim MJ (2001) Urachal remnant diseases: spectrum of CT and US findings. Radiographics 21:451–461